Praise for *The Cure for Women*

"Through brilliant and creative prose, Lydia Reeder brings to life the world of Mary Putnam Jacobi and other pioneering women who fought to be treated as equals in the American medical community, in turn revealing how the sexism they faced impacted doctors and patients alike. It's a story that's simultaneously enraging and inspiring."

—Catherine McNeur, author of *Mischievous Creatures*

"A fascinating history of the women who charged down medicine's 'forbidden path,' fighting not only for better care and opportunities for women, but so much more."

—Rachel Swaby, author of *Headstrong: 52 Women Who Changed Science—and the World*

"Reminds us of the state of unfreedom and constraint of women just 150 years ago, with its implicit warning not to take our rights for granted."

—Victoria Sweet, M.D., author of *Slow Medicine*

"Both a riveting and chilling story. The history of gynecology under men is barely distinguishable from quackery, revealing rampant abuse of the female body and psyche disguised as care. Women's very anatomy was used against them as a reason that they could not possibly become doctors themselves—or even use their brains at all. As we live in a time of the increasing trivialization of the health—and pain—of women, Reeder has found a heroine for our age."

—Catherine Prendergast, author of *The Gilded Edge*

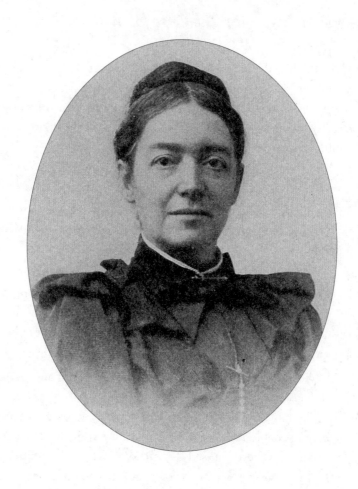

The
Cure
for
Women

Dr. Mary Putnam Jacobi and
the Challenge to Victorian Medicine that
Changed Women's Lives Forever

Lydia Reeder

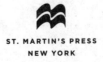

ST. MARTIN'S PRESS
NEW YORK

Frontispiece: *Portrait of Mary Putnam Jacobi, M.D., New York,* in M. T. Valentine, *The Biography of Ephraim McDowell, M.D.,* New York: McDowell Publishing Co., 1897

First published in the United States by St. Martin's Press, an imprint of St. Martin's Publishing Group

www.stmartins.com

Design by Meryl Sussman Levavi

The Library of Congress Cataloging-in-Publication Data is available upon request.

ISBN 978-1-250-28445-7 (hardcover)
ISBN 978-1-250-28446-4 (ebook)

Our books may be purchased in bulk for promotional, educational, or business use. Please contact your local bookseller or the Macmillan Corporate and Premium Sales Department at 1-800-221-7945, extension 5442, or by email at MacmillanSpecialMarkets@macmillan.com.

First Edition: 2024

1   3   5   7   9   10   8   6   4   2

For my great-grandmother Ellen Keith Babb
Beloved midwife and healer

Contents

Since 1848 [when the first women's rights convention
occurred in Seneca, New York] . . . the revolution in
public opinion about women has been so enormous,
that there is no century, nor five nor ten centuries of all
preceding European history, which can compare with it.

MARY PUTNAM JACOBI, M.D.,
"COMMON SENSE" APPLIED TO
WOMAN SUFFRAGE

I said I did not believe it was best either for the sick or
for society for women to be doctors; that, personally,
women lose something of the natural charm of their
sex in giving themselves either to this or to the other
avocations until now in sole possession of man.

SILAS WEIR MITCHELL, M.D., CHARACTERISTICS

The
Cure
for
Women

Prologue: a Desire to Heal

ONE AFTERNOON IN THE SUMMER OF 1985, MY GRANDMOTHER AND her four sisters, ages seventy-two to eighty-nine, gathered to celebrate their mother, Ellen Babb, who had passed away in 1953. They drank strong coffee, ate crustless sandwiches, and reminisced about being raised by a practicing midwife and healer who cared for the women and children in her rural Missouri community during the first years of the twentieth century.

Speaking into a tape recorder, they shared memories about her life. She'd run the farm and raised twelve children, all of whom went to college. She taught her daughters how to care for the ill and craft remedies from herbs gathered along the nearby Niangua River. Among her friends and neighbors, she was known to work miracles. The busy county medical doctor trusted her judgment and often referred his patients to Ellen. Neighbors sent their young daughters to learn about their monthly periods. She concocted remedies to cure cramps. She cooled fevers, calmed gout, and soothed anxiety among young expectant mothers, attending to their births when the time came. Once, she saved a premature baby by placing it in a homemade incubator: an insulated cabinet lined with hot-water-filled milk bottles that surrounded the infant, keeping it warm. Throughout the days and nights that followed, she and other family members replaced the water in the bottles as it cooled with water heated in a nearby kerosene fire. The baby lived.

But one particular story seemed to best describe Ellen's deep courage and quick thinking. One morning a panicked neighbor rushed over carrying her toddler, who had swallowed a safety pin. It had opened and was pointing upward in the poor child's throat. Without any hesitation, Ellen shoved two fingers down the child's throat, impaled her forefinger on the sharp pin, and removed her finger with the pin attached. The toddler was uninjured.

To keep up with the latest developments in medicine, Ellen read the medical books recommended by the county doctor. Deep down, she always wanted to be a doctor but had never gotten the chance.

A few years ago, after listening to the recording of my grandmother and great-aunts, the love for their mother shining forth in their voices, I became curious about the great-grandmother I had never known. Her medical skill was superb. Why hadn't she become a doctor? I performed a few haphazard Google searches, unwittingly planting the early seeds of this book as I soon discovered that, until the end of the nineteenth century, women had been barred from medical schools and higher education. I had heard of Elizabeth Blackwell, so I knew that women doctors existed then. But I was fascinated and chagrined that I did not know about the other pioneering women doctors who followed her—Emily Blackwell, Ann Preston, and Marie Zakrzewska, among others. In order to practice medicine and thrive as doctors, these women had to open their own medical schools and hospitals.

Yet women's struggle to become licensed physicians spurred a massive backlash. Using Charles Darwin as their guiding star, top scientists and professors of medicine—Oliver Wendell Holmes Sr. (famed author and dean of Harvard Medical School), S. Weir Mitchell (inventor of the rest cure for women), J. Marion Sims ("father" of gynecology, a man who tortured enslaved women to earn that moniker), and Edward H. Clarke (a Harvard professor who literally wrote the book on women's inferiority), among others—conspired to obstruct the advancement of women. They argued that a woman's inferior biology should prevent her from pursuing higher education or any other endeavor outside the home. If upper-class women—the only women for whom higher education was even a possibility—strained their delicate systems with too much brainwork, they'd become infertile, and the white supremacists at the helm of society just couldn't have that.

Fortunately, a hero arose and brought data-backed science to the fight. Mentored by Elizabeth Blackwell, the brilliant Dr. Mary Putnam Jacobi, in her scathing response to Clarke and the rest of the medical establishment, argued that women had the right to control their own physical and intellectual destinies. Most radically, she argued that men and women were not so different and that social restrictions, not biology, threatened female health.

In a Victorian culture that valued women as ornamental birthing machines, the cutting-edge, evidence-based medicine Jacobi practiced was an act of disobedience. Her scientific research dismantled the myths about women's bodies spread by men, transformed medicine, and laid the groundwork for the future advancements of women, including suffrage. It was a turning point for women struggling to be seen as fully human. Jacobi became one of the most important physicians, male or female, of the nineteenth century. Her amazing accomplishments remain mostly unrecognized today. Along with Elizabeth Blackwell and Susan B. Anthony, Mary Putnam Jacobi should be celebrated for her advancement of women's rights.

In the decades since the battle against medical men like Clarke and Mitchell, as women fought for the right to vote, own property, use contraception, get equal pay, play sports, et cetera, the white men in power have continued to use "science" and "biology" as ammunition against them. Former Harvard president Lawrence Summers reignited the 1874 controversy in 2005 with his infamous statement that women were less successful than men in science and engineering because of sex differences. Popular evolutionary psychologist Jordan Peterson, a modern-day Victorian and a champion of men's rights, has published three books arguing that women's capabilities are defined by their biology and their evolutionary ties to child-rearing, echoing Clarke and Mitchell.

During Hillary Clinton's presidential campaign, some people consistently questioned her ability to make decisions because they believed that her hormones would make her irrational, especially if she got her period. Apparently, some men still don't understand women's biology.

Disputes over a woman's capacity to live a fully human life despite her reproductive organs remain a central point of contention. It is imperative that we understand when and where these ideas originated so that we can determine how to defeat them.

As I write this, another profound backlash against women's fundamental rights and autonomy is underway. In 2022, the U.S. Supreme Court overturned *Roe v. Wade*. Justice Alito, in writing the court's majority opinion, ignored judicial precedent and cited the work of seventeenth-century witch hunter and defender of marital rape Sir Matthew Hale, a timeless authority on women's biology: "Two treatises by Sir Matthew Hale likewise described abortion of a quick child who died in the womb as a 'great crime' and a 'great misprision,'" Alito wrote.

Like Clarke and his associates, Alito believed that women would not fight back. All of them were wrong.

Part One

Beginning

**Unknown things want science
to make them known.**

Mary C. Putnam Jacobi,
"Theorae ad Lienis Officium"

1

A Moral Imperative

ELIZABETH BLACKWELL, M.D., PACED BACK AND FORTH IN HER DRAB Lower West Side apartment, stopping occasionally to glance through her parlor window at the blizzard swirling outside. The deepening snow had quieted the metallic clickety-clack of horse hooves and carriage wheels on the bumpy echoing cobblestones in front of her building at 44 University Place. On a typical day, she saw patients at this time, between ten a.m. and noon, but today, none had appeared. Even on fair-weather days, her landlady might chase them away. The woman, who kept raising the rent, spread terrifying gossip.

Thirty-year-old Blackwell had been called an abortionist and a prostitute and had been spit on, too, in the years since she had won her battle to attend medical school. She was rejected by twenty-nine medical schools before being admitted to New York State's Geneva Medical College in 1847. After receiving her application, the faculty decided to let the student body decide whether or not to allow Blackwell into their hallowed halls. The young men apparently thought that the members of the faculty were playing a joke, so they voted yes. From that supposed joke came Blackwell's opportunity, which she seized with determination. While earning her degree, she learned to be impervious to disparagements.

Adding more coal to her small iron furnace, Blackwell remembered the mortifications that she had endured to reach this point. With few exceptions, the citizens of the staid village of Geneva had regarded her as a wanton woman, utterly insane, and a traitor to her sex who would be a wicked influence on children. After all, in today's world, a proper lady did not lead an independent public life. Only poor and immigrant women who labored as servants, clerks, factory workers, or prostitutes were seen walking the streets. The refined upper- and middle-class women remained in the private sphere of home and hearth, cloistered and happy all their lives.

But Blackwell, against every custom, attended medical school with the smirking young men, more like boys, who, in her presence, whistled and catcalled to attract the high-school girls walking by on their way to class. These same rowdy young men robbed local graves for fresh bodies to use in their anatomy classes. But Blackwell's quiet determination, sober dress, and cool responses to the paper darts aimed at her in lectures eventually won the young men's grudging admiration.

Blackwell constructed an imaginary brick wall around her nerves, practiced superhuman self-control, and negotiated with her medical-school professors when they were angered or embarrassed by her presence. By the end of her two years—the standard length of medical school at the time—she had earned the respect of her instructors, and she graduated at the top of her class.

While attending the medical college, she had been invited by Elizabeth Cady Stanton to speak at the first women's rights convention held a few miles from Geneva in Seneca Falls during the summer of 1848. Blackwell refused, believing such efforts to improve the lives of women trivial. She had given up on the "sisterhood of suffragettes." They reminded her of the chickens on the farm who kept running around even after their heads had been chopped off: No direction, only frantic reaction, unlike Blackwell, who had taken bold action by confronting the system head-on and become the first woman to earn a medical degree in the United States. Nonetheless, she was blind to the fact that she treated the suffragists the same way the town of Geneva had treated her—as freakish.

Influenced by the charismatic Unitarian minister William Henry Channing and the transcendentalist writings of Margaret Fuller, Blackwell was deeply religious. She believed in the inherent goodness of people and nature, self-reliance, and intuition. In her daily struggle to become a doctor, she saw herself as a lone prophet, sympathetic and godly, someone whose message would one day be heard above the common babble, guiding men and women alike into a better world.

When she arrived in New York City after graduation, her overconfidence led her to believe that being first in her class along with her experience working in clinics in Paris and London would secure her a position at a prominent hospital or medical practice despite her being a woman.

Unfortunately, while feminists of the day were supportive of her cause, the patriarchal medical establishment was not.

The deep resentment felt by most physicians toward women becoming doctors surfaced soon after Blackwell graduated in the correspondence columns of the highly influential *Boston Medical and Surgical Journal*. One letter from an angry physician who called himself D.K. argued that women must remain the pride and glory of the race, "the sacred repository of all that is virtuous, graceful, and lovely." A woman should not dishonor her sex by "seeking laurels in forbidden paths." This letter was challenged by another pseudonymous correspondent, Justus, who pointed out that female midwives had been bringing babies into the world since time immemorial, and it would surely be better for everyone if they continued to do so after having been properly trained in modern scientific methods. But while the writer, a man, defended women's right to oversee a childbirth, he also wrote: "As to females engaging in the general practice of medicine, the idea is absurd; D.K. need have no fears of a rivalry, which he seems to dread." In the end, the medical establishment publicly condemned Geneva Medical College for its irresponsible action of admitting a woman into a man's profession. The college responded by immediately shutting its doors to all further women applicants.

After being rejected by every hospital and clinic in New York, Blackwell decided to open her own practice. She approached landlords about leasing offices, but they turned her away too. She finally obtained decent lodgings near Washington Square with enough space for consulting rooms. But even with nearly daily advertisements for her services in the *Tribune*, her patients were few and far between. Her practice was damaged by the cruel gossip, insolent letters, and frequent harassment from "unprincipled men," especially those who propositioned her when she was out alone at night visiting her patients.

Being the first woman in the United States to earn a medical degree was a lonely business. Blackwell had grown up with two older siblings and six younger ones; one of her younger brothers, Henry, had recently married the illustrious activist Lucy Stone. Blackwell was accustomed to the warmth and camaraderie of her well-educated family, and when she encouraged her sister Emily to study medicine, she feared that her primary reason was so that she would have a supportive companion to help her own practice succeed.

Still snowbound in her apartment, she heard her landlady's craggy voice direct someone toward her rooms. Blackwell opened her door to find a tiny Quaker woman brushing away the snow that had caked along the folding hems of her bell-shaped skirt and petticoat. Her pinched face, cheeks bright red from the cold, broke into a luminous smile when she saw Blackwell. Once inside and standing next to the stove, she removed her Quaker-style wool bonnet and cloak, embraced Blackwell like a sister, and introduced herself as Ann Preston from Philadelphia, a student of medicine.

Blackwell likely surmised that Preston was attending one of the many eclectic medical schools that had opened in response to the growing dissatisfaction with the so-called heroic medicine administered by regular physicians. Their strict regimen included bloodletting, sweating, and purging to shock the body back to health following an illness brought on by "humoral imbalance." The fact was, medicine in the mid-nineteenth century hadn't changed much since Hippocrates. The emerging health-reform movement flourished by promoting more humane methods, including public hygiene, dietary reform, temperance, hydrotherapy, and instruction on human physiology. New, gentler healing approaches had become enormously popular. Eclectic (sometimes called "irregular") medical schools had opened across the country and offered training in a wide variety of alternative health methods, including water cures, botany, and homeopathy. All of these eclectic schools welcomed female students. The American Medical Association had been formed in 1846 to counter these trends by advancing traditional medical science, raising the standards for medical education and licensing, and establishing an ethics board to enlighten the public about the so-called quack science practiced by eclectic doctors.

While Blackwell agreed with many of the new natural approaches, especially public health, hygiene, and disease prevention, she was firmly on the side of traditional medicine. It was all she could do to keep from rolling her eyes at Preston. Instead, she smiled and nodded.

Sensing what Blackwell was thinking, Preston assured her that she was part of an inevitable historic movement to educate women as regular medical doctors that was just beginning in Philadelphia. She felt that her news was so exciting and hopeful, she had to tell Blackwell in person, even during a blizzard. After all, nothing great was easily earned. As she spoke, her fragile demeanor resonated with such courage that Blackwell's initial misgivings softened.

Preston explained that a group of powerful Quakers, all wealthy Philadelphia abolitionists and philanthropists, including William Mullen, Dr. Joseph Longshore, and Dr. Bartholomew Fussell, felt that it was morally imperative for women to be educated like men as medical doctors. Many women who were suffering from severe illnesses could not bring themselves to violate the Victorian ideals of purity, chastity, and social propriety and expose their bodies to male physicians. According to Fussell's nephew Edwin, "Many sensitive women were seen suffering and dying rather than shock what they felt to be the sacredness of their womanhood."

Even worse, doctors heard that some husbands were refusing to permit the indecency of male doctors bringing their children into the world. The proper education of more women doctors would alleviate this tragedy and save the lives of countless loving mothers.

These Quaker men had applied for and received a charter from the Pennsylvania state legislature in May 1850 for the Female Medical College of Pennsylvania, making it one of the first institutions worldwide to grant women legitimate regular medical degrees. A member of the first class, Ann Preston was to receive her degree in December 1851. (The mayor of Philadelphia had to send fifty policemen to her commencement to ward off threatened disruptions.)

Eight years older than Blackwell, Preston had been involved in antislavery struggles from a young age. Inspired by the courageous escape in 1849 of Henry "Box" Brown, an enslaved Richmond man who shipped himself to Philadelphia in a small wooden crate, Preston published a popular abolitionist children's book called *Cousin Ann's Stories for Children*. "To My Little Readers," the book began, "I thought I would write a little book, and that would be a good way to speak with you, though I am far away." Cousin Ann advised her young readers to treasure freedom, abhor slavery, and treat others generously and honestly and encouraged them to avoid tobacco and alcohol and eat a healthy diet. Preston yearned to become a doctor; she had felt helpless during her younger sister's lengthy illness and painful death.

She assured Blackwell that things would get better. Women physicians would not suffer the fate of the midwives, who had nearly disappeared from cities after being replaced by male obstetricians. It was women's destiny to become doctors, she proclaimed boldly. They would thrive through institution building, constructing their own schools and hospitals.

Still, Blackwell's doubts remained a stone-cold weight inside her. It would take a monumental effort to change the culture. The lives of middle- and upper-class nineteenth-century women were deeply shaped by the popular "cult of true womanhood," set firmly in the private sphere of home and family. In a rapidly changing world where men were charged with forming an industrialized civilization from a vast wilderness, the true woman, the angel of the home, embraced her natural tendencies toward piety, purity, submissiveness, and domesticity and exerted a serenely moral influence over her husband. She and her children were the bright inner sanctum against a corrupt outer world.

Today, Preston had come to Blackwell with a solution to the predica- ment women doctors faced. It was simple: As professionals, they should embrace the moral ideal of "true womanhood" and adopt a narrative that connected home and hearth directly to the public office of a female phy- sician. Since mothers tended to sick children, Preston maintained that the practice of medicine was inherently female. More important, women healing other women was the moral choice. Unlike the masculine jobs that required hard labor, complex politics, or harsh business dealings, medicine was a viable part of the woman's sphere. By adopting preven- tive medicine and focusing on personal hygiene, women's reproductive health, and children's health, women doctors, like good mothers, would help manage the daily lives of their patients and teach them good habits. In other words, women were best equipped to care for the private lives of women and children.

Male doctors, even the forthright ones, could not hide their aversion to treating issues of breasts and vaginas. In fact, most examinations were done in the dark with the patient fully clothed. In order to preserve female modesty (and reassure husbands), the male obstetrician examined his pa- tients by touch. The whole process was less like the practice of medicine and more like spelunking. Though Preston would never criticize any male doctor—the success of the women's medical college depended on its male professors and benefactors—she did not hesitate to further her arguments by using their own words against them. For example, she often quoted Charles D. Meigs, a popular professor of obstetrics at Jefferson Medical College. He admitted to the difficulty of treating women in his renowned book *Females and Their Diseases:*

All these evils of medical practice spring not, in the main, from any want of competency in medicines or medical men, but from the delicacy of the relations existing between the sexes of which I spoke. . . . There are women who prefer to suffer the extremity of danger and pain rather than waive those scruples of delicacy which prevent their maladies from being fully explored.

If women were meant to remain separate in their own feminine world, Preston argued, why should men be allowed to treat them at all?

In the days after Preston's visit, Blackwell felt revitalized by their new-found professional sisterhood. She agreed that virtuous women belonged in the medical profession because of their God-given talents for nurturing and healing. In fact, women were most radically feminine as doctors. Like Preston, Blackwell needed to see her professional advancement as inevitable because the future well-being of women and children depended on their success. Most important, as Preston had cautioned, female physicians must not suffer the same fate as midwives.

Back in 1820, an esteemed doctor from Boston wrote an essay so controversial that he decided to publish it under the name "Anonymous." He titled his work *Remarks on the Employment of Females as Practitioners in Midwifery.*

"The question is," he wrote, "can the practice of midwifery be carried on with equal safety by female as by male Practitioners?" The simple construction of his sentences hid the fact that his proposals were meant to upend centuries of tradition and terminate the practice of midwifery.

Members of a highly respected profession, midwives had long cared for women and children in America and Europe. All births occurred at home and were overseen by the midwife and her network of attendants, who provided comfort, nourishment, and nurturing while patiently waiting for the wholly natural process of labor and birth. Together, women endured the pain and dangers, looked to one another for support, and shared the happiness of successful deliveries and the devastation when a child or mother was lost.

The midwife's specialized skill complemented women's duties at home, which strengthened her position as a legitimate, socially acceptable professional woman. For generations, midwives had successfully bridged the gap between public and domestic life for women.

In addition to birthing duties, midwives also acted as nurses, morticians, and pharmacists for entire families, and those who could did pay well for their specialized skills. They helped men and women prevent pregnancy with the use of condoms made from animal intestines, cervical sponges, and douches. They also performed abortions, allowed under common law and widely practiced. Most eighteenth-century Americans considered abortion to be a normal part of life. In fact, Benjamin Franklin included a recipe for an abortifacient in a book he published titled *The American Instructor or Young Man's Best Companion*, a manual to teach useful skills, including mathematics:

> For this Misfortune, you must purge with Highland Flagg, (commonly called Belly-ach Root) a Week before you expect to be out of Order; and repeat the same two Days after; the next Morning drink a Quarter of Pint of Pennyroyal Water, or Decoction, with 12 Drops of Spirits of Harts-horn, and as much again at Night, when you go to Bed. Continue this 9 Days running; and after resting 3 Days, go on with it for 9 more.

The author called the recipe a solution to "the misfortune" of an unwanted pregnancy for "unmarry'd women." Franklin was following the English and European tradition in which abortions were legal up to quickening, meaning when a pregnant woman felt the fetus moving.

Consequently, a good midwife was able to carve out a significant economic niche for herself. Even though she made sure that physicians and surgeons were notified for difficult births, in reality, she was a formidable competitor for their patients. Custom and superstition continued to bar men from the lying-in chamber, except when the surgeon's tools were needed to extricate a dead fetus. Rural communities could support two midwives but only one physician. Moreover, early eighteenth-century ignorance of anatomy, physiology, and surgery put physicians and midwives on equal footing when it came to managing childbirth.

During the final two decades of the eighteenth century, the prestige midwives enjoyed began to diminish. Technological developments, such as the invention of the forceps, a corrected understanding of the anatomy of the birth canal, and the use of ether for anesthesia and opium and laudanum to ease pain and quiet nerves, transformed the way babies were born. Skilled mechanical intervention shortened labor and sometimes saved the lives of the mother and child. Doctors promised patients that the use of forceps, therapeutic drugs, and especially ether and chloroform would protect against the overwhelming pain and terrors of birth. Doctors also began to institutionalize the practice of medicine by requiring appropriate formal licensing.

By the mid-eighteenth century, the few hundred formally trained American physicians sought to improve their professional status by studying abroad in the hospitals and medical schools of England, France, and Germany. Astounded by European advances in medical science and by the elite professionalism of European publications, societies, and hospitals, these doctors returned home ready to guide the institutional development of the medical profession in America.

In colonial America's villages and cities, opportunities for building a reputable medical practice multiplied. Benjamin Franklin helped to found the Pennsylvania Hospital in 1751, the first hospital in America, and patterned it after European models. Serving both rich and poor, the institution provided new clinical opportunities to medical students. Fourteen years later, the Pennsylvania Medical School opened, followed by King's College (later Columbia) medical school in 1768 and Harvard's medical school in 1780. These schools provided education for the few hundred elite physicians who practiced in urban areas. The hundreds of rural doctors, like midwives, received no formal training and learned their skills through apprenticeship and direct experience.

In urban areas, practicing midwifery provided the means for a struggling young doctor to introduce himself to respectable clients. Sometimes the fierce competition for patients between midwives and physicians resulted in mutual disputes and verbal attacks.

In the end, the cries of immodesty made against physicians were no match for the charges of incompetency hurled at the midwives. The only hope for the continued existence of female midwives, especially in urban areas, was for midwives to gain access to the mechanical instruments and scientific knowledge necessary to advance their skills. That's why, when the anonymous Boston physician set out to discredit women as midwives in his essay, he focused not only on their lack of medical education but also on why they should not be educated at all.

"It is obvious that we cannot instruct women as we do men in the science of medicine," he wrote. Females should never be allowed to enter the dissecting room or the hospital except as patients because their refined sensibility and delicate bearing would be completely destroyed. It was difficult enough for the men, who had to subdue their own shock and distress while helping patients. A doctor's methods of treatment—bleeding and purging—were painful and dangerous. The possibility of inflicting extreme pain on patients was part of the daily reality of the heroic medicine in professional practice and, arguably, an integral part of the masculine self-image. A woman entering their field was simply unimaginable. The midwife, who experienced birth, death, and the expelling of blood, feces, phlegm, and all known bodily fluids on a daily basis, was too delicate to learn dissection or surgery.

"It was one of the first and happiest fruits of improved medical education in America, that . . . [women] were excluded from practice," the anonymous writer continued. Thus, the answer to his opening question—"Can the practice of midwifery be carried on with equal safety by female as by male Practitioners?"—was obviously no.

Remarks on the Employment of Females as Practitioners in Midwifery sold out quickly and was reprinted again and again. The author was eventually revealed to be Walter Channing, M.D., professor of midwifery at Harvard Medical School and founding editor of the *New England Journal of Medicine and Surgery*. The esteemed professor's arguments against women in medicine became the standard view of all medical schools. Almost overnight, women, the traditional health-care providers in the home for centuries, were barred from being educated as doctors.

At the time that Channing wrote his essay, the new field of obstetrics was struggling to find legitimacy. Young medical students considered midwifery to be an old woman's kind of business, and many women continued to employ midwives in a desire to preserve modesty.

In response, medical-school professors went to great lengths to help their male students learn the proper method needed to soothe a female patient into compliance. The most famous of these was Charles Meigs, professor of obstetrics and diseases of women at Jefferson Medical College, who trained some of the most respected doctors in America. Full of charisma, Meigs had the soul of a performer, which made his flamboyant lectures memorable. In each of Meigs's skits, the hypothetical female patient, chaste and reluctant but also a dimwit, would be lured into an examination by the heroic male physician's delicately manipulative rhetoric.

He always entered his classroom with his back straight, eyes forward, like a polite visitor to a lady's parlor. He would introduce the topic and proceed to act out his case in a highly entertaining performance. Attending a Meigs lecture was like reading a romance novel.

Today's imaginary patient, a pregnant twenty-two-year-old woman, was unable to urinate due to retroversion of the uterus. Clearing his throat, Meigs said in his deep, doctorly voice, "Will you please inform me what it is that has induced you to call for me, madam?"

Changing position, he crouched down to look shorter and fluttered his eyelashes. "I am in great pain, sir," he wailed in a high-pitched tone.

Meigs's doctorly voice grew stern as he began questioning the woman about her symptoms. After this verbal examination, he explained that her womb had gone "topsy-turvy."

"What in the world is to be done?" Meigs cried in the young woman's shaky voice.

He answered: "You are to allow me to remedy the difficulty."

Now as his female patient: "How?"

"By replacing the womb in its natural position."

"But how can you do that?"

"With my hand."

Meigs's face looked shocked, and he shuddered for effect. "I can't think of such a thing," he replied in his young female patient's voice.

Meigs, once again as the doctor, grew silent; his face turned dour. His students held their breath and waited, excited for what they knew would be a brilliant reprimand of the puerile woman.

"Very well, madam, I shall have to bid you a good afternoon, for I can't think of anything else. In fact, there's nothing else to be done for you."

"Why, I'd rather die."

Meigs's students all rolled their eyes at the woman's ridiculous behavior.

"As you please, madam; you are the mistress; *ce que femme vent, Dieu le vent*; but I hope you will permit me to say it would be very silly of you to die, for want of the power to make water, when there's a physician at hand, who can put you so easily in the way to do it easily."

To the joy of his students, Meigs, as the fragile woman, began to cry real tears. Finally, in a quivering voice, Meigs asked, "Will it hurt me, sir?" And with that, in a most dramatic fashion, he proceeded to save the woman and her future child.

Meigs's students were entranced.

Meigs was America's expert on women's health. In his bestselling book *Females and Their Diseases*, published in 1848, he wrote that woman "has a head almost too small for intellect but just big enough for love." She was "queen of the loves." He informed his students that by studying female sex organs, they would have expertise over a woman's whole being.

Yet these tactics, fated to be used by an army of doctors for decades to come, alarmed many women and men and provided strong ammunition in their arguments for educating women as doctors. In the early days, before Elizabeth Blackwell was accepted into regular medical school, a middle-aged woman named Harriot Hunt led the charge to fight for educating women as doctors. In the late fall of 1847, she applied to the dean of Harvard Medical School, Oliver Wendell Holmes, asking to attend lectures. A resident of Boston, Hunt had been trained in herbal medicine, water cures, and human hygiene a decade earlier when her sister, who had suffered through treatments with mercury, leeches, purging, and bleeding by conventional doctors for a debilitating illness, was cured by the eclectic remedies of fresh air, herbal tinctures, diet, and exercise.

Known as the first woman in America to practice medicine professionally, Harriot Hunt treated women of all classes who were drawn in by her caring bedside manner and gentle cures. Her experience confirmed her theory that "concealed sorrows" were often the root of physical ills. As she listened to her patients' "heart histories," she was repeatedly exposed to horrifying scenes of domestic suffering.

Hunt taught women about their own bodies, purposely removing their dependency on male doctors and husbands who wanted to keep them ignorant. She showed them how to prevent illness through proper exercise, rest, diet, and hygiene. She advised them to learn to dance and demonstrated a few steps to illustrate how healthful it could be. To bring her self-help principles to a wider audience, she organized the Ladies' Physiological Society of Boston, holding meetings in the homes of middle- and upper-class women, including her own home. She proved to be a powerful public speaker.

Hunt's eclectic medical practice eventually made her wealthy. Nearly everyone in New England knew her name. To keep up with advances in science, she studied and memorized medical textbooks on her own, but she yearned for the credibility that medical doctors enjoyed, so she applied to Harvard. At first, she was hopeful about being admitted. Dean Holmes said that he admired Hunt's zeal for science. Moreover, due to her mature age (forty-one) and general unattractiveness, she might be "dobly [*sic*] trusted, so far as appearances go," Holmes said, meaning that she would not distract the male students from their studies. But despite Holmes's encouraging comments, her application was rejected.

Compelled into action by Harvard's rejection, Hunt, along with her life partner, activist Sarah Grimke, began a series of free lectures in Boston's North End to educate the public about the fight for women's rights. Even though her wealthy clients and friends warned her against becoming associated with the suffrage radicals, Hunt gave a blazing speech advocating for more women doctors at the national women's rights convention held in Worcester, Massachusetts, in 1850.

Hunt loved being in the thick of the struggle. When she met Lucy Stone and Lucretia Mott, she felt that she had at last found her home with the founding mothers of America's women's rights movement. Her eyes were opened to the power of women working together. She vowed to dedicate her life to helping deserving women become medical doctors. As a first step, in 1850 she applied to Harvard Medical School a second time, claiming that, with the graduation of Elizabeth Blackwell from medical school, public opinion was turning in her favor. Three African American men requested admission at the same time as Hunt. Two of them were sponsored by the American Colonization Society and would serve as missionaries in Liberia, and the third was abolitionist Martin R. Delaney. Faced with racial and gender challenges to the status quo, Harvard initially agreed to let all four of them attend lectures, but their prospective classmates, all white males, threatened to ruin Harvard's reputation by exiting for other schools, ones that showed more respect for their white male students.

Fearing open mutiny, Harvard reversed its decision and stated that it would not allow any women or "colored students" to intermix with the white males. To frighten away other women applicants, Harvard made sure that Hunt was ridiculed in the press. One newspaper excoriated her for violating "God's truth" that women were subordinate to men.

A furious Hunt responded, "When civilization is further advanced, and the great doctrine of human rights is acknowledged, this act will be recalled and wondering eyes will stare, and wondering ears will be opened, at the semi-barbarism of the middle of the nineteenth century."

In 1851, the case for women physicians won an enormous victory when

Sarah Hale, the influential editor of *Godey's Lady's Book*, the most popular women's magazine in the country with a subscription base of 150,000, published a series of editorials extolling the virtues of female physicians, noting they were, "by nature, better qualified than men to take charge of the sick and suffering." They were best suited to treat children and were the only "proper attendants for their own sex in the hour of sorrow." Hale praised Elizabeth Blackwell and Ann Preston and applauded the opening of the Female Medical College of Pennsylvania. Boldly, she argued that half the physicians in the United States should be women. After reading Hale's editorials, more women began asking for female doctors.

In 1852, energized by her newfound friendship with Ann Preston, Elizabeth Blackwell delivered a series of lectures in New York City church basements and living rooms to audiences made up mostly of Quaker ladies on the proper spiritual, intellectual, emotional, and physical care of girls. Many of these women became her patients, and her lectures were so popular, G. P. Putnam published them that same year as *The Laws of Life, with Special Reference to the Physical Education of Girls.*

Harriot Hunt joined with philanthropist and activist Caroline Severance and other wealthy donors to establish the Ohio Female Medical Loan Fund Association. Its primary purpose was to grant prospective female medical students across the country interest-free loans that they would repay once they graduated and their practices were established. Ohio had several eclectic medical colleges that accepted women, and Elizabeth's sister Emily Blackwell graduated from the regular medical college of Western Reserve University in Cleveland in 1854. That same year, Hunt toured Ohio lecturing on medical education for women; she received enthusiastic public support and favorable press coverage.

With grants from the state and donations from the wealthy, Blackwell opened the New York Dispensary for Poor Women and Children, a free clinic. She wanted independence and a way to use her skills as a physician, but she ended up in a small damp room in the heart of Little Germany near the tenements on East Seventh Street. Here, she made available to the seamstresses, factory workers, domestics, and their children basic medical care, gave advice on proper hygiene, diet, and home ventilation, and offered instructions on the best way to find a job.

Poor women had never experienced the "cult of true womanhood," nor did they have anything resembling the "private sphere of hearth and home." A crowded tenement room could never be called private. Because they lacked the means to pay, poor women received little attention from the medical profession. They routinely experienced injury, illness, and exhaustion, especially when pregnant. Employers provided no paid time off for pregnancy or illness. Absences from work could cost a woman her job.

Just as the dispensary opened, Dr. Emily Blackwell arrived in New York from Cleveland; she was on her way to Scotland to study obstetric surgery under the illustrious physician James Young Simpson, chair of midwifery and diseases of women at the University of Edinburgh. Five years younger than Elizabeth, Emily felt liberated by her own success. While Elizabeth had sailed through life, buoyed by her utter self-confidence, Emily, although equally intelligent, often stewed in self-doubt. Her brother Henry, in a letter to Elizabeth, described Emily as shrewd and full of productive energy. "She is possessed of a most admirable *balance* of physical and mental qualities—strong but not heavy, with clear definite common sense, quick prompt, decided, quiet, cheerful & self possessed."

After helping Elizabeth for three weeks, Emily sailed for Europe. With more than a twinge of jealousy, Elizabeth watched her sister go. "This medical solitude is really awful at times," she confided days later in a letter to Emily. But her spirits were lifted when she received news that Ann Preston had been appointed professor of physiology and hygiene at the Female Medical College of Pennsylvania. She would be the first woman professor of medicine at an accredited college in America. The same college also awarded Harriot Hunt an honorary medical degree.

Elizabeth made plans to expand the dispensary and open a hospital dedicated to women and children that was staffed by well-educated women doctors. The problem was, highly trained women doctors were scarce, and her sister Emily would not finish with her studies in Scotland until 1856. Elizabeth searched for another physician but was not satisfied with any of them until, one day, a young redheaded German showed up at her clinic. Soon, she realized that this woman was the answer to her prayers.

A Tale of Two Hospitals

IN 1840, TEN-YEAR-OLD, AUBURN-HAIRED MARIE ZAKRZEWSKA WAS living with her mother at the Charité, a prominent teaching hospital and midwifery school in Berlin. Her father, a man of "revolutionary tendencies," had been dismissed from his position as a military officer, and to help support her family, Marie's mother was training to be a midwife at Charité. The courses required her to reside in the hospital for several months and receive clinical training along with the male medical students. At first, Marie was sent to live with an aunt, but a short time later, Marie's eyes "became affected with weakness so that [she] could neither read nor write." Marie's mother received permission for her daughter to stay with her at the hospital while receiving treatment for her eyes. Dr. Müller, Marie's physician, was so charmed by the girl's cleverness that he began taking her with him on his rounds. With her eyes bandaged, she listened to his lectures with such focused attention that he began calling her his "little blind doctor."

One day, after her eyes had healed, Dr. Müller entertained young Marie by describing how the corpse of a young man who had died of poisoning had turned completely green. The body was now resting in the deadhouse, the hospital's morgue and pathology laboratory. Marie was astonished. She asked if she could see the man's body, but the doctor was too busy to take her.

After finishing rounds with Dr. Müller, Marie, who had grown more curious throughout the day, decided to view the body on her own.

When she entered the deadhouse, she was surprised to find the room filled with living people—the mourning relatives of the deceased were adorning the body with flowers. To pass the time until the relatives were finished, she walked through the nearby pathology rooms, where other dead bodies were waiting to be examined. She wrinkled her nose at the sour smell of formaldehyde. More than a dozen corpses, all dressed in white gowns, were laid out on boards attached to the newly painted milk-white walls. A dissecting table stood in the center of each room. She was tall enough to see over the tables, but she could not reach the cutting instruments.

After examining the pathology rooms, she saw that the corpse's relatives had left, so she went to look at the body of the young man who had been poisoned. His skin was a dull, dark green, similar to the stain left on fingers from copper rings. His face wore its death mask, still grimacing from pain. His icy-cold skin amazed her. She found a chair, pushed it over, and climbed up so she could see the entire body. He was very young, not more than twenty. She felt sad for his relatives but not for him. Not now. She knew that he was beyond any pain. The more she looked, the more she saw. Finally, her curiosity fully satisfied, she climbed down from the chair.

That's when she noticed that the morgue had grown silent. Everyone was gone. The doors were all locked. She banged on the doors until the sun disappeared. The deadhouse was now pitch-dark.

Exhausted, Marie decided to sit on the floor and wait. She knew she would be found eventually. She fell fast asleep. Her frantic mother did not find her until close to midnight. A few days later, Dr. Müller, impressed by Marie's fearless behavior, gave her two books: the *History of Midwifery* and the *History of Surgery*. She found the books so interesting that Dr. Müller could not pry her away from them to join him on his morning and evening rounds. She would later say that this was when she began her study of medicine.

In the fall of 1849, at age twenty, Marie Zakrzewska was accepted into the Charité's school of midwifery, where she studied for the next three and a half years under the watchful eye of her mentor Joseph Herman Schmidt, associate professor of obstetrics. She learned about the natural sciences and acquired excellent obstetric skills, delivering thirty babies per year herself and assisting in numerous other births. She also learned that in a battle between a physician and a midwife, the physician always won. Nevertheless, the education Zakrzewska received at the Charité was equal to or better than that of American medical students. At the time, few American medical schools offered bedside training or clinical instruction in gynecological-speculum use. Since Zakrzewska's midwifery professors also taught at the University of Berlin, her obstetrical training differed little from what the male medical students received. When she graduated, she was appointed head midwife.

Zakrzewska, the star pupil, was extremely self-confident. She never hesitated to state her opinion but had to learn over time the advantages of diplomacy and negotiation. One leading physician at the Charité, Ernst Horn, complained that "Marie had shown a hint of snappish nature, impudence, and a lack of control." Zakrzewska found Horn to be equally insufferable.

Because of Zakrzewska's clashes with Horn, her tenure as head midwife lasted only six months. More than anything, she wanted to be the doctor who gave the orders. She had heard that in America, "women will now become physicians, like the men." She had read about Elizabeth Blackwell. Restless and ambitious, Zakrzewska decided that she would go to America to study medicine. When she told her father that she wanted to emigrate, he said he would not help her unless she took along her younger sister Anna. On March 13, 1853, they left home. Three weeks after that, they sailed from Hamburg in the clipper ship *Deutschland*, experiencing "excessively stormy" seas before arriving in New York forty-seven days later.

In New York, Zakrzewska discovered that, in fact, American men were doing all they could to bar women from practicing medicine. Further, since midwives had been replaced by male obstetricians, she could not find a job. She spent her last few dollars setting up a business knitting worsted wool into fancy wares to sell in the marketplace.

It turned out that she was a gifted businesswoman. At one point, she had thirty women working for her. She persisted in her attempts to become a doctor, though, and as luck would have it, a connection she made with the manager of a homeless shelter brought her to Elizabeth Blackwell. Elizabeth was very impressed by her training and ingenuity.

"I have at last found a student in whom I can take a great deal of interest," Elizabeth wrote to Emily about Zakrzewska. "There is true stuff in her, and I shall do my best to bring it out." Nicknaming her Zak, Elizabeth immediately asked her to start assisting at the dispensary. She also hired a tutor to help the young midwife become more proficient in English and promised to find Zakrzewska the medical education that she was searching for.

In 1854, Elizabeth succeeded in getting Marie accepted at Cleveland Medical College, where her sister Emily had just received her medical degree. Just four years later, with mounting pressure from male students and donors, the college would stop admitting women.

Because Zakrzewska's business customers no longer wanted items made from worsted wool, her income declined, and she could not afford to pay for her education. So Elizabeth arranged financing through a newly formed women's scholarship fund. One of Zakrzewska's benefactors, Caroline Severance, was a suffragist who was elected vice president of the recent National Woman's Rights Convention in Syracuse, New York.

Zakrzewska's meeting with Severance at her home in Cleveland marked the start of her political awakening. A new world appeared, full of abolitionists, spiritualists, free-lovers, women's rights advocates, Quakers, and Unitarians. She met William Lloyd Garrison, Ralph Waldo Emerson, Frederick Douglass, and the Grimké sisters, Sarah and Angelina, to name a few. And no one seemed to be more influential than Harriot Hunt, who, along with Severance, had organized the special fund to pay for Zakrzewska's education. When the forty-eight-year-old Hunt met the young Zakrzewska, they felt "an electric communication" instantly between them, "a combination of head and heart," as Hunt wrote in her memoirs. And it was through Hunt that Zakrzewska began to understand how her own struggles to pursue a medical career related to the battle to gain legal rights for women. In 1856, when she returned to New York with her medical degree at the age of twenty-seven, she was more than ready to help the Blackwells open a women's hospital in New York.

~

The Blackwells' infirmary was not the first hospital in New York City that catered to female patients only. On May 18, 1854, Elizabeth, who was contemplating the idea of expanding her small dispensary into a large infirmary, attended a public lecture by J. Marion Sims, a self-promoting surgeon who had recently moved from his home state of Alabama to New York City. His open smile, gentle Southern accent, and self-described achievements impressed her. Exhibiting the agile storytelling ability of P. T. Barnum, Sims conveyed his life story in breathless details that lionized his own character. Like Elizabeth, he professed to be doing God's will by helping women. She held great hopes that she and Sims could work together.

Unlike Elizabeth, Sims had become a woman's doctor by accident. After graduating from Pennsylvania's Jefferson Medical College, he set up a practice near his home in Montgomery, Alabama. Known throughout the state as a highly ambitious young surgeon, he performed "all sorts of beautiful and brilliant operations," as he later wrote in his memoir.

One morning after rounds when he was about to get into his buggy, Sims was asked to attend to a local woman who had been thrown from her pony. "She fell with all her weight on the pelvis. She had no broken bones. She was in bed, complaining of great pain in her back, and a sense of tenesmus in both the bladder and rectum. . . . If there was anything I hated, it was investigating the organs of the female pelvis. But this poor woman was in such a condition that I was obliged to find out what was the matter with her."

He discovered that the fall had caused a retroversion of her uterus. Like most doctors of his time, Sims had no specific gynecological training, but since he thought he knew what was wrong, he decided to try an obscure treatment that he had heard about in medical school. He placed her on her knees and elbows, covered her with a sheet, inserted two fingers into her vagina, and moved them up and down; this, he wrote in his autobiography, allowed air to rush in and forced the displaced uterus back into position. During this procedure, the mechanics involved interested him so much that he forgot about his aversion to feminine physiology. He needed a better way to see the uterus. Later, an idea occurred to him that was so simple, it almost made him laugh. "Introducing the bent handle of a spoon [into a subject's vagina], I saw everything as no man had ever seen before. . . . The speculum made it perfectly clear from the beginning. . . . I felt like an explorer in medicine who first views a new and important territory." At that moment, he decided to claim that territory for himself.

Sims immediately thought of vast possibilities for the speculum, especially for his cases of rectovaginal fistula, a debilitating tear between the rectum and vagina that often occurred during childbirth and caused continual urine and feces leakage into the vagina. Women suffering from this condition always smelled like an outhouse. He "ransacked the country" for cases from which he could learn and develop new surgical techniques. From 1845 to 1849, he performed experimental operations on at least ten enslaved women without their consent and without using anesthesia, even though chloroform was introduced for surgery in 1846. Sims's operating table was a small wooden structure four feet high and two and a half feet wide. His instruments were—like the pewter proto-type speculum—self-constructed.

He operated on eighteen-year-old Lucy first. He positioned her, com-pletely naked, on her knees and elbows with her head resting in her hands. With a dozen other doctors either watching her or holding her down, Lucy endured an hour-long surgery, screaming and crying out in pain. As Sims later wrote, "Lucy's agony was extreme." Due to his mishandling of a sponge to drain urine away from the bladder, Lucy developed blood poisoning and became extremely ill.

"I thought she was going to die," he wrote. But she survived.

For four years, Sims kept experimenting on enslaved women. After thirty operations on a young woman named Anarcha, he finally "perfected" his method. Afterward, he began to practice on white women, using anes-thesia. That's when he moved to New York, hoping to continue his experi-mental surgeries, increase his wealth, and become famous.

Knowing very little about his background, Elizabeth saw herself in Sims, an ambitious outsider who wanted to build a hospital to treat women's dis-eases. She expected him to seek her out because of her unique expertise in women's medicine. When he did not show up at her infirmary, she decided to pay him a call to offer her support.

"He is thoroughly in favor of women studying, and will treat them *justly*, which is all we want," she later wrote to Emily, who was still in Edinburgh. "He is a most fiery man, but with much sweetness nevertheless, honorable and a gentleman." She hoped that his hospital would offer clinical training to female medical-school graduates.

At the time Sims was promoting the opening of a women's hospital, he was probably the only surgeon in America with a practice devoted exclu-sively to the diseases of women. Charles Meigs, who taught obstetrics at Jefferson Medical College, Sims's alma mater, backed him, saying that his success "entitles him to the praise and gratitude of our whole profession."

Yet even with Sims's illustrious background and unique salesmanship, prominent New York surgeons and physicians balked at the idea of a hospi-tal for women only. In response, Sims recruited thirty prominent women, many of whom were married to the resisting doctors, to influence their wealthy husbands in favor of his plans. He received the women's backing by promising to create a women-run board of managers at his new hospital.

After weeks of reading about Sims in the newspapers, Elizabeth had realized that he was not interested in her at all. His Woman's Hospital, located in a four-story brownstone on Madison Avenue, held forty beds and would be staffed entirely by male doctors beholden to Sims. She was not fooled by women managers either. "Half are doctors' wives, the stiffest of the stiff," she complained, "the rest the richest & best known New Yorkers, but all of the fashionable unreformatory set."

When the Woman's Hospital first opened in 1855, it was not an immediate success. Most women gave birth at home, and few saw the need for a hospital devoted entirely to women. Only half the beds were regularly filled. Since surgical gynecology was in its infancy, Sims had to promote his services. With that goal, he built a special arena for surgical demonstrations where he could fine-tune his own technique while entertaining his professional colleagues. This time, instead of practicing on enslaved women, Sims performed his experiments, often without anesthesia, on destitute Irish immigrant women whose fistulas and general health were so bad, they were willing to stay at the hospital indefinitely. Mary Smith, one of the first Irish women to receive surgical treatment, underwent thirty operations between 1856 and 1859, the same number Anarcha, one of Sims's enslaved experimental subjects, endured between 1845 and 1849. Sims made his money by applying the hospital discoveries to his private practice, where he charged astronomical fees. All of these surgeries were performed years before Joseph Lister's antiseptic surgical technique was adopted. Until it was, surgical infection was more dangerous than the surgery itself.

In 1856, Emily Blackwell returned to Elizabeth's dispensary with better training than most surgeons in America, including J. Marion Sims, had. She had cultivated the reserved, clinical detachment evident in highly skilled surgeons, confessing to her sister, "The blood affected me no more than so much warm water." Professor Simpson was a rare supporter of women's medical education. "As this movement progresses, it is evidently a matter of utmost importance that female physicians should be fully and perfectly educated," Simpson wrote to Emily after her training ended. "I have had the fairest and best opportunity of testing the extent of your medical acquirements during the period of eight months when you studied here with me and I can have no hesitation in stating . . . that I have rarely met with a young physician who was better acquainted with the ancient and modern languages, or more learned in the literature, science, and practical details of his profession." High praise indeed.

Not long after Emily returned to New York, Sims's Woman's Hospital was rumored to be searching for a female surgeon. Apparently, the same lady managers whom Elizabeth had disparaged as socialite hacks had included in their bylaws a clause that required Sims to hire a woman as an assistant surgeon. The obvious candidate was Emily Blackwell. She had apprenticed with Simpson, one of the most celebrated surgeons in Europe, and was the most qualified—in fact, the only—female surgeon in New York.

At the time, Sims's surgical demonstrations were a booming success. Attracting physicians, medical students, and other qualified observers—all men except for the occasional nurse and, of course, the patient—the procedures entertained as well as informed. Sims would perform a series of surgeries on different patients that could last all day. He had someone run a stopwatch timing his surgeries to make it even more interesting. Spectators frequently erupted in boisterous applause and cheers, as if they were at a sporting event.

Since she was a practicing surgeon, Emily might have attended one of Sims's surgical demonstrations. An adoring audience of professors of medicine and their students always filled the room, and on hot days, the pungent smells of body odor, urine, and blood thickened the air.

When Sims strode into the arena, arms outstretched, the audience applauded wildly. Young medical students called Sims the "architect of the vagina" and compared him to the frontiersman Daniel Boone and James Fenimore Cooper's protagonist Hawkeye. The trembling female patient was usually positioned naked on the operating table, covered by a thin sheet when possible. She might not have been etherized because an awake patient screaming in pain was much more entertaining than an operation on a patient quietly sleeping.

Emily, who had built up an immunity to charismatic medical men while working with Dr. Simpson, was not impressed. She understood that Sims's bravado concealed the limits of his skill and drew attention away from the number of patients he had maimed or killed.

While the voyeuristic nature of Sims's surgical theater might have dismayed Emily, she still wanted the job of assistant surgeon at his hospital and was disappointed when he rejected her application. Instead, out of pure cynicism or as a joke, Sims appointed Mrs. Brown, the widowed sister of a friend and not a doctor at all, as a "matron and general superintendent." Six months later, he told his board of lady managers that he needed an assistant and chose Thomas Addis Emmet, a well-connected young surgeon whom he knew socially. The Blackwell sisters would not contact Sims again.

The success of the Woman's Hospital made another one of Sims's dreams come true. He was allowed entrance into the inner circle of the most influential businessmen in New York. In 1857, the New York legislature granted the hospital its charter and ten thousand dollars. The new act of incorporation removed any female influence by taking control of the hospital away from the original board of lady managers and giving it to a male board of governors that included a who's who of the wealthiest men in New York, among them John Jacob Astor, Theodore Sedgwick, J. P. Morgan, Henry J. Raymond (founder of *The New York Times*), and shipping magnate Robert Minturn. The lady managers occupied a subordinate position, focusing on so-called moral and domestic issues.

As time passed, Sims became so wealthy that he opened an additional office in Newport, Rhode Island. He threw lavish parties for hundreds of guests. The *Newport Daily News* called the wedding of Sims's fourth daughter "the great social event of the season." And he continued to display his surgical prowess, once performing a series of gynecological operations on destitute women that lasted several days to display his talents to the ovarian surgeon John Light Atlee, a founder of the American Medical Association. Ovariectomy was the surgical removal of one or both ovaries. Usually performed to treat an ovarian cyst or cancer, the procedure was quickly becoming a popular remedy for women's perceived mental illnesses, such as hysteria and nymphomania. Since these doctors believed, with no scientific proof, that the full spectrum of women's illnesses emanated from their sex organs, removing them seemed laudable.

Years later, Dr. Mary Putnam Jacobi wrote of Sims and his failure to acquaint himself with Elizabeth and Emily:

> Suffering womanhood undoubtedly owes much to Marion Sim's [sic] inventive genius. But, on the other hand, Sim's [sic] fame and fortune may be said to have been all made by women, from the poor slaves in Alabama who, unnarcotized, surrendered their patient bodies to his experiments, to the New York ladies whose alert sympathies and open purses had enabled

him to realize his dream, and establish his personal fortunes. It would have been an act both graceful and just on his part, at this crisis, to have shared his opportunities with the two women who, like himself had been well buffeted in an opposing world, and whose work and aspirations were so closely identified with his own. But this he failed to do; and the lost opportunity made all the difference to the pioneer women physicians, between brilliant and modest, between immediate and tardy professional success.

While Sims was performing experimental surgeries that attracted donors to his hospital, the Blackwell sisters and one of their protégées, the newly graduated Zakrzewska, were busy finding investors for their own infirmary. Elizabeth wanted to build a medical palace for women that would also offer clinical training. Zakrzewska, while applauding Elizabeth's vision of a healing mecca for women, suggested a more practical plan: a modest "nucleus hospital." Elizabeth and Emily eventually agreed with Zakrzewska, noting that she was the only one with successful business experience.

To campaign for her cause, Elizabeth held a drawing-room talk for a small group of wealthy sympathizers. "The most serious difficulty to be overcome by women students is the closure of all avenues of practical instruction to them," she explained. She also outlined the ethical benefits of a hospital run by women for women. Medicine would be a broad new field of endeavor for unmarried ladies. As physicians, these women would train a better class of nurses. Most important, women doctors would save sick women from the "bitter mortification" that came from being used as case studies for male medical students and physicians.

The well-connected Harriot Hunt referred many potential donors to Elizabeth, including educator Elizabeth Peabody, sculptor and poet Anne Whitney, and famous abolitionists Sarah and Angelina Grimké. Other valuable aid came from the Blackwells' sisters-in-law Lucy Stone and Antoinette Brown Blackwell, the first ordained woman minister in the United States. More influential women joined to form a social circle to fundraise for the new hospital, among them women journalists, artists, the highly fashionable, spiritualists, philanthropists, abolitionists, and socialists.

Still, the idea of a woman physician practicing in a hospital, much less an all-women's hospital, was a hard sell, so in addition to fundraising, the founders added a board of consulting male physicians, all highly skilled and well-respected doctors.

As Zakrzewska predicted, the three women were not able to raise enough funds for an expansive hospital. A modest-size, more intimate hospital, the New York Infirmary for Indigent Women and Children, opened on 64 Bleecker Street on May 12, 1857, which happened to be Florence Nightingale's thirty-seventh birthday. The Dutch-style, red-brick four-story building was originally the residence of James and Harriet Howland Roosevelt, great-grandparents of future president Franklin Delano Roosevelt. At the opening ceremonies, the Reverend Henry Ward Beecher, Quaker Dr. William Elder, and the Reverend Dr. Tyng gave rousing speeches. Zakrzewska suggested that Elizabeth should address the crowd too, but the patrons rejected that idea, fearing that she would speak "like a Woman's Rights woman."

The infirmary sat on the dividing line between New York's wealthiest and poorest neighborhoods. To the west lay the pristine Washington Square. To the south and east was Five Points, home to thousands of Irish, German, and African American immigrants who lived in ramshackle tenements in the most notorious urban slum of the antebellum period. Five Points housed the urban workers whose labor would fuel the rise of the city's industrial order.

Two months after the infirmary opened, *The New York Times* reported enthusiastically that the "homelike" establishment was "as fresh and clean as if just swept by the proverbial new broom" and that, judging by the faces of the "motherly-looking dames," the nursing must be unusually skilled. The *Times* noted that the front entrance hall and waiting room were nicely appointed with rugs, sofas, and other furniture. It was an entirely comfortable and intimate setting perfect for women in need.

The second floor contained two wards with six beds each. Maternity patients were housed on the third floor, which also had a sitting room for the physicians. Open coal grate fires provided the only heat throughout the hospital. The student doctors resided on the fourth floor. Recent graduates from the Female Medical College of Pennsylvania learned to practice medicine at all hours of the day and night. Policemen walking the beat would escort the doctors and their students into the nearby slums to care for women in labor.

The Blackwells and Zakrzewska depended on their private practices to make a living. The medical students received only room and board. As Zakrzewska said, "Only the brave, the courageous, the determined, and the financially equipped women could remain and weather the stormy days of their student life."

Visitors curious about women physicians came from all parts of the United States and Europe to view the New York Infirmary. After the excellent publicity it received, demand for services ran high. During the first year, nearly a thousand women and children were treated. Dr. Emily Blackwell performed thirty-six operations. The infirmary's success attracted patients who otherwise might have gone to the New York Woman's Hospital. Consequently, a certain number of wealthy male physicians resented the Blackwells' triumph. Rumors, possibly instigated at Sims's hospital, started circulating about the quack women doctors putting innocent female patients at risk, sparking fear in the patients and their families who lived in the tenements south of the infirmary. In one particular case, the gossip might have put the women doctors and nurses in grave danger.

During the infirmary's first year, as a patient lay dying after giving birth, the doctors used cold-water compresses to ease her pain. A female relative of the patient—her mother or sister—sat at her bedside for many hours until she passed away. A woman dying in or shortly after childbirth was, unfortunately, not uncommon. In the nineteenth century, there were almost a thousand maternal deaths for every one hundred thousand births. And women gave birth to an average of seven children. In the late stages of pregnancy, during childbirth, and immediately after, many things could go wrong. Women died of puerperal fever (also called childbed fever or postpartum sepsis; it was caused by an infection of the uterus), other infectious diseases, hemorrhage, eclampsia (dangerously high blood pressure and seizures), and obstructed labor.

Less than an hour after the woman's death, her distraught male relatives carrying pickaxes and shovels appeared at the infirmary's front door demanding admission. The angry men kept shouting that "the female physicians who resided within were killing women in childbirth with cold water." Their yells attracted an immense crowd that filled the block between the infirmary and Broadway.

The neighborhood police, now accustomed to escorting the hardy women physicians through the neighborhood to patients' sickbeds, arrived swiftly to the riotous scene. After hearing the men's complaint, they ordered the crowd to disperse, saying that they knew the doctors in that hospital "treated the patients in the best possible way, and that no doctor could keep everybody from dying sometime."

Despite that bumpy start, the infirmary expanded rapidly and experienced no further violence. By 1859, the founders had raised enough funds to move to a larger building, this one at 126 Second Avenue. During this time, and especially after Elizabeth left for an extended trip to England, Emily and Zakrzewska began to clash. The two both had extremely forceful personalities, and neither wanted to give in when they disagreed about a case or the business of the infirmary. Feeling a growing discontent, Zakrzewska started searching for her next place of employment. Later that same year, she accepted a position as professor of obstetrics and diseases of women at Boston's New England Female Medical College, founded in 1848 by Dr. Samuel Gregory to train women doctors.

Nevertheless, Zakrzewska and Emily had the same professional goals: to succeed as practicing physicians and educate other women in medicine. And so they and other women labored on in their institution-building, the Drs. Blackwell in New York, Dr. Zakrzewska in Boston, and Dr. Ann Preston in Philadelphia. One more pioneer was destined to join their ranks, but she was still a teenager searching for direction. Like Zakrzewska, she would find a mentor in Elizabeth Blackwell.

3

Awakening

Seventeen-year-old Mary Corinna Putnam adjusted the tie on the waist apron of her floor-length muddy-gray uniform as she brushed by the other busy nurses, all with their hair pinned up beneath white caps. Elizabeth Blackwell, director of the New York Infirmary for Women and Children, had recently returned from a monthslong trip to England, and she made sure that their uniforms were just like the one worn by her new friend Florence Nightingale.

Because her chestnut hair was very thick and she had a sensitive scalp, Mary refused to wear the bonnet-like headpiece of her nursing uniform. Besides, she was not really a nurse, just a recent high-school graduate who was spending a few months at the infirmary to learn about medicine.

The eldest of eleven children, Mary was the daughter of publishing magnate George Palmer Putnam and his wife, Victorine Haven Putnam. Her Putnam ancestors had arrived in New England in 1642 and were, famously, among the notorious accusers in the 1692 Salem witch tragedy. Mary had been interested in science and medicine for as long as she could remember. At age nine, she discovered a recently deceased rat in the family barn and asked her mother if she could slice open its abdomen to observe its heart, lungs, and stomach contents. Disgusted, her mother forbade her to touch the disease-carrying animal. But Mary, who also showed a talent for literature, writing, and teaching, remained fascinated with animal dissection.

In 1854, when Mary was twelve years old, her father published Elizabeth Blackwell's first book, *The Laws of Life*. Its success allowed Blackwell to build her practice and got her invited to Putnam family gatherings. Putnam regularly published single women authors. His inclination to help these "literary domestics" was also good business, since their books had a growing audience of literate middle-class women.

Like most Victorians, Putnam considered the practice of medicine to be an improper profession for ladies. He had published Elizabeth's book because he liked her ideas about hygiene and public health, not because she was a trained doctor. Even so, because he admired and loved his gifted daughter more than he disapproved of women doctors, he let Mary work at the clinic. But when he observed the Spartan living conditions at the infirmary, it took great restraint on his part to keep from escorting his daughter straight back home. During her time there, Mary slept in a tiny room on the top floor of the infirmary with another teenage girl who was also interested in medicine. The Blackwell sisters and three or four interns—recent graduates of the Female Medical College of Pennsylvania—lived in the attic rooms as well. They all shared a tiny bathroom the size of Mary's closet at home.

Starting at 8:00 a.m. every day except Sunday, dozens of patients, all women and children, began lining up for care at the dispensary, an outpatient clinic for the poor and working class. Some had fevers; some had infected wounds, dysentery, or croup. Others needed gynecological care or were experiencing the first hints of pregnancy. If they were able, the patients paid a trivial sum for their care, but payment was never expected. The annual report from 1861 for the infirmary counted 4,792 patients.

After days spent on her feet working in the dispensary, Mary felt exhausted, but she finally got used to the smell. Dozens of patients waiting together, especially in the warmer months, stirred up pungent odors. Soap and hot water were luxury items to those living on the poverty line. The sicker patients often stank like rotted pumpkins or wool socks dipped in sour milk. The younger ones carried the odor of their children's soiled diapers. Those who worked at the factories smelled like their products: wood pulp, linseed oil, or tobacco. The ones from the nearby fat-rendering establishment reeked of roast mutton.

One day, Emily Blackwell was in charge of seeing patients, and Mary was assisting. One woman was so pregnant that her growing stomach had torn through the seams of her worn cotton dress. She had tried to cover up her fierce body odor with the scent of bergamot, but Mary still turned away and dabbed a bit of camphor beneath her nose. Many of those who worked at the clinic kept a bottle of the pungent oil in their skirt pockets.

The woman nervously dipped her chin and lowered her gaze, apologizing for not bringing along her marriage license. Dr. Emily informed her that, unlike the other New York hospitals, the infirmary did not require a pregnant woman to have one. The young woman's face relaxed and her fists unclenched with relief.

In the examination room, Mary recorded the woman's name, height, weight, exact symptoms, and any medications prescribed. After a brief examination, Emily admitted the woman to the hospital. Mary then went to find the next patient, and the next.

Today, Mary was filled with anticipation. Emily had invited her to observe a surgical procedure that only promising interns were allowed to attend. Elizabeth Blackwell herself had called Mary "a very talented girl." And her praise did not come easily.

Dr. Elizabeth Blackwell was thinking about opening her own medical school. She envisioned a three-year course of study even more stringent than the medical colleges that men attended. Her lectures would build progressively from year to year, and a board of examiners would test students yearly. Her school would be the first ever to feature a professor of hygiene—Elizabeth herself. She wanted Mary to be her first student. Mary told Elizabeth that she was not sure of her plans but would think about her generous offer. Throughout Mary's life, her intelligence combined with excellent manners and a charming demeanor attracted mentors and opened doors closed to most other girls.

Growing up, Mary was always the cleverest person in the room. Although she was nicknamed "Minnie" because of her size, her view of the world was as tall, wide, and clear as if she were gazing from a mountaintop. Her parents encouraged Mary's vivid imagination. Evenings at the Putnam house were spent entertaining professors, ministers, scientists, and authors, including Edgar Allan Poe, Washington Irving, and Elizabeth Barrett Browning. One friend of the family wrote that "you would see Thackeray one night, and Lowell another; and run the risk of being asked (as I was) by George P. Marsh, just back from foreign duty, 'what I thought of the state of Europe?' Poor young me!—I didn't know Europe had a 'state'!"

Mary, aged ten at the time, would put a sign on the front door just before the first arrivals that read "Nobody admitted who cannot talk." One time, though, her overconfidence almost killed her. Mary and her brothers and sisters liked to play in the shallow parts of a nearby lake, sometimes paddling out on boards. One day, Mary kept paddling. She felt strong and brave, like a soldier at sea. She heard her sister shout a warning that she was out beyond her depth. Mary retorted that her sister was mistaken, and to prove her point, she rolled off her board. She was startled to discover that she had been wrong. She tried to push upward through the murky water but couldn't reach the surface. She tried two more times before realizing that she was drowning.

"Tomorrow I shall be thrown upon the shore, just like the drowned kittens," she thought. She pictured herself stretched out limp and unmoving on the sand. But as she was going down for the fourth time, someone lifted her out of the water and carried her, coughing and sputtering, to shore. Her rescuer, a tall workman from the nearby window-glass factory, could easily wade through the very water in which she had been drowning.

When he set her down on the sand, her legs felt wobbly, her head was spinning, and she almost blacked out—an astonishing fact, because she had never fainted in her life. Seeing that she was not well, her rescuer carried her home and all the way up to her bed, where she fell asleep immediately. When she finally woke up to find the family doctor smiling down at her and her mother holding her hand, she did not feel shocked by her life-threatening experience, only flabbergasted that she had been wrong. To Mary's chagrin, her mother kept her in bed for the rest of the day. When her father came home from work and heard the story of her near drowning, she saw the fear and emotion in *his* eyes.

The next day, her father purchased a handsome silver watch, and he and Mary walked to the factory, where he presented her rescuer with the gift as a token of his deep gratitude. Still confused by her shocking error in judgment, ten-year-old Mary could not understand what the man had done to deserve this gratitude. As she grew older, though, she made a serious effort to overcome her selfishness. At age fifteen, she wrote to a friend, "But I am so unaccustomed to be with any people but those whom I like . . . that I am entirely unfitted for general society." She looked to religion for guidance and grew closer to her paternal grandmother by promising to accept God's will and join her grandmother's evangelical Baptist church. Mary was searching for a touchstone, something that would inspire her heart and drive her forward. She hoped that it would be God.

Until 1857, the Putnams were moderately religious Episcopalians. While George Putnam's mother had always preached the Gospel to her grandchildren, historically, his family had devoted more of their energy to literary, political, and cultural interests. But this all changed when the economy collapsed in the Panic of 1857. Many businesses at the time, including Putnam's publishing company, had overextended credit. His financial manager had also used the company's funds for personal investments. When the man's embezzlements came to light, he drowned himself. Forced to declare bankruptcy, Mary's previously secular father sought consolation in religion. The 1857 revivals in downtown Manhattan, which attracted struggling businessmen eager for spiritual guidance in a time of desperate uncertainty, came to be known as a "masculine millennium" and the "great awakening."

The revivals were also popular because of their youthful, charismatic leader, Abner Kingman Nott, who projected a robust, manly sincerity in his Christian spirit. The Putnam family traveled from their home in the Bronx to Lower Manhattan every Sunday to hear Nott preach. Through his earnest eloquence, dignified bearing, and upbeat sermons, the young pastor of the First Baptist Church on Broome Street "ushered the entire Putnam family into the revivals."

At age sixteen, Mary developed a crush on the charming Pastor Nott. During his visits to their home in the Bronx, the two spent hours together discussing her spiritual development and other theological topics. She felt closer to God while talking to Nott and hoped for a spiritual enlightenment that would also reveal her true purpose in life.

One day, he did not appear for their talks, and the family soon received news that Abner Nott, age twenty-five, had drowned while swimming with friends in the waters between New Jersey and Staten Island. Heartbroken, Mary felt the shock and sorrow for Nott that she never felt for her own escape from a watery death. She began questioning her faith and soon left the church altogether. Instead of religion, she focused on her studies and wrote essays critical of the constraints placed on women. She expressed growing frustration with society and the "cult of true womanhood."

Mary's father encouraged his daughter's brilliance and adored her for it, but there was a limit to even his progressive attitude. That threshold was reached when Mary became interested in medicine. Even though George Putnam had helped single women like Elizabeth Blackwell by publishing their writings, he did not want that life for his daughter. He directed Mary toward proper feminine professions. Unlike the "spinster" Blackwell sisters, many women who were teachers and writers also attracted husbands and raised children. Putnam feared that if Mary became a doctor—considered to be a highly masculine profession—her soft femininity would harden, her ability to have children would diminish, and he would lose his wonderful daughter. He had reluctantly encouraged Mary's apprenticeship at the Blackwells' infirmary because he expected her to become bored with doctoring.

But Mary's fascination with medicine grew even stronger. At the procedure that Mary had been invited to observe, she watched closely as Emily performed surgery. Standing a few feet away from the operating table, she could imagine herself holding the scalpel, cutting through flesh, and risking the life of her patient to cure her pain. The whole thing took nerves of steel. Unlike male surgeons, who reused their white surgical aprons over and over until they were stiff with dried gore, Emily wore a clean white uniform for each procedure. Once the patient was sufficiently unconscious from the chloroform mask, Emily's small hands moved quickly and accurately, and she made the incision with minimal blood spatter. When she was finished, she saved the removed specimen in a glass jar.

The next morning, Mary entered the hospital lab for the first time. At the beginning of the nineteenth century, the word *laboratory* meant a general workspace or workshop. By midcentury, the term *laboratory* referred to an institution for scientific, especially experimental, practice. The Blackwells made sure that the New York Infirmary had the most innovative equipment and processes. In addition to dozens of chemicals and hundreds of glass vials, their workroom doubtless contained at least one compound microscope. Compared to the simple microscopes comprised of a single magnifying lens, compound microscopes had two lenses that increased magnification at least a hundred times. Mary had likely peered through simple microscopes at school and observed the crisscrossed veins on leaves or the eight bulging eyes of a deceased spider. But she had never looked through a powerful, properly adjusted compound microscope at slides of human tissue. The miniature universe that appeared before her left her speechless. The hundreds of magnified cells looked like worlds within worlds. She literally stopped breathing when she realized that she was looking at the most basic form of life.

Suddenly, she was filled with a galvanizing desire to know more.

In the days and weeks that followed, she spent hours analyzing specimens in the lab. She studied the periodic table of elements and pored over biology textbooks, reading Virchow's cellular theory, first proposed in 1855, that all cells came from existing cells. She realized that the cells that formed a woman's body were no different than a man's. Superficial boundaries such as those subjecting women to cloistered lives dissolved in her mind. They meant nothing. Science was freedom. She was reborn a scientist.

Ever practical and methodical, drawing strength from her robust self-esteem, Mary now craved legitimacy in the medical profession and decided that, as a woman, she had to graduate from a proper medical college. Although she greatly admired the Blackwell sisters, Elizabeth had not yet built a school with an accredited curriculum and was basically offering Mary a lengthy internship. Mary declined Dr. Blackwell's offer and continued to search for legitimate medical education. Her pursuit finally led her to the New York College of Pharmacy. Taking advantage of the fact that the school was struggling with financial problems and desperately needed students, she talked her way into becoming the first woman in the United States to attend pharmacy school.

Mary's decision produced a panicked response from her father. He begged her to come home to assist her mother and teach her younger siblings, especially since a civil war was brewing. "What possible evil can result from your suspending those medical studies, entirely, except general reading at home, for the space of two years?" he asked her in a letter. He never outright forbade her to go, but he did offer her $250—the amount of her tuition—to stay home. At first, Mary gave in to his pleas, but her restlessness soon caused her to change her mind, and even as the Confederates fired on Fort Sumter, she continued to study cell theory, organic chemistry, and materia medica at the pharmacy college.

~

In April 1861, the war broke out, and Northern women wanted to help. With the best intentions for their sons, husbands, and brothers in the fight, they mailed homemade jam in glass jars that shattered and cooked meat that spoiled before reaching its destination. They knit socks and sewed coats but did not know where to send them, so some regiments were flooded with warm clothing and others went without. Quilts were sent to Louisiana when the demand was for mosquito netting. Mothers, sisters, and daughters rushed to volunteer as nurses, but the skills needed to care for sick children did not translate to the battlefield. The military allowed only male nurses and untrained, recuperating soldiers to care for its sick and wounded, and it took enormous public pressure to convince the War Department to train women as field nurses.

Seeing the chaotic nature of this response, Elizabeth realized that the Union army needed to properly organize all of this feminine energy and goodwill. On April 25, 1861, she and Emily called an informal meeting at the infirmary. To their surprise, dozens of women and a few sympathetic men showed up to discuss the situation. They decided to organize a bigger meeting at the nearby Cooper Union's Great Hall and printed an advertisement on April 28 in New York newspapers:

"To the Women of New York and especially to those already engaged in preparing against the time of wounds and sickness in the Army," the ad in the *New York Daily Herald* began.

The next evening, arriving in fancy carriages, horsecars, and on foot, three thousand "brave and philanthropic ladies" and a few hundred men crowded into the nine-hundred-seat Cooper Union hall for the unprecedented event. The largest secular meeting room in New York was usually filled with men, but tonight, a flood of colorful bonnets worn by well-dressed women in rustling silk and cotton dresses with wide hoop skirts transformed the enormous room. Most of them carried fans or handkerchiefs with flowery scents of rose, violet, or lavender. The mumbled chatter of thousands of feminine voices echoed off the three-story-high brick-and-mortar arched hall. Patriotism and the fight for freedom had finally called the women out of their private homes and into the bustling public sphere of men.

"God bless you, women of New York!" cried Vice President Hannibal Hamlin, who had made a surprise appearance at the event. A dozen speakers followed, all prominent men, including ministers, physicians, and a surgeon who had witnessed the recent skirmish at Fort Sumter. By the end of the evening, the Woman's Central Association of Relief (WCAR) had been formed, and Elizabeth Blackwell was named chair of its registration committee. Its crucial task was to screen the multitudes of women who wanted to become new Florence Nightingales.

Wartime physicians and surgeons, however, claimed that women did not have the constitution and hardiness to care for wounded soldiers and follow the strict military protocols. Furthermore, where would they live? No one had the time to build separate accommodations for women. But with the outbreak of the Civil War and the ever-increasing number of wounded and dying soldiers, the need for nurses on both sides became desperate. The War Department began assigning qualified female recruits to nursing duties. Women who were considered qualified ranged in age from thirty-five to fifty, were "plain-looking," in good health, obedient to regulations, and willing to take orders from superiors. They had to commit to training at qualified hospitals and to at least three months of service.

Even though Elizabeth had initiated the formation of the WCAR, her authority was limited. The president (Dr. Valentine Mott), vice president (the Reverend Henry Bellows), and at least half of the board members were men. Out of the WCAR initiative grew the highly effective United States Sanitary Commission (USSC), endorsed by President Lincoln on June 13, 1861. Thousands of women volunteers organized under the USSC to develop a centralized system that collected and distributed bandages, blankets, food, clothing, and lifesaving medical supplies from women's charities and aid societies.

Elizabeth's position was further undermined when the government appointed Dorothea Dix as superintendent of army nurses. A fifty-nine-year-old Boston schoolteacher with no formal medical training, Dix had made powerful friends in Washington, DC, through her successful campaign to improve conditions for the mentally ill. At the war's outbreak, Dix hurried straight to Washington and lobbied for the establishment of an army nursing corps under her leadership. Elizabeth was understandably bitter: "The government has given Miss Dix a semi official recognition as meddler general—for it really amounts to that, she being without system, or any practical knowledge of the business."

Although working in a reduced capacity, Elizabeth and her committee poured themselves into processing the hundreds of applications they received from aspiring nurses. Although the youngest age for acceptance was thirty-five, younger women and even teenage girls tried to fake their way into the service. The committee ended up selecting ninety-one nurses, women who were trained at either Bellevue or New York Hospital and then sent—under Dix's supervision—to a military hospital. The Blackwells' infirmary was noticeably excluded as a training center for nurses. The army surgeons and regular hospitals refused "to have anything to do with the nurse education plan 'if the Miss Blackwells were going to engineer the matter,'" Elizabeth wrote to a friend. These were the same hospitals that refused to hire Elizabeth or allow any woman medical student to receive clinical training.

Over fifteen thousand women on both sides served as nurses during the Civil War. They left their paneled drawing rooms, country home kitchens, and cabins out west to care for wounded soldiers and risk their lives for the war effort. In addition to overcoming the contempt of the male surgeons and military officers, war nurses had to adapt to a military setting. Most women had never experienced a military hospital, but they eventually got used to the morbid piles of amputated limbs and the acrid smell of festering wounds. They soon learned to choke back their tears. They fed, clothed, and bathed patients, changed bandages, and dispensed medicine. They offered emotional comfort to soldiers by praying with them, reading to them, and writing letters home for them. Nurses managed supplies, operated hospital kitchens and laundries, emptied bedpans, and kept the floors clean.

Besides the constant dangers of serving during wartime, nurses were exposed to infections and illnesses such as strep, typhoid, and smallpox. Many succumbed to these diseases. Numerous nurses, including Black women such as Harriet Tubman, became heroes and earned a place in history. Stationed on the front lines, Clara Barton cared for the wounded on the battlefield. After the war, women would continue to work in health care, and by 1900, they represented 91 percent of U.S. nurses. Opportunities for women to work in medicine had suddenly exploded, and the nursing profession would be forever changed.

～

The Civil War sparked an outpouring of patriotism and a feeling that great things were afoot because everything was changing. There was a sense that self-determination was at hand for everyone, including the women who fought for suffrage. Dr. Harriot Hunt, who, through her smart real estate investments, had become one of Boston's most affluent citizens, hoped that the Civil War would initiate "a struggle for a higher perception of freedom . . . when bondage after bondage is being removed."

Almost a decade earlier, in 1853, when the Massachusetts Constitutional Convention refused to enfranchise its female citizens, Hunt began to publicly protest having to pay taxes while also being denied the right to vote. Year after year, she purchased newspaper advertising space in every state and eloquently described how she was being taxed without representation. Married women were required to give all earnings to their husbands, but a single woman's income was always burdened with taxes. In 1861, her advertisement in Boston newspapers stated that she looked forward to the day when the freedoms promised in the Declaration of Independence would no longer be limited to white men.

In addition to the Blackwell sisters, other prominent women doctors contributed to the war effort. At the beginning of the Civil War, in 1861, the Female Medical College of Pennsylvania founded an affiliated health-care center, the Women's Hospital of Philadelphia, directed by Dr. Ann Preston.

In 1862, Dr. Marie Zakrzewska opened the New England Hospital for Women and Children, a teaching institution where female medical students could receive clinical training. She was adamant about improving the lives of the impoverished, pledging to provide a homelike environment during times of need. Some of Boston's most prominent physicians supported the hospital, among them Henry Bowditch, Walter Channing, John Ware, and Edward H. Clarke, all Harvard graduates. A few years later, Zakrzewska's hospital established the first formal nurse-training program in the United States. Linda Richards, the first graduate of the intensive sixteen-month program, went on to work at Bellevue Hospital in New York, where she invented the charting system for patient medical records. Her system would be widely adopted both in the United States and England.

～

At the start of the Civil War, New York City boiled with tension. Most of the abolitionists lived in the northern part of the state. The city's wealthy merchant class had close business ties to Southern slaveholders, and Confederate sentiments ran strong. To demonstrate his sympathy for the South, outspoken New York City mayor Fernando Wood called for New York to secede from the Union. As the war intensified, the federal government instituted a draft, and those who could not pay the three hundred dollars needed to escape conscription were forced to join the military. Working-class men who feared job competition from newly liberated enslaved people began to tear apart Lower Manhattan. They shot, burned, and hanged African Americans in the streets. Taking advantage of the chaos, white gang members rampaged, killing police and many Black citizens. To stop the violence, President Lincoln ordered regiments to leave Gettysburg, Pennsylvania, and go to New York. It took thousands of Union soldiers to finally restore the peace.

A Republican gentleman and abolitionist, Mary's father, George Putnam, had voted for Abraham Lincoln and volunteered for public service at the start of the Civil War. He witnessed the First Battle of Bull Run and published harrowing accounts of the Confederacy's bloody victory. Other members of the Putnam family did their part too. Eighteen-year-old Haven, the eldest son, enlisted in the Union army, and Mary's younger sister Edith signed up to teach the freedmen and freedwomen.

Haven registered with the 176th New York Infantry Regiment in December 1862 and was detailed as assistant to the quartermaster in New Orleans, a Union foothold in the Deep South. The capture of New Orleans on April 29, 1862, had been a turning point in the war and gave Union forces control of the Confederacy's largest port on the Mississippi River and of the lower river valley. There was a constant threat of Confederate attacks, and the Union soldiers stationed in the mosquito-infested swamps surrounding New Orleans often suffered from malaria. Fully one-quarter of all illnesses reported in the Union army were malarial, resulting in over 1.3 million cases and 10,000 deaths by the end of the war.

Haven's worried family felt blessed relief each time they received one of his letters. But in late May, the letters stopped coming. The family soon learned that he had malaria. Everyone felt helpless except for twenty-year-old Mary, who had just graduated from pharmacy school. She decided to go to New Orleans, find Haven, and nurse him back to health. Traveling alone to the front lines of the Civil War was a bold move even for Mary. But she worked up the courage to ask her father's permission, and to her surprise, he immediately consented. Sending Mary to the battlefront seemed justified to a man deeply afraid for his eldest son.

Through her father's many connections, she received permission to join a federal transport going south via rail and steamship to the Port of New Orleans. On June 5, her steamship chugged into the harbor packed with clipper ships, steamboats, and schooners, and she wondered how many had been used to transport enslaved people. Since President Lincoln's issuance of the Emancipation Proclamation on January 1, 1863, all Black people living in New Orleans—and everywhere else in the Union—were free. New Orleans, the sixth-largest city in the country and the largest in the Confederacy, was the central point for the slave trade. After the Union army took over, slavery in Louisiana was crippled; over 24,000 Black men, more than from any other state, enlisted in the army.

Even though she had hardly slept during the uncomfortable journey south, Mary was focused and determined to find her brother. Immediately after departing the ship, she was required to sign a formal oath of allegiance to the U.S. government, pledging to perform all the duties of a "true and loyal citizen." Then she searched for her military contact.

Quartermaster general Samuel B. Holabird informed her that her brother had been released from the hospital and had gone back to his regiment, which was stationed somewhere among the lakes, marshlands, and bayous surrounding New Orleans. She realized that her most difficult journey was still ahead. Wandering through the bustling city that housed Union soldiers, resentful Confederate citizens living under martial law, and formerly enslaved people, Mary knew she had entered the heart of the Civil War. She could barely contain her excitement.

During her first few days in New Orleans, she lived with Colonel Holabird and his family, who were social acquaintances from New York City. The family, impressed by Mary's fearlessness, eagerly helped her search for her brother. Military records did not exist, so no one knew exactly where he was stationed. Mary put a large advertisement in the local paper using the name of one of their childhood ponies, Guyascutas, to attract Haven's attention, but it did not get a response. Finally, after following several false clues, a young friend of the Holabird family, Lieutenant Taylor, traced Haven's regiment of New York volunteers known as the Ironsides to a camp near the Atchafalaya River town of Brashear City, about eighty miles west of New Orleans. Mary convinced a guide to accompany her on the train to Brashear and then help her safely navigate the snake-and-alligator-filled bayou to the front lines of the Civil War. Rumors of attacks were numerous. If the Confederates were able to retake Brashear City, they would threaten the Union's hold on New Orleans.

Mary purchased mosquito netting and Wellington boots for the journey. When she and her guide arrived at the small Union garrison, she looked a mess in her mud-splattered dress, her hair parted in the middle and haphazardly pulled up beneath her bonnet, and a handkerchiefed hand dabbing away her perspiration. She found the entrance gate, and, noting that she was the only white woman within miles, she calmly introduced herself to the gaping soldier and asked where she might find her brother, recently promoted to sergeant. Her matter-of-fact way of speaking convinced the

officer in charge that she was on a legitimate mission, and he let her inside the compound, which was filled with orderly tents, temporary wooden
buildings, and busy soldiers.

She went to the hospital tent, expecting to find Haven inside, but he
wasn't there. Every soldier she asked about her brother's whereabouts
pointed her in a different direction. She began to think they were playing
a joke on her. On her own, since she had released her guide, she wandered
the camp, earning surprised looks from the men wherever she went. Purely
by accident, she found Haven, recovered and hard at work digging a drain-
age ditch. The troops at Brashear City had trouble keeping their camps dry,
and many succumbed to malaria.

When Haven caught sight of Mary, he gasped with surprise. The first
words he said to his dear sister Minnie were that she should reprimand
their father for allowing her to come. But then they laughed, embraced
each other, and enjoyed a happy reunion.

The first order of business was to find her decent living quarters. Officers outfitted Mary with her own tent and assigned her a Black woman
servant. Eventually, this woman would accompany her north and become
known to the family as "Sarah Contraband." Since Haven had fully recovered and did not need Mary's nursing skills, she went in search of ways to
be useful. Once, she spoke to a group of freed and runaway enslaved people
at their camp meeting. She remained with the army for two weeks, but then
news of a Confederate assault drove her back to New Orleans.

Mary spent the rest of the summer living with the Holabirds and tutoring
their young son. She also volunteered at the hospital and the Freedmen's
Commission, a government agency established to help feed, educate, and
provide medical care and general support for freed slaves. She directly witnessed the brutal consequences of slavery and war. Observing hundreds of
deaths from injury and disease at the hospital, she realized the vital importance of medicine and how the advance of science could save lives. Becoming a doctor would allow her to join the public fight for social reform. By
the end of summer, she was ready to pursue a medical degree at the Female
Medical College of Pennsylvania.

She wrote her father about her decision, and he wrote back, "Now Minnie, you know very well that I am proud of your abilities and am willing
that you should apply them even to the repulsive pursuit . . . of Medical
Science. But don't let yourself be absorbed and gobbled up in that branch

of the animal kingdom ordinarily called strong minded women! . . . Don't be congealed or fossilized into a hard, tenacious, unbending personification of intellectual conceit, however strongly fortified you feel sure that you are. . . . I do hope and trust you will preserve your feminine character. . . . Be a lady from the dotting of your i's to the color of your ribbons—and if you must be a doctor and a philosopher, be an attractive and agreeable one."

On her journey back to New York, Mary prepared herself for the possibility that her father might change his mind again. But this time, it was not George Putnam who threatened her success but rather, ironically, the Female Medical College of Pennsylvania.

4

Setbacks

THE PALE BLUE FLAME OF THE BUNSEN BURNER EMITTED JUST enough light for Mary Putnam to finish writing her thesis in the otherwise darkened laboratory of the Female Medical College of Pennsylvania. Surrounded by glass beakers and dancing shadows cast by the burner flames, she sat in the one place at school where she felt at home. She needed peace and quiet to do her best work because she was planning to graduate two years early.

Even though she had not attended the full three years of courses that the college required, she believed that the scope of her writing plus credit for the courses she had taken at pharmacy school would prove to administrators that she was ready to be a physician. Ignoring her growing hunger—she had skipped dinner—she dipped her fountain pen into the inkwell and kept writing. Her thesis was due to the college dean, Dr. Edwin Fussell, first thing in the morning.

Mary Putnam had made the unprecedented choice to leave the Female Medical College of Pennsylvania because, as each day progressed, she discovered that she knew more about medicine than most of her instructors. Well-intentioned but unqualified men gave rambling lectures to female students whose previous education, unfortunately, had left them ill-equipped to be physicians. While Putnam appreciated that Dr. Ann Preston was a superb lecturer and a nurturing teacher, she felt that the professor was not sufficiently schooled in her subject of physiology. From Putnam's reading and classes at pharmacy college, she had gained a better understanding of human physiology than Preston had. And the fact that Preston and the young women attending the school referred to themselves as "hen medics" caused Putnam to grit her teeth. She would never refer to herself as a female chicken.

As far as she was concerned, only one of her professors had any real ability: Emeline Horton Cleveland, who had recently finished postgraduate work in obstetrics at Maternité de Paris. After a year of study, she received her diploma along with special awards for excellence in clinical observation. Cleveland returned to Philadelphia with advanced clinical training and experience in hospital management. Putnam considered her a woman of real scientific ability. She had other talents as well. After class, Cleveland made a beeline for the kitchen to bake bread for the students' meals, supplementing the college's meager resources.

Putnam would have liked to travel to Europe for a medical education too. But first, she had to graduate. To demonstrate her mastery of science, she was writing her thesis, "Theories with Regard to the Function of the Spleen," entirely in Latin, the root language of medicine. The fact that a number of her professors could not read Latin was not her concern. Her father would have chastised her for being overly vain and ambitious. *Don't make a spectacle out of yourself*, she could hear him say. But Putnam was determined to meet her own high standards. While most students at the female medical college chose thesis topics on general health or hygiene, Putnam focused on a specific organ and its diseases. She had selected the spleen because she wanted to elevate the organ's scientific status. The size of a fist and full of blood, the deep red, squishy organ had a sour reputation.

"When dealing with physiology," she wrote, "there are no more unsettling and absurd ideas than those which have tried to explain the function of the spleen." It was thought that if someone was feeling low, it was because the spleen was overproducing "black bile." But the spleen could also cause happiness and laughter because it cleaned the bile. In women, due to their supposed physiological weakness, the spleen caused hysteria, sometimes called "vapors," and produced frenzied symptoms such as a vast outpouring of tears. Putnam rejected these outdated concepts. She then presented an overview of what she called the "whole recent controversy" about the spleen, including debates over its role in the manufacture of blood.

She continued working until she couldn't keep her eyes open. The next morning, Putnam collected the pages of her thesis, penned the title in her most beautiful handwriting, punched two holes into the left-hand margins, and bound the pages into a notebook. Feeling absolute confidence in her work, she put on her coat and walked the half mile from her boarding-house to the school.

On the way, she passed a classmate taking in the crisp, cold winter air. They barely exchanged glances. Putnam had not made friends with any of her fellow students. In fact, she considered most of them illiterate. On the whole, she decided, women were not accustomed to the absolute discipline required for scientific research.

In addition to Putnam, only a dozen or so students were currently attending classes. The Civil War had disrupted colleges all across the Union and had even caused a few to shut down. To attract more paying students, American medical schools had stopped requiring previous degrees or prior training. To graduate, students worked in the hospital for three years under the direction of a qualified physician, attended two four-month terms of lectures, and sometimes wrote a thesis. Many students could barely write, so most schools required only oral examinations. Failing the oral exam rarely kept a student from graduating. Yet even though regular medical schools were facing financial obliteration, they stood fast in their refusal to accept female students.

Once she reached her destination, Putnam pushed open the heavy double doors leading into the main building and scanned the hall for Dean Fussell. A restless man who often roamed the school greeting students and professors, Fussell was usually absent from his office. His uncle Bartholomew Fussell was a famous abolitionist who participated in the Underground Railroad, providing refuge to at least two thousand runaway slaves at his safe houses throughout Pennsylvania and Ohio. Bartholomew and other Quaker physicians were the founding fathers of the Female Medical College of Pennsylvania. Edwin Fussell, unlike them, could be summed up as an unambitious man.

Today, Putnam was surprised to find him seated at his desk and writing notes in a journal. She considered the slightly bug-eyed Fussell to be a simple but well-meaning bureaucrat. Feeling her presence, he glanced up and frowned at the interruption. When she attempted to hand him her thesis along with tickets indicating the classes she had attended, he looked confused. When she told him that she wanted to graduate early, his confusion turned to shock.

Why hadn't she conferred with him? he sputtered.

Putnam calmly replied that she had informed the entire faculty, with Dr. Cleveland's blessing.

Only candidates who completed the full three years of courses were qualified to graduate, Fussell snapped. Dr. Cleveland should not have allowed Putnam to hope for special treatment.

Confident that her expertise would shine through, Putnam urged him to accept her thesis and then decide about her qualification to graduate. Finally, he acquiesced and took her bound writing. Her thesis and tickets would be included with the other students' work being evaluated by the faculty for graduation, he grudgingly assured her. At most medical schools, students bought tickets for a professor's lecture at a cost of ten to fifteen dollars each, and those fees helped pay the speaker's salary.

When Fussell told her that she would receive notice of the faculty's decision in two weeks, Putnam thanked him and said that was all that she asked. She spent those weeks working in the lab, attending classes, and reading medical books. She was confident that she would have her degree by March.

On February 3, 1864, the faculty reported that all student theses except for two met the prerequisites for graduation. Unfortunately, Putnam's was one of the two not accepted.

"Miss Putnam's tickets were found deficient by ones for Practical Anatomy—for Chemistry—the Practice of Medicine & Physiology." Her thesis was excellent, but her coursework was incomplete. Furthermore, she lacked the required clinical experience.

Dean Fussell cheerfully notified Putnam of her ticket deficiencies. He also demanded that she rewrite her thesis in English so that faculty members who did not know Latin could read it.

Putnam followed up with a note to Fussell stating that she held no ticket for chemistry, physiology, or the practice of medicine from the New York Medical College because during the year in which she bought the tickets for those courses, they were taught by amateurs who were replacing the appointed professors. Further, she refused to rewrite her thesis, noting that the faculty's deficiency in Latin was not her concern.

Fussell wadded up her note and pitched it in the trash. Then he notified her that she was required to appear before the meeting of college administrators to further explain herself.

Three weeks later, Putnam stood before Fussell, Preston, Cleveland, and other college faculty members. Raising his chin and pressing his lips together to keep from smirking, Fussell said that Putnam had failed to convince the committee of her qualifications to graduate. In fact, they were unsure why she was even there.

Putnam could not believe that she had to explain herself. When she felt steadier, she said that the reason she did not want to attend all the lectures required by the Female Medical College of Pennsylvania was that she had already gained the knowledge from her years at pharmacy college in New York. Why should she be required to pay for courses that she had already completed? In addition, she had obtained months of clinical experience while working for Elizabeth Blackwell in the New York Infirmary. If Dean Fussell would contact these institutions, they would verify her experience and course completions. Finally, she suggested that she be examined to test her knowledge for graduation.

When Putnam finished speaking, Ann Preston thanked her for her detailed explanation and then made a motion "that Miss Putnam be admitted to an examination."

Putnam's face relaxed and she said that she would be happy to participate in examinations, tomorrow if necessary. Preston and the rest of the faculty except for Fussell looked completely satisfied. Next, Preston turned to Fussell and, after pointing out that he should have already done this, asked him to find out the exact history of Putnam's attendance at the schools and hospitals in New York.

Fussell reluctantly agreed, and in the meantime, Putnam easily passed her examinations and continued to prepare for graduation.

Two weeks later, Fussell reported that, while the New York professors involved seemed evasive, they did confirm that Putnam had legitimately completed the courses she had described. Putnam was vindicated.

Fussell grew more disconcerted. He was seen pacing the hallways, shaking his head and mumbling that Putnam's behavior was elitist and wrong. He led a protest against her graduation. He accused her of initially lying about her intentions. When he accused her former teachers at the pharmacy college of fraudulently representing her coursework, other faculty members secretly warned him against denouncing New York physicians with sterling reputations. But he would not be dissuaded. He claimed that allowing Putnam to graduate would "degrade the college."

Nevertheless, on March 12, the faculty members voted six to one to allow Putnam to graduate, ranking her third highest of eight candidates. Putnam received her diploma, signed, as required, by Edwin Fussell.

Still angry, Fussell resigned, stating, "I think the College is disgraced &

I should feel myself degraded did I remain longer in connection with it." Neither the faculty nor the board wished to lose Fussell, so they approved changes in the bylaws in order to retain him. Reluctantly, he withdrew his resignation.

In 1866, Dr. Ann Preston was elected the first woman dean of the Female Medical College of Pennsylvania, and in 1867 she joined the college board of directors. Determined to improve the educational opportunities of her students and the school's reputation, she changed the college's name; now it was the Woman's Medical College of Pennsylvania. The school's annual report explained the name change as "a simple recognition of the growing purity of our English tongue, which demands that terms shall be distinctive in their signification; and of an increasing regard for the dignity of woman—the co-worker with man, and his companion in the noblest thoughts and pursuits."

That same year, Rebecca Cole became the first Black woman to graduate from the Woman's Medical College. Born in Philadelphia, Rebecca Cole attended the Institute for Colored Youth, the only school for Black children in Pennsylvania. Ann Preston sponsored Cole in medical school and mentored the bright young student until she graduated. Dr. Cole next went to work at Elizabeth Blackwell's New York Infirmary as an assistant physician. Blackwell assigned her the job of sanitary visitor for her tenement-house service, caring for poor patients in their own homes, providing practical instruction on managing infants and preserving the health of families. In her autobiography, Blackwell wrote that Dr. Cole was an "intelligent young coloured physician" who carried out her work "with tact and care." Dr. Cole eventually founded the Physician Woman's Directory, an organization that offered both medical and legal services to destitute women. In addition to providing health care, the directory challenged discriminatory housing practices and fought against the unhealthy living conditions that led to the spread of diseases. Dr. Cole inspired generations of Black doctors to work within their own communities.

By 1900, the Woman's Medical College had graduated approximately a dozen Black women doctors, including Caroline Still Wiley Anderson, Georgianna E. Patterson Young, Verina M. Harris Morton Jones, Juan Bennett-Drummond, Halle Tanner Dillon Johnson, Alice Woodby-McKane, Lucy Hughes-Brown, and Lulu Matilda Evans. The college also graduated the first woman doctor from India, Anandibai Joshee (1882); the first Native American woman doctor, Susan La Flesche Picotte (1889); and other women M.D.s originally from China, Syria, and South America.

And finally, in 1867, the students at the Woman's Medical College of Pennsylvania stopped calling each other hen medics.

After graduating, Putnam considered her options for continuing her medical education. Since she had no savings, she could not travel to Europe like Emeline Cleveland. Her father could not afford to help her; he still owed creditors from his bankruptcy back in 1857. To obtain clinical experience in America, she could work in the Blackwells' New York Infirmary or the New England Hospital for Women and Children. She applied to the latter.

With the magnetic charm of a stage actor, thirty-three-year-old Zakrzewska towered over Putnam as she welcomed her to the New England Hospital. She gestured dramatically while explaining that skilled women physicians providing medical care to their own sex saved many lives. Her German accent, with "vhat" for "what" and "somezing" for "something," added even more depth to her rough charisma. Zakrzewska taught her interns that medicine played a critical role in women's struggle for equality. Moreover, almost all of the hospital's staff had studied in Europe.

Among the most influential physicians at the hospital besides Zakrzewska was Lucy Sewall, chief resident. Her father, Samuel Sewall, was a renowned judge, a prominent abolitionist, and a strong financial supporter of the hospital. Lucy Sewall had the distinction of being the first socialite to study medicine in the United States. She had just completed training in Paris and London, making her one of the best educated doctors in Boston.

Unfortunately, Zakrzewska had little time for teaching Putnam. The hospital was full to capacity, and many patients required house calls. Zakrzewska always seemed to be out on emergency visits, sometimes walking as far as Cambridge, West Roxbury, and Brookline. But the bulk of the patients came to the hospital's dispensary. In 1864, Zakrzewska and Sewall treated nearly two thousand patients. They did have help from Henry Bigelow and the surgeon Horatio Storer, both prominent Boston physicians. But Zakrzewska had recently received complaints against Storer concerning poor surgical outcomes, and relations between the two were strained. In addition, the women had to fundraise. Society ladies often dropped by to donate food and old linens, and the hospital was continuously holding events to raise money.

Putnam trained as an intern under Lucy Sewall, who lived at the hospital. Interns entered training at the New England Hospital for a period of twelve months, spending three months each in the medical, maternity, and surgical wards and three months in the outpatient dispensary. Their lives were highly regulated: meals at 7:00 a.m., 1:00 p.m., and 6:00 p.m. and a 9:00 p.m. bedtime. They could not leave the hospital without Sewall's permission.

A typical day started before breakfast when they attended rounds with the resident physician. During these rounds, each intern wrote prescriptions, prepared medications, and labeled bottles. Interns visited their wards two more times each day to record each patient's pulse and respiration. Twice a week, they charted fevers, symptoms, and treatments for each patient in the ward. The New England Hospital was the first in Boston to keep routine fever charts. In addition, surgical interns cleaned and straightened the operating room. They organized the instruments and handed them to the surgeon as needed during surgery. The maternity intern recorded patient arrivals and ordered enemas, and the dispensary intern ordered medicine, managed prescriptions, and maintained daily accounts. It was exhausting work.

After a few months of treating the constant flow of patients suffering from every form of illness she could imagine, Putnam decided that she was not cut out for hospital work and wanted to focus on research in a quiet laboratory. She asked to be released from her internship. She could hardly wait to return to New York to study chemistry. But before she left, Sewall and Zakrzewska sat her down and explained that if she was serious about becoming a prominent physician, her next step should be studying in the clinics of London, Edinburgh, Dublin, Paris, or Vienna. These cities housed the medical centers of the world. Putnam's success as a "scientific" physician depended on her traveling across the Atlantic.

But before she could heed their advice, she fell in love.

After returning home to live with her parents in August of 1864, right before General Sherman's occupation of Atlanta, she plunged back into her chemistry studies. She could read the textbooks herself, but she needed to find a laboratory where she could work on experiments. One of her professors at the New York College of Pharmacy, Ferdinand Mayer, maintained a small private laboratory where he conducted experiments and offered tutoring. Putnam had been one of Mayer's favorite students partly because of her sharp intellect but also because she was an attractive young woman among the bearded apothecaries and naive assistant druggists.

Professor Mayer was delighted to have Mary Putnam back in his laboratory. To pay for her studies, she set up a small medical practice. She refused to ask her father for money. As a passionate Union supporter, he was a member of the Loyal Publication Society of New York, a group that strengthened Union support by distributing pro-Union news stories and commentaries to newspapers around the nation. In addition, he had suspended his business at the start of the Civil War, in 1863, to become the U.S. government's collector of internal revenue in New York City. He would continue that role until the war ended, in 1866. Mary Putnam's father permitted her to study in the lab on one condition—she had to take her younger brother Bishop with her. He would learn chemistry while keeping an eye on his sister. So fifteen-year-old Bishop accompanied twenty-two-year-old Mary to her tutoring sessions and acted as chaperone.

Apparently, he was terrible at his job.

At least a decade older than Mary, Ferdinand was handsome in a dark, Heathcliff sort of way, with wild, curly hair and deep-set eyes that often clouded with pain because he suffered from bouts of neuralgia. Ferdinand moved around his lab with catlike agility. Mary loved to watch him work, skillfully fastening a semipermeable membrane filled with plant extract to a delicate, long tube or transferring alkaloid derivative from the experiment to an evaporating dish. Sometimes while they worked, their hands touched, causing Mary to feel electrified.

"See how the water column has risen," Ferdinand remarked, turning to Mary as though she deserved credit for osmotic pressure. She hoped that Bishop did not notice her bright red cheeks.

Mary started wishing that Bishop would leave the room. When he finally did get up to stretch his legs and relieve himself, Ferdinand Mayer asked her to marry him. And she answered, "Yes." But before she could tell her family, a series of misfortunes occurred that required her complete attention.

In October of 1864, Mary's brother Haven was captured during the siege of Petersburg and incarcerated in the bowels of a ship in the port of Richmond, Virginia. Rumors spread that the prisoners in these ships were crammed together with little room to lie down and hardly any food or water. Food and clothing sent from home never reached Haven or any other prisoner. Instead, the Confederates kept these supplies for themselves. Mary and her family grew sick with worry.

Then Mary's sister Edith, who had traveled to Norfolk, Virginia, to teach the formerly enslaved, caught typhoid fever. In the same way that she had rushed to Haven's side, Mary hurried to her sister. Edith badly needed the care. Mary stayed with her through Christmas and until she was recovered enough for the train ride back home to New York. They arrived in time to receive the news that Haven was still alive. The entire family rejoiced. In March, he returned home in a prisoner exchange. Finally, with the family back together, Mary felt that it was time to let them know that she was engaged.

Her family was stunned. Mary had passionately denounced the idea of marriage most of her adult life, so her sudden about-face left everyone confused. No one had expected independent Mary to become the first Putnam child to get married, much less to a poor, nervous scholar, not to mention a foreigner, both a German and a Jew.

When Ferdinand came to the Putnam house to meet Mary's enormous family for the first time, her youngest brothers and sisters—Irving, Ruth, and seven-year-old Kingman—would not sit still and roughhoused the entire time. Ferdinand seemed astounded. He was not accustomed to a family with so many children. When Mary mentioned how delightful youngsters were when they had not been stifled by too much discipline, poor Ferdinand shuddered.

"It's only the excitement, and being so upset at the thought of having our circle broken," she said apologetically. Ferdinand gallantly replied that he could appreciate how they must feel about the prospect of losing their oldest sister.

The wedding was set for September 1865. Her entire family celebrated because Haven was now engaged to be married too. The Union was winning the war, and a lightness seemed to take hold throughout the household. And then the greatest tragedy of the age happened: On April 14 at Ford's Theatre in Washington, DC, President Lincoln was assassinated by John Wilkes Booth. Even though the war was almost won, her family, along with the entire Union, mourned. Mary's father felt like he had lost a close friend.

Not long after the president's assassination, Mary began to quietly dread the approach of September. She was having doubts about her engagement. When she was with Ferdinand, she felt attracted to him, but when they were apart, Mary simply forgot that he existed. Even worse, her parents did not like him. The fact was, they felt uneasy about the idea of their English and Dutch daughter marrying a German Jew.

Even though anti-Semitism had pervaded American culture, during the war, Lincoln appointed army chaplains to serve Jews in the military. After the 1860s, with the beginning of the influx of millions of Jewish immigrants escaping persecution in Eastern Europe, anti-Semitism escalated in America. The Shylock image became popular in political cartoons, the quintessential parvenu who wore vulgar, glittering jewelry, lacked table manners, attracted attention with his raucous behavior, and forced his way clumsily into elite society.

Mary's parents would have considered it poor taste to judge someone by his ancestors or his religion, but they felt that he was not good enough for their brilliant daughter. Still, George Putnam trusted Mary to make her own choices.

While Mary held her fiancé's character in the highest regard, as she learned more about his personality, she started to feel that he was somehow narrow-minded, and his desire for her admiration seemed childish. Every time they were together, even in the lab, he asked her if she loved him. She would always say yes, and he would smile and tell some story about his day that bored her into yawning. Even worse, he was moody. She hated adjusting her own state of being so that he felt at ease.

Confused about whether everyone felt this way before getting married, she wrote a long letter to her father that spelled out all of her lackluster feelings toward Ferdinand. She received a reply almost immediately that read: "The whole thing must end now! Once and for all, unconditionally." Every word was underlined. With great relief, Mary called off her engagement, and her father delivered the message to Ferdinand. Heartbroken, he disappeared without contacting Mary again. He was last seen by a coworker from pharmacy college in 1869; he had suffered a nervous breakdown.

Freed of her engagement, Mary decided on a different future. She would go to Paris, but not to learn obstetrics in the Maternité de Paris hospital, as Emeline Cleveland and Elizabeth Blackwell had. She set her sights on the best medical school in the world, the École de Médecine at the Sorbonne.

When she told her parents, they were calm and supportive. As long as she was a doctor, George Putnam said with a smile, he had no objection to her being an outstanding one.

Now Mary needed to figure out how to pay for her trip. Her father offered to borrow the money, but Mary refused to let him go into more debt on her account. Instead, she contacted the Holabird family in New Orleans, with whom she had stayed during her visit with Haven at the start of the war, and secured a tutoring position with them to earn her travel money. Once in Paris, she would find other jobs to keep her going financially.

During the winter and into spring and summer of 1866, she lived in New Orleans tutoring the Holabird children and writing articles for the *New Orleans Times*. Finally, in September, with her twenty-fourth birthday behind her and sufficient savings for her great adventure, she returned to New York and set sail for France.

Revolutionary

MARY PUTNAM ARRIVED IN PARIS MID-SEPTEMBER OF 1866. THE
French administrator and city planner Baron Haussmann had just
begun the third phase of city renovations that started when Napoléon III
declared himself emperor in 1852. The massive urban-renewal project de-
molished the overcrowded, ancient buildings in neighborhoods that were
deemed unhealthy and built wide avenues, new parks and squares, and
waterworks that included sewers, fountains, aqueducts, and public urinals.
Thousands of artful gas lamps transformed Paris into the City of Light.
Bustling department stores and haute-couture shops allowed more women
to dress in the highest fashions, featuring expansive crinolines, varnished
boots, and colorfully designed hats, cementing Paris as the most modern
city in the world.

On her first official day of sightseeing, Mary Putnam traveled by train
to Rouen, where she gawked at the towering abbey of Saint-Ouen, the first
Gothic church she had ever seen. The decorative weave of the S-curved
flames carved into stone that magically entwined the structure like thick,
gray vines combined with the ornate stained glass reflecting the sunlight
left her giddy. Tracing the footsteps of Joan of Arc, she visited the Palace of
Justice, the bridge of the patron saint, the tower where Joan was confined,
the place where she was burned, and the ugly modern monument erected
to honor her memory.

Never before had Putnam felt so wide-eyed. In Paris, even the ancient
structures seemed new. She toured the city during the day and after dining
stayed up late in her hotel room reading Rousseau's *Émile*, his treatise on
the nature of education.

With the help of Elizabeth Blackwell, who had come from London
to visit friends, Putnam found an excellent French teacher and a place to

live: a tiny room on the fifth floor of an immense Parisian-style apartment house that seemed to hold an entire village of people. Although small and without a stove for heat, her room was in a choice location near Sorbonne University, established in 1253 and one of the first institutions of higher learning in the Western world. Situated among the narrow, winding cobblestoned streets of the Latin Quarter, the building was a ten-minute walk to the Luxembourg Garden.

She shared her apartment with Mademoiselle Hartung, a middle-aged single woman who reminded Putnam of a character in one of Elizabeth Gaskell's macabre *Gothic Tales*, the old nurse Hester who had protected her young charge from the evil ghosts trying to lure her to her death. The living arrangement gave Putnam an opportunity to practice her French, and Mademoiselle Hartung's fierce respectability guaranteed Putnam a propriety of her own.

Now happily situated, Putnam began the difficult task of gaining access to the hospital clinics, a central feature of French medicine and medical education. Armed with letters of introduction from Blackwell and Lucy Sewall, both of whom had attended the clinics at the Maternité de Paris hospital, she walked five or six miles a day visiting hospitals and socialized at night, making new friends and networking at dinner parties to gain patronage and political support.

After weeks of disappointment, she finally met someone who would be a key ally: Dr. Benjamin Ball, an English physician working in Paris. Through his influential connections, he finagled internships for her at two hospitals, Lariboisière, a general hospital, and Salpêtrière, the hospital for the insane. She was one of twenty interns at the Lariboisière on the service of Dr. Hippolyte-Victor Hérard, who often kept her by his side during rounds because she was a woman, and a petitely feminine one at that. She also began attending lectures at the museum of the Jardin des Plantes and, in December, at the College of France.

After two weeks at the Salpêtrière, she wrote her parents that whatever tiny inclination she had had to believe in spiritualism had been swept away. She'd found a perfect explanation for all supernatural phenomena: they were simply the delusions of the mentally ill.

Typically, instructors and students at the teaching clinics observed and examined patients together. Putnam felt that she performed as well as or better than the male students who were graduates of regular medical schools. She bragged in a letter home, "Friday I was particularly exultant at the fact that in our auscultation class at Lariboissière [*sic*], I was in the right three times, when everyone else was wrong."

Despite her pride of accomplishment, she complained to her mother, "I have been much exasperated lately by the difficulties I have encountered in finding a laboratory where I can pursue certain chemico-medical analyses." None of the hospitals she worked at, including Dr. Hérard's, allowed women to access their labs. Additionally, she could not afford to purchase her own microscope, and thus she remained entirely without access to the work she loved the most.

Putnam's service to Dr. Hérard, however, proved to be a vital link into the centers of Paris medicine. By May of 1867, after intense study and practice, she was speaking fluent French and had acquired a full schedule of hospital visits, spending three to five hours a day in clinics studying topics ranging from specific diseases to practical diagnosis. Dr. Hérard offered to introduce her to a fourth clinic at a hospital for diseases of the larynx.

Eager to secure funds for her education, Putnam used her growing access to clinics and hospitals to become the Paris correspondent for the *Medical Record*, a highly respected American journal. Speaking to the American men of medicine in a column titled "Medical Matters in Paris," she described her observations of working on clinical rounds with Hérard and other instructors. She wrote about Bright's disease, tracheotomies, ovarian versus renal cysts, cholera, thyroid function, and lithotomies. Disguising her gender, she signed her articles P.C.M. (a reversal of her actual initials). Later, she would secure correspondence positions with the *New York Evening Post* and her father's own *Putnam's Monthly*.

Yet even after gaining all of this clinical experience, she was no closer to being admitted to the École de Médecine at the Sorbonne. The fact was, prejudices against educating women in medicine were worse in France than in America. Putnam had begun to suspect this after reading Rousseau's *Émile*.

The revered philosopher saw women as voracious temptresses, much like the Catholic Church fathers, whose teachings Rousseau professed to abhor. To the famous author, men risked annihilation because of their inability to resist women. So it was for good reason, according to Rousseau, that France's civil code enshrined the power of the husband over his wife and children and stipulated that the wife must submit to her husband.

Furthermore, under an 1810 Napoleonic law, a man could freely murder his adulterous wife if she was caught in the act at home.

In a letter to her mother discussing the supposed power of French women over men, Putnam wrote, "French prejudices rest upon an entirely different ground from those that obtain in England or America. An Englishman would say that it was indelicate to admit women to study medicine, a Frenchman, that it was dangerous."

Luckily for Putnam, she happened to be a cold-tempered, earnest American. "I knew well enough I was not 'dangerous,' and that Frenchmen would instantly perceive that I was not, and when once that first difficulty was overcome, that I could be much more at ease here."

She knew that her acceptance as the first woman at numerous hospital clinics could be attributed to her Americanism and also to the fact that she purposely wore dark-colored clothes. She had even dyed her favorite red skirt a murky brown to attract less attention. She wore her chestnut hair parted in the middle and pulled back into a neat little bun, never indulging in the popular hairstyles that featured complex braids or flowing curls.

Putnam once described herself as a short, thick-set Dutch-built figure with large hands and feet and a certain tendency toward overweight kept down only by much activity of mind and body. She wrote that she had a square and massive face with a big nose and large, dark eyes below black eyebrows that made her look almost Egyptian. To receive special treatment and meet important people, she played up her persona as a plain-looking, passionless foreign woman who posed no temptation for any man. It seemed to be working.

～

Putnam smiled when Dr. Montard, another connection from her mentor Dr. Hérard, suggested that to blend in and be treated equally, she should wear men's clothing when she worked in the clinics. But he was quite serious.

Putnam politely thanked Montard for his unexpected suggestion. "Why, Monsieur, look at my littleness! Men's clothes would only exaggerate it; I should never be taken for a man, and the objection to mixing with the students would be increased a hundred fold."

Montard, who openly admired Putnam as one of his smartest students,

said that he had only wanted to be helpful. She assured him that, by allowing her to attend his clinics at Beaujon Hospital, he was already being most
obligeant.

Dr. Montard ran his student clinic differently from the others that she
had attended. At the other hospitals, patient examinations took place
during rounds. Each student was asked to express an opinion in turn and
had to make a quick response. Under the direction of Montard, the students examined the patients before the *visite* and then reported on the
cases. Montard had helped Putnam by securing her the special privilege
of visiting patients in the afternoon by herself. This meant that, while the
other interns worked one case at a time, she could go at her own pace and
interview many patients.

On Thursday, May 2, 1867, she examined an even dozen of Montard's
patients. Recording all of these cases took a while, and Putnam found herself unable to leave until 8:00 p.m. She filed her final report and then made
her way out of the hospital. Beaujon had many floors, and she had to cross
through several wards, some darkened and others so bright that she had to
squint. Just before she reached the exit, she passed through another darkened ward. She paused, blinking. When her eyes had fully adjusted, what
she saw stopped her breath.

The scene before her resembled those in the popular Gothic novels by
so-called literary physicians describing macabre cases with exceptional
gore or full of supernatural and unexplainable events meant to arouse sus-
pense, horror, and astonishment in the reader. The patients on this ward
were in beds that lined the room and were situated behind flowing white
draperies casting fantastic shadows against the wall. In the middle of the
ward, a solemn group gathered beneath the night lamp that shed a dim
light on a woman stretched, unmoving and apparently lifeless, on a litter.
A young man wearing a *paletôt*, a double-breasted overcoat, stood guard
over the woman. To Putnam, the flowing overcoat on the heroic young
physician, the seemingly acute nature of the patient's disease, the dim lamp,
the moving attendants—all suggested something military, as if the patient
had been shot in a battle raging outside the walls of a besieged fortress. It
resembled a beautifully staged opera.

Tragedy was always picturesque to the bystander, Putnam thought.

Just then, the young physician seemed to recognize her. When he came
forward with a certain pleased surprise, her heart beat faster. He had an

earnest face and an honest intelligence that worked through all of Putnam's defenses. She had to make herself listen as he described what was indeed a ghoulish case. The unfortunate patient had attempted to poison herself by drinking sulfuric acid. He asked Putnam if she wanted to observe the patient's continued deterioration and death. As a medical student, Putnam had a perfect right to stay, but suddenly her growling stomach and tired feet, blistered from walking all day, urged her to flee. Making a quick excuse and sacrificing a portion of her reputation for medical enthusiasm, she hurried from the scene in search of home and sustenance.

That night, she dreamed about the doctor. The next morning, any memory of him vanished because she was finally getting to do what she loved most: scientific research. Every day for a couple of hours, she would work for Louis-Antoine Ranvier, an assistant to the French physiologist Claude Bernard, and his partner André-Victor Cornil in their innovative laboratory.

In 1865, Bernard had published *An Introduction to the Study of Experimental Medicine*, the foundation for medical reform in Europe and America. Known as one of the greatest men of science, Bernard called for the experimental methods used in physiology, chemistry, biology, and microscopy to be applied to clinical medicine. Putnam had arrived in Paris just in time to help invent scientific medicine.

This morning, she found herself gazing at a chemical palace. Numerous large, arched windows allowed bright sunlight to illuminate the work area. The room was filled with rows of laboratory benches, each supplied with gas and water taps, tiers of bottles, and a washbasin. There were separate darkrooms for spectroscopes and polarimeters, and open-air balconies for conducting dangerous experiments. Through forced ventilation, fume cupboards, and plumbing, all laboratory waste was swept out of the room and into the sewer or atmosphere.

Professors Ranvier and Cornil were charming French gentlemen who took pride in the safety of their laboratory. Ranvier bubbled over with an airy, lighthearted humor. The French managed to say so much with tones and gestures that, to Putnam, their wit was like the rustling of butterfly wings. They were nothing like the English, whom Putnam found to be insipid. She wrote to her mother that she "encountered frequently along the rue de Rivoli whole families of English girls, all dressed alike, all wearing the same expression, all meek, subdued, conventional as a pack of sheep.

In my anatomical class is a young Englishman who is the centre of amusement for the whole class. . . . He seems a good innocent youth, too, but so daisy-like, sandy and English. I am always imagining him on his return to London seated at his father's substantial mahogany dining table, surrounded by his four well educated sisters, and relating his terrific adventures in Paris,—and how finally he will say, as he tries to eye a glass of port with the air of a connoisseur, 'Oh, by the way, there was a woman in our class—Yes there was, 'pon my honor, and by Jove she always answered just as well as us fellows.'"

While working for Ranvier and Cornil, Putnam began writing a thesis, hoping that it would help her chances at being accepted into the Paris medical school. Based on several of her chemical experiments using human livers from autopsy subjects and animal livers from rabbits, pigs, and cats, she examined how the fatty degeneration of tissue cells resulted from failed nutrition (cellular absorption and breakdown of food materials). Her thesis addressed the physiological impact of cellular degeneration and how cellular nutrition altered a body's general health and vitality. Putnam believed that such investigations were essential for diagnosing and curing illnesses.

On Monday, she rose at 5:00 a.m. and studied for two hours before leaving for Dr. Hérard's clinic at Lariboisière. She inhaled the sweet springtime air as she hurried past the Luxembourg Garden, where she waved a greeting to the statue of a duchess of Orleans, whose ringlets reminded her of her mother's. The familiar clatter of horses' hooves along the cobblestones jostled Putnam out of her thoughts as she climbed the steps to the hospital.

The lecture room was packed with students. Hérard was presenting a case of leprosy, and everyone wanted to observe. Putnam tried pushing her way through the crowd of men, to no avail. She looked for a chair to stand on. Just then, Hérard stopped his lecture and demanded to know the whereabouts of Miss Putnam. She called out from her position in the rear. Hérard expressed his irritation at the ill manners being displayed and gestured for the male students to clear a path to a spot where Putnam could see. The men stepped aside for her in waves until she reached the front of the room. Putnam wrote to her mother about Hérard: "A man who can think of other people in such ways must have an immense amount of kindness of heart, I think."

A few days later, her friend and teacher Ranvier secured for her the privilege of using the great library within the medical school; she would be permitted to read privately in the office of the librarian in chief. Her presence at the library became routine. Next, Dr. Hérard obtained permission from the dean of the faculty for Putnam to attend a surgical class in the fall at the École Pratique des Hautes Études. This was one of the institutions that Elizabeth Blackwell had prophesied that Putnam would never be allowed to enter.

Every day she gave thanks for her gallant mentor Dr. Hérard. Each step into uncharted territory meant that she was getting closer to her goal of acceptance into the École de Médecine. Yet the risk of self-sabotage was around every corner. She had to keep reminding herself to stay focused and grateful.

∾

On a cool evening in October, Putnam sat chatting with Emily Blackwell at a reception held for Emily by her older sister Anna. A famous spiritualist, natural health practitioner, and intellectual, Anna lived in Paris and worked as a newspaper correspondent. Many well-connected Parisians attended her social gatherings, hoping to rub shoulders with illustrious mesmerists, psychics, and mediums. Putnam liked the intellectually flamboyant Anna despite her delusional claim that she communicated with the recently deceased.

Tonight, Anna was on her best behavior, cordial and pleasant, showing little of the critical temperament her sister Elizabeth found distasteful. Putnam was glad to have been invited, especially since Emily introduced her to Dr. Ulysse Trélat, a military surgeon who currently practiced at Salpêtrière hospital and had previously been minister of public works and a cabinet member in the French government. Putnam's stories about her work with French doctors at the hospital clinics and her valiant quest for admission to medical school charmed him so much that he introduced her to his wife, Madame Trélat, a prominent Paris socialite. Throughout the rest of the evening, Putnam entertained Madame Trélat with delightful conversation about her love of France and her new life in Paris.

A week later, Putnam entered the office of the secretary to the faculty of medicine to obtain an admittance card for her course starting at the École Pratique des Hautes Études. Expecting resistance, she had spent the morning worrying over how to persuade the secretary to give her the card.

It took an hour for her to pick out the right dress to wear, something dull yet attractive, an impossible decision. Her trepidation made her feel uncomfortably vulnerable.

When Monsieur Forget, the secretary of the faculty, introduced himself, she thought that he looked familiar. She inquired if they had had the pleasure of meeting. He responded that yes, he had observed her at a *cours* they had taken together. They chatted a few more minutes about her current research in Ranvil's laboratory. Then, squaring her shoulders and preparing for an argument, she asked for the admittance card. When he handed it over without question, she was surprised. She expressed her thanks and commented on how simple it had been for her to obtain this card. Then, feeling more confident and genuinely curious, she asked why her admission to École de Médecine was so out of the question.

Monsieur Forget smiled at her knowingly. "If you wish yourself to take out inscriptions and graduate with our degree, nothing is easier!" he replied.

Putnam was stunned. "But sir, last year I applied merely for permission to attend the lectures, and the dean refused me."

"Yes, yes, I know, it was I that refused. [The dean] consulted me, and I advised him not to allow a lady to enter among the students."

"You have then changed your mind?" Putnam could not hide the rising excitement in her voice.

To this, the secretary shrugged. It was not a problem. He would begin preparing a formal request for her entry into École de Médecine as a foreign physician and obtain a certificate of citizenship from the American ambassador. Her American medical diploma would be converted to a bachelor of science. On payment of a fee, about five hundred francs, preliminary examinations would be waived; the later five examinations required for graduation would cost three hundred francs each.

She left his office walking on air. Feeling pride mixed with an overwhelming sense of relief and sheer joy, at home, Putnam sat down and wrote to her parents about her victory even before she received her official acceptance.

What Putnam did not know at the time was that Forget's enthusiasm masked his political ambition. Empress Eugénie, wife of Napoléon III, had expressed interest in opening a French medical school for women, and the dean at the *école*, afraid of the competition and wanting to please his empress at the same time, had suddenly become fascinated with women doctors. Secretary Forget *was* acting on behalf of the dean.

Three miserable weeks passed before Putnam heard about her application from the faculty of medicine. The decision was devastating. On November 23, 1867, they voted to deny her request. Only one member spoke in her defense. The reasoning of the faculty was that a woman could not enter the main amphitheater, a masculine domain, in safety. The uproar at her presence among the students would be so great that it would be impossible for the professor to protect her from insult and abuse.

Putnam was furious at herself for being so naive as to think that her acceptance would be this easy. Secretary Forget had not merely overstated his power; he had spoiled any chance she had had to simply attend a single *cours* at the medical school. She wrote to her parents explaining the situation, apologized for raising their hopes, and promised that she would do her best to enjoy the upcoming Christmas celebrations in Paris.

Three weeks later, she received an invitation to dinner from Madame Garnier, the widow of a prominent professor of metaphysics at the Sorbonne and a very influential woman in Parisian society. On the invitation, Putnam was referred to as *protégée par Mme. Garnier*. Apparently, Madame Trélat, whom she had met at Anna Blackwell's party, had endorsed her to Madame Garnier. Being a favorite of someone in the upper tiers of French society was like receiving a magical key to the kingdom—all doors could be opened. Putnam would never forget how these so-called powerless women, through lasting connections built on respect, created invisible webs of support that elevated those deemed worthy.

The attendees were listed on the invitation. It would be a small dinner party of seven or eight people that included Joseph-Arsène Danton, the secretary to France's minister of education, Victor Duruy. Duruy was known for establishing the "Duruy law," which gave girls' primary schools legal equality with boys' schools. He was currently attempting to build a system of public secondary schools for girls. Justifying his plans to the Empress Eugénie, Duruy argued that the education of women and girls would build a stronger France and enhance family life, allowing mothers to educate their sons. Putnam immediately recognized that Danton could be recruited as an ally to her quest and sent Madame Garnier a note saying that she would be pleased to attend.

Understanding the importance of appearance, Putnam put as much thought into choosing her outfit as she did in planning her laboratory experiments. She chose a burgundy silk evening dress that enhanced her pale skin, deep brown eyes, and chestnut hair. At dinner, Madame Garnier seated her next to the secretary, and he and Madame Garnier complimented her on her excellent French. They begged her to tell them about her medical training in France, the clinics where she worked, and the instructors she liked best. In the course of the conversation, Putnam happened to mention that she was bored with her current courses and suggested that, with Danton's assistance, she might attend a histology *cours* taught by Charles Robin in the grand amphitheater at École de Médecine. Her request was risky. In the six hundred years since the university was established, no woman had entered the grand amphitheater as a student.

To her surprise, Danton was perfectly agreeable. "Write me a letter making this demand, and I will present it to the Minister," he replied.

Putnam left the dinner party full of renewed hope. Few young physicians could have received a better opening. But, she reminded herself, it was just an opening, not an acceptance. It seemed that men in power always overestimated their actual capabilities when speaking to women.

In the days that followed the party, a wave of frigid weather took hold of Paris. For Putnam, they were the coldest days of her life. The Seine froze hard enough for her to walk across it. Her tiny room was not heated even with a fireplace, and everything froze—water, oil, ink. Friends from home wrote asking if she was ready to leave. After all, she'd had more than a year of studying at the clinics, enough to establish a thriving practice. But even though she had given up hope of hearing from Danton about attending the course, she would not consider leaving Paris.

On New Year's Day, she sat in her apartment with Mademoiselle Hartung mending old clothes. In the evening, she played chess with a neighbor. A few days later, the weather warmed, and she felt more comfortable in her frigid room. Soon, she was back to her full schedule attending hospital clinics. At this time, she received an invitation from Madame Garnier to a second dinner party in the coming week, but she sent a refusal, feeling too busy to go. The next day, she was dressing for supper at home when she heard the distinct rustle of silk in the passage outside her door, a very narrow one and pitch-dark at that hour. Then she heard someone calling out, "Miss Putnam, Mary Putnam." It was the soothingly delightful voice of Madame Garnier. Putnam rushed to open the door, and sure enough, the woman, who was well past fifty years old, had walked up the five flights wearing a bustle with numerous petticoats and now stood, winded but smiling, on her doorstep.

Madame Garnier greeted her by kissing each cheek and handing her a neatly folded note. Putnam opened it right away and found a cordially written rejection of her refusal. The note also listed the names of the people expected at the dinner. One stood out: Monsieur Danton, secretary to the minister of education. Madame Garnier said that Putnam would miss out on the conversation of a lifetime if she did not come.

Of course Putnam agreed to attend. She grew so excited that night, she barely slept. The next evening at dinner, too excited for small talk, Putnam blurted out her question to Monsieur Danton: Would she be allowed to enter the grand amphitheater and take the course?

With a knowing smile, Monsieur Danton assured her that her histology *cours* had been satisfactorily settled. Sure enough, three days later, she received an official authorization. The authorization included strict instructions on how she could safely enter the room: by a side door, separate from the students' entrance; a chair would be reserved for her near the professor.

On her first day of class, she half expected the entire faculty of the École de Médecine plus riot police to be waiting in the wings, ready to swoop in and save the damsel in distress from rampaging men. What actually happened could not have been further from that scenario. The male students, who by now knew her from clinics and classes, did not lift an eyebrow at her appearance, taking it as a matter of course. Feeling like she had been doing this her entire life, she pulled out her inkstand and proceeded to take notes. But inside, she glowed. A woman student had entered the amphitheater of the École de Médecine for the very first time, and the world had not ended.

In a letter to her parents dated January 25, 1868, she announced her groundbreaking news: "For the first time since its foundation several centuries ago, a petticoat might be seen in the august amphitheater of the École de Médecine. That petticoat enrobed the form of your most obedient servant and dutiful daughter!"

Many less stubborn people would have accepted this historic victory, finished the course, and secured passage back home. Instead, Putnam plotted her next bold move: to take the entrance exam for official acceptance into the school. Contacting the administrators who had encouraged her advancement, she took brave steps on her own behalf. She wrote to Monsieur Danton, her champion, requesting to take the entrance exam and warning that she would appeal to the faculty or the education minister himself if necessary. Knowing full well that Putnam would receive more support from the minister than from the faculty members who had denied her previous application, the dean of the faculty, the chemist Adolphe Wurtz, suggested that she not wait for Danton's response but contact the minister directly. Taking his advice, Putnam submitted a request to education minister Duruy and then began studying for her exam.

For the next four days, she waited for the response. What was taking so long? Finally, her patience was gone. She tromped down the five flights from her apartment and marched toward the Sorbonne to demand an answer to her request.

As she hurried across the street, someone called out her name. It was the secretary of the faculty, Monsieur Forget, the same gentleman who had initially promised her, falsely, that he alone could gain admittance for her. He was rushing to meet her.

Smiling sincerely, he said that he had news and he was not able to keep it a secret any longer. His hands shook nervously as he revealed a folded note.

"I have been asking everywhere for you and nobody knew what had become of you," he said, flustered. Then he handed her the note.

Putnam's heart raced as she read through the letter. She read it again and again. When she finished, she almost started dancing. Her face broke out in a radiant smile.

The official note conveyed the decision of Minister Duruy and stated that it was he who granted Putnam permission to take her entrance exam. The faculty, upon his recommendation, would officially accept her degrees from the Woman's Medical College of Pennsylvania and the New York College of Pharmacy. All of her credits from these schools would count toward her graduation from the École de Médecine. The highest ranks of the French empire—the empress and the Ministry of Education—had just enforced her deepest aspiration. A young woman who had begun her medical career in Paris as a freakish outsider had just sparked the acceptance of women physicians in the Paris clinics.

Forget then invited her to stroll with him around the Luxembourg Garden. Surprised, Putnam accepted. As they walked, she drank in the evident astonishment of the numerous bands of male students that watched them take what was obviously a victory lap. She was thrilled by the open gesture that assured the other students that France was on her side.

During the first months of 1868, Putnam continued her work in the laboratories of Cornil and the highly regarded anatomist Marie Philibert Constant Sappey. She prepared for her examinations, worked on her thesis, and attended Professor Robin's course on histology. Her social life in Paris had always been busy, but now she received invitations daily from society women and intellectuals who wanted to get to know her better. At one of these social outings, she struck up a conversation with Élisée Reclus, a charming, middle-aged man with kind blue eyes. Her host had described Reclus as the most outstanding French scientist in the field of physical geography.

Talking to Reclus, Putnam discovered that they had more than science in common; he was an ardent abolitionist who was thoroughly familiar with the causes behind America's Civil War. Most Parisians Putnam talked to had either never heard of the war or tended to favor the Confederacy. One educated Frenchman thought the Civil War had been fought on the isthmus of Panama between North and South America. Reclus, however, had written a series of articles on the war titled "La Grève d'Amérique" for the magazine *Le Travailleur*. Putnam was surprised to learn that he had spent more than two years in New Orleans, from 1853 to 1855, tutoring the children of the proprietor of a sugar plantation. Excitedly, Putnam shared with Reclus her own adventures in New Orleans, and by the end of the evening, they had developed a genuine friendship. Over the next few weeks, she would meet his entire family and receive an invitation to spend the summer at their country home in Normandy.

ↄ

Ninety-two-year-old patriarch Dumesnil, the grandfather of Élisée Reclus's wife, had been ill for several weeks, and he died the day following Putnam's arrival in Normandy. In the next few weeks, she attended his funeral, two weddings, and many dinner parties held by the Dumesnil family. The father, Alfred, was Élisée's brother-in-law. Other family members included his older brother, Élie; Élie's wife, Noémi; and their two sons, Paul and André. Ardent feminists, they were all delighted to meet the courageous and famous woman scholar Mary Putnam.

Putnam soon learned that the Recluses were French radicals who regularly entertained anarchist sympathizers from all parts of the world. Élie and Élisée Reclus helped create an international network of socialist militants and scholars fundamentally opposed to colonialism and European empires. Their scientific and political theories offered the ideological underpinnings for social change in France. The Reclus brothers were also fascinated by volcanoes, seeing the explosive mountains as symbols of not only the revolution but also the aggressive impulse, which they suppressed within themselves by becoming teetotalers and, later, nudists.

For Putnam, the Recluses were cultivated, charming, and virtuous men from a large Protestant family like her own. A renowned geographer and gifted speaker, Élisée could motivate revolutionaries in the same way a popular minister attracted followers to God. Believing that humanity was nature becoming self-conscious, Élisée insisted that communities should have natural, not political, boundaries. Each geographical region had a right to determine its own fate. He applied the scientific method to his study of geography using a positivist approach that Putnam admired.

As a friend of the Reclus family, Putnam met prominent members of leftist politics in Paris and listened to their ideas about religion, the bourgeoisie, feminism, and the value of socialism. She absorbed the radical idea that everything, even science and medicine, was political. In a letter home, she described them as "red-hot republican reformers." Their support for women's rights and education along with her own academic pursuits affirmed her both personally and intellectually. She pored over the writings of Auguste Comte and the utopian socialist Charles Fourier, who believed humanity was evolving toward a harmonious state that was characterized by, among other things, equality between the sexes. Putnam described people who would die for a cause as the "salt of the earth."

Putnam also spent her school break earning the two hundred francs per month that she needed to live on by writing stories for the *New York Post* and *Putnam's Monthly*. She arose at dawn and composed stories in her room until breakfast at eight and then again until lunchtime. In the afternoon, she sat by a stream and read. She got her exercise by going for walks through the pristine countryside and teaching the Dumesnil children an energetic form of calisthenics. In the evening, she and the Recluses and Dumesnils continued a more animated version of the conversations they had started at breakfast about such topics as the materialistic orientation of French bourgeois culture, Napoléon's evil regime, and the absurdity of marriage for women unless it was a union of "free will."

The Recluses' simple way of life shined with authenticity. In America, Henry David Thoreau advocated for living modestly in nature without superficial luxuries and presented similar radical ideas in his book *Walden* and the essay "Civil Disobedience." Since the Recluses were too poor to hire servants, Élie's wife, Noémi, did most of the cooking. The children helped with all household chores. Their library overflowed with books, and every child was educated. But the meals were sometimes meager, and the rooms, though clean and comfortable, were sparsely furnished. Yet everyone was so friendly, witty, and intelligent. Putnam felt more content with her new friends than she had with her own parents or even her brother Haven. The Recluses admired Putnam *because* she was a brilliant student, a feminist, and a pioneering doctor. Her own family loved her *in spite* of those qualities.

Every few days, Putnam had a visitor who made the children giggle and Noémi wonder how a young woman could be so smart and yet so naive. Putnam's guest was a thoughtful young man, the intern she had met when he was caring for the dying woman that spooky night at Beaujon Hospital. He had begun calling on her in Paris, and now they were taking long walks together in the countryside. Putnam insisted that they were just friends, but after he left, she would remain flushed for hours. When she finally wrote about him to her sister Edith, she never referred to him by name but only as "Monsieur M." When her mother saw Putnam's breathless writing, she recognized her daughter's infatuation and asked in a letter if Putnam was considering marriage. Putnam, who was twenty-six, replied, "As to my marrying, even at forty, it is absurd, it would be horribly inconvenient." And yet she continued to meet with Monsieur M. throughout the summer.

⤸

Back in Paris after the break, Putnam felt relieved and proud finally to be enrolled as a real student at École de Médecine. She had moved out of her room with Mademoiselle Hartung and into a vacant room in the large apartment of Élie and Noémi Reclus that she rented for one hundred francs a month. Coming from a sizable family, she felt right at home living in this bustling household. All she needed now was a microscope.

When her father sent her a gift of money, she thought her wish for a microscope had been granted, except for one thing: he wanted her to use it to buy a dress. Her father's greatest fear was that she would become dowdy and humorless. Promptly, she wrote him, "Thank you very much for the handsome present. Would you greatly object if I put it into a microscope instead of clothes? . . . I will not buy it till I hear from you, but I rely upon your consent."

Of course she got the microscope, and now she had everything she wanted. "My only trouble," she wrote her mother, "is a chronic perplexity as to why I should nearly always have what I want, when hardly anybody else has. I certainly do nothing to deserve such superior prosperity, and if anything should happen suddenly to cut me off or cripple me or make me an invalid for the rest of my days, I should feel that it was only fair balance for the uninterrupted happiness that has been granted me."

Yet despite her happiness, after two years abroad, she was surprised by her sudden yearning for home. As soon as she received her degree, she vowed to travel back to New York like an arrow. By November 1869, Putnam was preparing for her third oral examination and attending clinics at the Hôtel Dieu, the famous hospital adjacent to the Notre-Dame Cathedral. The expansive hospital seemed like its own municipality, with subterranean passages and physicians who crossed into each other's wards like warlords clashing over scientific theory and its application to medicine, cementing its reputation as one of the great research hospitals of its time.

For weeks, Putnam studied with a private tutor to prepare for her third examination. This oral test covered topics most students hated: chemistry, natural history, and physics. She must do her best on the subject of chemistry because she hoped to teach that subject after graduating. Wishing to gain prestige among her professors by outperforming her male colleagues, she worked day and night practicing her answers.

On Friday, December 24, she sat on a bench outside the arena with two other students who both seemed very nervous. She went last. The six professors dressed in black silk gowns with scarlet satin lining and hats shaped like pies sat in judgment before her. The room was filled with students invited to watch and others interested in the proceedings, including the Paris correspondent for the *New-York Tribune,* who wrote that the American woman was "dressed with an absolute plainness . . . and with a certain quaint, scholastic air that contrasts oddly with her fresh girlish face. . . .

The young American, with all her unconsciousness, is a character that must one day take its place in history."

The first professor to question her, Monsieur Gavarret, had a reputation for always asking the same question: "*Et bien, Monsieur, qu'avez vous étudié?*" What subject had the pupil studied?

She ignored the noisy cordon of youth two deep about her and said in a conversational tone, "Sir, I studied the things we're supposed to know to pass this exam. But a subject that left me particularly interested is that of the solenoids."

Upon hearing her answer, the professors looked astonished. Her fellow students applauded her response. She had purposely chosen a topic that other pupils had never even thought about but that she knew Monsieur Gavarret valued.

Another professor questioned her about botany, and she had no difficulty answering. Finally, Monsieur Wurtz, the renowned chemist and dean of the faculty, asked her about tannin. At her reply, he said, "*Ah, c'est très bien.*" Putnam continued by giving the specific chemical formula for tannin. He laughed and said, "Well, I couldn't have asked you that, because I forgot it myself."

She continued answering his questions perfectly, and the professor sat bemused as well as pleased because she remembered his writing better than he did. After several minutes, he closed the examination with remarks of great satisfaction. Putnam withdrew to wait with the other students for the results.

The *Tribune*'s Paris correspondent captured the entire event. It constituted news because not only was Mary Putnam being examined; so was Elizabeth Garrett, the English woman doctor and protégée of Elizabeth Blackwell; she was taking her fourth exam in a different room. Since she had years of clinical experience in England, she had come to Paris only for the required examinations and thus was on track to graduate after taking the fifth and final exam in a few weeks. Even though she had started at the school after Putnam, she would become the first woman to graduate. Garrett was staying with Putnam at the home of the Reclus family, and they had become fast friends.

The *Tribune* correspondent was astonished by Putnam's performance. He wrote that the young woman had sailed past her two male companions "as if she were born to the water, and they were canary-birds. . . . One stuttered and stammered so that it was heartbreaking to see. Finally, tears coursed one another down his innocent nose. He could not describe a potato. . . . He could not describe anything. His tongue cleaved to the roof of his mouth."

The professors and their fellow students offered words of encouragement to the two male examinees, but they were of no use. "The first had failed when brought up to the standard of potato; the second succumbed when asked to tell what he knew about opium. . . . Then came the lady's turn and how easily she did it! . . . Perfect self-possession with perfect modesty—a born lady. . . . At the end, when the Dean of the Faculty, who had not attempted to conceal his satisfaction at the failure of all his efforts to stump the American girl, rubbed his hands, and turning to his colleague, said, aloud, '*Oh! Très bien! Très bien!*'"

Finally, the students rushed to the courtyard to hear the attendant read the decisions. The verdict for the two young men: *Passable*, a very low mark. Elizabeth Garrett received a *Bien satisfait*, the second-highest mark available.

"*Très satisfait*," the usher called out to Putnam—the highest mark possible, a grade that had not been awarded to any student in two years.

Putnam easily passed her fourth exam in May, and by June 1870, she was preparing for her fifth and final examination and the completion of her thesis. She planned to be home by Christmas, although she was dreading a stormy voyage across the Atlantic in December. However, the political climate in France was turning equally tempestuous.

In a letter to her mother, she wrote, "The revolution is advancing rapidly. . . . I should be much disappointed not to be here to see it." Workers everywhere were on strike. Even the students at the medical school had rioted against an instructor who had served as the medical expert at the infamous murder trial of Pierre Bonaparte, Napoléon's nephew. In a fit of anger, Pierre had shot and killed Victor Noir, a journalist for the leftist newspaper *La Revanche* whose recent articles had been highly critical of Emperor Napoléon. Pierre claimed it was self-defense, but it was obvious to the medical students that he was guilty. At the trial, the professor, a noted imperialist, "cooked the facts" in favor of the scamp Pierre and got him off. The medical students resolved to teach the professor a lesson. The first time he attempted to deliver his lecture, they erupted in a perfect storm of hisses and insults that chased him out of the classroom. The students repeatedly disrupted classes until finally the minister of education closed the school for a month.

Then, in July 1870, France declared war on Prussia. When anger toward the imperial French government swelled with that declaration of war, Putnam joined the Recluses in rejoicing over the prospect of social revolution ignited by an unpopular conflict with Prussia.

By August, France's defeat was imminent. The army was struggling and had suffered severe losses. Apparently, Napoléon III was so fearful of internal revolution that he kept thousands of troops in Paris instead of sending them to the front. In Paris, people grew impatient with the emperor and his incompetence. In the evenings, Putnam strolled the Latin Quarter with Élie Reclus observing the French soldiers stationed with arms lining the boulevards like treacherous statues ready to fire on the people.

One morning when Putnam arrived for work at the hospital, she saw her friend Monsieur M. waiting for her near the door. She noticed the bright morning sun reflecting off the brass buttons of the soldier's coat he was wearing. Suddenly, her throat felt dry and she was shocked by a wave of dread. When he told her that he had joined the reinforcements and was leaving for battle, she almost fainted. In the midst of war, with life and death only moments apart, their friendly relationship turned deeply romantic. She begged him to stay. He said that only a coward would not fight for his country. But he told her that he loved her too. Feeling a frantic desire never to separate, they promised each other that, upon his return, they would get married. Then, after a final long embrace, he bowed to her, turned on his heel, and disappeared. As she watched him leave, she realized that she had been overcome by passion. The experience felt earth-shattering. She had never felt more alive. Even though she did not believe in God, she prayed every night for his safe return.

On September 4, 1870, Napoléon III was taken prisoner by the Prussian army. It was the end of the Second Empire. In Paris, Putnam and her friends celebrated. In a joyous letter to her father, Putnam announced: "I write the date to my letter with precision, for it is a great day. I have heard the Republic proclaimed in Paris!" Her father published that letter in the November issue of his magazine, enabling Putnam to become a wartime correspondent. In her accounts, she described herself as being part of the effort to establish a republic in France, an American witness and ambassador.

When the Prussian army threatened to seize Paris just two weeks after the proclamation of *Vive la République!*, the provisional government ordered all noncombatants to leave. Dr. Emily Blackwell, who was in Paris visiting clinics, caught the last train out of the city before the gates closed on September 18, shutting out some 240,000 German troops, and trapping inside over 500,000 French soldiers, mostly national guardsmen, in addition to the entire population of Paris, nearly two million. The sole means of transportation to or from the French capital was gas balloons, which were launched at night to avoid being shot down. Prussian lieutenant general Philip Sheridan advised Chancellor Otto von Bismarck to cause the French "so much suffering that they must long for peace and force their government to demand it. The people must be left with nothing but their eyes to weep with over the war."

Determined to finish her studies, Putnam, along with 250 other Americans, stayed in Paris during the siege, suffering all the hardships that ensued. If she had left the city in September, she would have been forced to abandon her degree and return home.

It was a cold winter, and the Reclus family, like everyone in Paris, was short on fuel and had a limited supply of food. Walking was the only way to get around because most of the horses had been killed for food. Mules, dogs, cats, rats, and, eventually, all of Paris's zoo animals were also on the menu. Putnam continued her work at the hospitals and witnessed considerable suffering. Via the gas balloons that left the city at night, she sent long letters home describing the siege. She was never sure if they reached her family. In January 1871, the Prussians began a bombardment of Paris, lobbing twelve thousand bombs into the city over several days. These bombs exploded all around the Recluses' home, killing a number of people in the neighborhood and forcing Putnam and the Reclus family to decamp. One night, along with five hundred others, she slept in the vaults of the Pantheon. "It was singularly dramatic, the tombs of Voltaire and Rousseau sheltering the victims of the Prussian barbarians," she wrote in her letter home.

With the city's population starving and some freezing to death, on January 19, the national guardsmen made one last, valiant attempt to break the German siege. A failure, it resulted in high French casualties. Three days later, a new protest calling for the end of bread rationing was held outside city hall by leftist supporters, including friends of Élisée Reclus. When someone in the crowd shot an officer of the guard, the guards returned fire, killing five and wounding eighteen. A week later, France and Prussia agreed to a cease-fire. After 132 days of siege, the war had ended.

The national guardsmen, who had been denied food and shelter while on duty, joined the radical faction of revolutionary socialists known as the Commune, which continued to push its demands even as some aspects of city life returned to normal.

On March 18, guardsmen at Montmartre refused to fire on an armed barricade and instead collectively declared allegiance to the Commune. The next day, the government of national defense fled to Versailles. Vowing to protect the city, the central committee of the national guard claimed power. Executions began, and there were threats against the remaining Americans until more responsible members of the Commune gained control. During its short-lived reign in Paris, the Commune tried to enact democratic reforms—to separate church and state, educate women, and expand workers' rights—but on May 21, Versailles attacked. In what came to be known as the Bloody Week, French soldiers executed thousands of insurgents in the streets, and the government took brutal action against the Commune, arresting thirty-eight thousand, including Élisée Reclus. The Reclus family began to campaign endlessly for his release.

As the new republican government faltered, Putnam wrote that "the crowning defeat of the Provisional Government lay in the inadequacy of its conception." After providing detailed biographical information on each leader, she attacked them all, criticizing their weak commitment and lack of vision for the republic. Her story was published in *Scribner's Monthly* in 1871. While Putnam's reporting from Paris was noted in newspapers across America, she was not the first American woman to act as a war correspondent. Margaret Fuller, American journalist, editor, feminist, and leader of the American transcendentalism movement, became the first woman war correspondent when she reported on the 1848 Italian revolution for the *New-York Tribune*.

In the midst of the chaos surrounding the fall of the Commune, Putnam's fiancé returned. She had warned herself that he would be changed, but when she first saw him, she did not recognize him. Terribly thin, withdrawn, and cold-eyed, he seemed like a stranger. They took walks trying to get to know each other again. Putnam assumed that, because of the war and devastation, he would want to come live in New York, away from the air still poisoned by the Prussian bombardment. But he refused. They would stay in France, he insisted. She tried to imagine herself living there as his wife, away from her own family in New York, and felt a desperate sense of confusion and loss. As a last resort, she consulted Noémi Reclus, who was like a mother to her.

"You have reached an impasse," Noémi said. "If you should consent to stay in France, you would be simply the wife of Monsieur M., which would not suit either your ambitions or your scheme of life." With tears flowing, Putnam said that she was in love and that she could fix it somehow. Noémi comforted the young woman and recommended that she accept the invitation she had received from a friend and go to London to recover.

After ending her second engagement, Putnam took Noémi's advice and traveled to London, where she spent the next two months getting over the end of her romance and waiting for the École de Médecine to reopen. She urgently wanted to finish her degree, graduate, and go home.

In July, a month before her twenty-ninth birthday, Putnam returned to Paris and easily passed her final exam. She was "now *docteur en médecine de la Faculté de Paris.*" After completing all five required exams and receiving top marks while also living through the Paris siege and the fall of the Commune, she submitted and defended her thesis on the nature of fatty acids: "De la Graisse Neutre et des Acides Gras."

Praising her thesis for its extraordinary research and eminently scientific tone, her examiners gave her the highest award, a bronze medal.

Le Figaro, the French newspaper of record, reported on her commencement, noting her astounding achievement and unique appearance among the crowd of male graduates. Both the *New York Evening Post* and the *New-York Tribune* reprinted the article from *Le Figaro*. The *Archives de Médecine*, the eminent medical journal in France, proclaimed that a "doctress has had her name inscribed on our registers." Her academic success was "proof that women are not only fitted for learning but also for the application and practice of medicine."

In the fall of 1871, Putnam left Paris, a city in both physical and political turmoil. It was not the magical city that had greeted her when she first arrived five years ago. She described the situation in her letters home as full of misery, noting that her friends the Recluses were in as much disarray as the city. Élisée was in prison and the rise of conservative forces gave little hope for his release. With the defeat of the Commune and repression of socialism, Putnam worried about the future of women's rights in France. But her own success had proved that cultural change was possible.

As she sailed across the Atlantic, Putnam carried more than a diploma from the École de Médecine. Her research and education made her one of the best educated doctors in America and placed her at the forefront of scientific medicine. Further, she had been radicalized by Élisée's feminist ideals and the understanding that the advance of science and the advance of women were one and the same. She vowed to undertake a new mission: to teach at Elizabeth Blackwell's recently opened medical school for women and instill in her students a robust scientific spirit.

Part Two

Backlash

It is inevitable that the old doctrine of the mental inferiority of women should be defended . . . on a new basis; a basis organic, structural, physiological, hence inconvertible; on an analysis, not of her reasoning faculties, her impulses, her emotions, her logic, her ignorance, but of her digestion, her nerves, her muscles, her circulation.

MARY C. PUTNAM JACOBI, "MENTAL ACTION AND PHYSICAL HEALTH"

A Mistaken Ally

In 1863, about a year before twenty-one-year-old Mary Put- nam joined the New England Hospital as an intern, Dr. Marie Zakr- zewska was making her rounds when she received word that a gentleman had arrived and was insisting on seeing her. Full of curiosity, Zakrzewska quickly finished her rounds and went to her office. Her visitor stood at once, shook her hand, and gave her his card, which read H. R. STORER, M.D. Zakrzewska blinked with surprise because she recognized the name. She was even more astounded when he told her that he wanted to apply for the attending surgeon position she had only just posted.

Horatio Storer had an exceptional reputation. His father was the dean of the faculty of medicine at Harvard Medical School. Horatio graduated from Harvard Medical School in 1853 and then, like Emily Blackwell, studied surgery with James Young Simpson in Edinburgh. He returned to Boston in 1855 and began practicing medicine, with an emphasis on obstetrics and gynecology, and lecturing at Harvard. He had also worked as an attending physician at the Boston Lying-In Hospital until it was forced to close be- cause too many women were dying from postpartum infections. Although he was in private practice and taught a gynecology class at Harvard, Storer wanted to make use of his surgical talents. Zakrzewska hired him on the spot.

In addition to working as a physician, Storer had spent years building a reputation as a moral crusader. In 1857 (the same year Elizabeth Blackwell opened the New York Infirmary for Women and Children), he uncovered statistics revealing that abortion was more prevalent among married Prot- estant white women in Boston than unmarried single and poor women. These findings shocked him to his core. At the time, women could obtain abortions legally until quickening, the stage when fetal motion was felt, usually sixteen to twenty weeks into a pregnancy; most religions believed that this was when a fetus was ensouled. Quickening was a subjective marker that could be judged only by the pregnant woman herself. Even so, no one worried about a woman ending her pregnancy before the fourth or fifth month. Many physicians performed surgeries to "restore stopped menstruation," while the *scandalous* women abortionists plied their trade in bigger cities.

Storer was so outraged by his findings—that married white women were avoiding the duties of childbirth—he persuaded the American Medical Association to research the number of abortions performed in the United States.

Since its founding in 1847, the AMA had struggled to be taken seriously. The editor of the *Cincinnati Medical Observer* described the medical association as "a body of jealous, quarrelsome men whose chief delight [was] in the annoyance and ridicule of each other." The organization was desperate to improve its reputation. Stirring up moral outrage against abortion seemed ideal, so the AMA appointed Storer to chair the Committee on Criminal Abortion, a group made up of strident antiabortion activists.

Broadening his campaign, Storer wrote to physicians throughout the country arguing (without any scientific proof) that human life began at conception rather than at quickening and pushing for legal restrictions on abortion. He proposed incarcerating the women who sought abortions as well as their doctors or abortionists and recommended even harsher sentences for married women. It was the first time a doctor had publicly elevated the fetus above the mother's well-being.

Storer's moral argument was drawn from racial fears that eventually inspired what was known as the "science" of eugenics: a social movement aimed at perfecting the human species by increasing the population with "desirable" genetic traits and reducing those with "undesirable" traits by forced sterilization. In their attempts to control the birth rate, safeguard the racial health of white people, and purge society's defectives, eugenicists primarily targeted women. Storer asked whether the United States would "be filled by our own children or by those of aliens? This is a question that our own women must answer; upon their loins depends the future destiny of the nation." Criminalizing abortion would put control of women's reproduction in the hands of male doctors and politicians and tip the racial balance in the white man's favor.

Physicians from across the country sent letters to Storer thanking him for alerting them to the dangers and the need for action. In 1859, Storer authored the committee's report, which recommended a strong antiabortion position. The AMA adopted this position as its official stance at its national convention that year, and the physicians' crusade against abortion was born. In 1860, J. B. Lippincott published the report under the title *On Criminal Abortion in America*. The doctors' crusade against abortion would finally knock out what the AMA considered its competition: amateurs, midwives, and female abortionists. And the AMA's poor reputation would begin to improve.

Despite Storer's reputation as a moralizer, Zakrzewska was grateful that a man of his prominence, connections, and ability was interested in working as an attending surgeon at her hospital. She had labored endlessly to gain the support of Boston's leading male physicians. Her favorite colleague and champion, Henry Bowditch, had introduced inductive reasoning to American medical science and pushed for public health by chairing the Massachusetts State Board of Health. He also encouraged the education of women as physicians, even at Harvard. In a letter to Zakrzewska, he wrote that women physicians and surgeons should be allowed to work in all hospitals and that hospitals should open their clinical instruction to both men and women.

Even though she welcomed prominent physicians as consultants, Zakrzewska had not intended to hire a man to work with the women physicians at her hospital. But she needed an attending surgeon and had scoured the region in vain for a qualified woman—a shortage she blamed on Harvard and the other regular medical schools that continued to exclude women—so she was willing to make an exception in Storer's case. It was a decision she would come to regret.

⁓

Within a year of moving from New York to Boston, Dr. Marie Zakrzewska bought a large home at 139 Cedar Street in Roxbury, a respectable middle-class neighborhood. Although at first she lived alone, her household grew into a communal refuge for like-minded companions. The family she attracted, however, had little to do with the idealized household of husband, wife, and children. Like the Blackwell sisters, she never considered marriage. In fact, she often compared it to prostitution.

Zakrzewska's sisters Minna and Rosalia lived with her for a few years before moving out, and shortly thereafter Karl Heinzen; his wife, Louise; and their sixteen-year-old son, Karl Friedrich, moved in. Heinzen was a German radical, an author, journalist, and lecturer who immigrated to America with other German Forty-Eighters to escape oppression after the democratic revolutions of 1848 that they supported failed. Through Heinzen, Zakrzewska became a member of the local German radical community devoted to social justice.

Heinzen, who paid for his family's room and board with proceeds from his newspaper *Pionier*, helped Zakrzewska care for the property's towering elms, woody shrubs, and flowers. So many rocks dotted the area that Zakrzewska and her family began calling their home "Rock Garden." Groups of hospital directors, doctors, and interns, as well as other friends, often gathered there. Zakrzewska would sit in the garden and write hundreds of letters to keep in touch with all the doctors and students who had been connected to her hospital. Christmas at Rock Garden became the trendiest party in Boston.

Two years after the Heinzens moved in, Julia Sprague, a women's rights activist and founding member of the New England Women's Club, also joined the household. Sprague and Zakrzewska established an immediate friendship and eventually became lovers, sharing a long-term romantic relationship.

From a young age, Marie Zakrzewska felt uncharacteristically shy around girls and spent more time roughhousing with boys. At age eleven, she met twelve-year-old Elizabeth Hohenhorst, a sweet Catholic schoolgirl who told vivid adventure stories that won young Marie's heart. "My love for her was unbounded," Zakrzewska wrote in her memoir. Even though she was Protestant, young Marie accompanied Elizabeth to her Catholic church and even received religious instruction to become a nun. This lasted until Elizabeth went to confession for the first time. After hearing about Elizabeth's adoration for her Protestant friend, the priest forbade her to continue the relationship. The separation broke young Marie's heart.

Now she surrounded herself with interesting women. Her circle of friends included Caroline Severance, Harriot Hunt, Anna Freeman Clarke, Lucia Peabody, Ednah Dow Cheney, and Lucy Goddard. Julia Ward Howe, Boston socialite and renowned lyricist of the "Battle Hymn of the Republic," often attended Zakrzewska's parties to read her most recent poems. Some of these women also invested in Zakrzewska's hospital and joined its board of directors. They weren't just her friends and business partners; they were her protectors too.

Zakrzewska's first job after moving to Boston was as a professor of obstetrics and diseases of women at the New England Female Medical College. The institution had been founded as a school of midwifery in 1848 by Samuel Gregory, an eccentric health reformer with no formal medical training. Gregory was able to secure the funding for his medical school by asserting that, for morality's sake, only women should assist other women during childbirth. Its board of lady managers consisted of some of the most prominent women reformers: Lucy Goddard, Harriet Beecher Stowe, and Ednah Dow Cheney. These women, not Gregory, had enticed Zakrzewska from New York to Boston, and the young doctor entered her new position full of energy and hope.

However, it soon became apparent that Gregory's unstable temperament and old-fashioned ideas about treating disease conflicted with Zakrzewska's scientific approach to medicine. She believed he had driven the school into quackery. The college offered only four months of study and without a standardized, graded curriculum. Zakrzewska received no support when trying to raise the school's standards. Worst of all, Zakrzewska later wrote, Gregory consistently antagonized Boston's elite physicians by accusing them of "the grossest indelicacy, yes, even criminality, in their relations with their [female] patients." In turn, Boston physicians refused to support the school, and women physicians who trained at other medical schools kept their distance. Zakrzewska realized that working for Gregory could result in the death of her own career. The final blow came when he denied her requests for thermometers, microscopes, and test tubes on the grounds that these were "new-fangled European notions." After that, the eminently scientific Zakrzewska resigned. She left with several top students and trustees, including Cheney and Goddard.

Zakrzewska envisioned building her own medical school, one that would be guided by the highest standards of excellence. To achieve her vision, she scoured Boston for funding. But even the charismatic Zakrzewska, who had attracted seemingly unlimited funds for the Blackwells' infirmary, could raise only pennies for a women's medical school. Refusing to admit defeat, she decided to open a hospital for women and children operated by women only. That endeavor proved to be extremely popular.

Women provided the backbone of Zakrzewska's support, but she also depended on the goodwill, encouragement, and active participation of men in Boston's inner circle of male reformers, including William Lloyd Garrison, the abolitionist Frederick W. G. May, and the wealthy state senator and judge Samuel Sewall. In addition, a number of physicians were willing to stake their reputations on a separate institution for women doctors. Drs. Henry Bowditch, Samuel Cabot, and Benjamin Jeffries were among twenty-six men who served as consulting physicians to the new hospital.

With the blessing of prominent Boston men and the help of Harriot Hunt's network of activists, Zakrzewska purchased used hospital equipment and rented a "sunny, airy house with a large yard at No. 60, Pleasant Street." On July 2, 1862, in the midst of the Civil War, she was ready to open the New England Hospital for Women and Children. She widely advertised that the institution would provide medical aid for women by competent physicians of their own sex, assist educated women in the practical study of medicine, and train nurses for the care of the sick. Lucy Sewall, Senator Sewall's daughter and a protégée of Zakrzewska's who had studied medicine in Europe, became the hospital's first attending physician. Lucy and Zakrzewska were close friends and often rounded together in the morning and evening, greeting patients, answering questions, calming worries, and establishing a nurturing environment. Women patients wanted to be cared for by other women. Some had complained to Zakrzewska that at the other Boston hospitals, the male practitioners treated them with open hostility, calling them names and blaming them for their own botched procedures.

By contrast, Zakrzewska required all of her employees to exhibit empathy toward patients and follow the Golden Rule: treat others as one wants to be treated. At the New England hospital, the doctors and nurses were less hurried and less interventionist in deliveries, and they performed practical charitable functions, such as finding housing and employment for their indigent patients.

Zakrzewska's hospital was very clean and well organized. Each room contained a sink with a bar of soap so doctors and nurses could wash their hands. Freshly laundered and vividly white hospital gowns, sheets, and towels were stored for easy access. Even the nurses' laced boots were perfectly white. Zakrzewska required her practitioners to keep written records on all patients, an extraordinary request back then. At the time, no other hospital in Boston kept any patient records at all. Commenting on this fact,

Zakrzewska mocked the male doctors by saying that perhaps important patient details remained permanently inscribed in men's large brains.

The lying-in center at the hospital provided care for impoverished women and women experiencing complications that prevented them from safely giving birth at home. Zakrzewska cared for the patient population that she deemed most vulnerable, including prostitutes. While most hospitals required proof of marriage from pregnant women, Zakrzewska never turned away a woman in need. "Let he who is without sin throw the first stone," she told her staff.

In fact, the New England Hospital proved to be better at caring for women than their competitors, especially when it came to the most dreaded infection plaguing mothers and newborns: puerperal, or childbed, fever. This infection occurred within ten days after delivery, and it almost always resulted in sepsis and death for the mother. Because it killed at the cruelest moments, the disease felt supernaturally evil. Doctors believed that the dead woman's internal organs were engulfed in milk, so many blamed the woman, saying that the putrid uterine discharge was caused by "milk metastasis." Eventually, scientists discovered that the fluid was pus, not milk.

Puerperal fever was epidemic at lying-in hospitals. In the first half of the nineteenth century, about five women in a thousand died from childbirth at home. Death rates in maternity hospitals could be ten times that number.

Even with so many women dying from puerperal fever, physicians ignored the emerging science explaining its cause. After attending a lecture in Paris that demonstrated how doctors themselves were spreading puerperal fever, Oliver Wendell Holmes published a report in 1843, "The Contagiousness of Puerperal Fever," in which he begged physicians to wash their hands, which would stop the spread of infection. He spoke in public on the subject but was often shouted off the stage. In fact, he was ridiculed by many of his colleagues.

"Doctors are gentlemen," said the eminent Charles Meigs of the Jefferson Medical College in Philadelphia. And "gentlemen's hands are clean." Years later, Meigs's imprudent statement returned to haunt him when it was proven that obstetricians who went from dissecting dead bodies to delivering babies without washing their hands spread the fatal infection over and over again.

But the New England Hospital for Women and Children seemed to exist in a protected world when it came to puerperal fever. The facility was among the first in America to introduce the sanitary and sterilizing methods that Holmes recommended, although the theory that disease was caused by microscopic organisms called "germs" was still up for debate. In addition, all nurses and doctors working for Zakrzewska washed their hands in a solution of chloric acid before examining patients. Taking cleanliness and hygiene ever further, she isolated patients with septic wounds and fevers. Zakrzewska implemented sterile technique before it was officially invented.

Into this environment of profound care for women came antiabortion crusader Horatio Storer. In 1863, when he began working with Zakrzewska, the other hospitals in Boston had banned surgery on women's reproductive organs and any surgeries of the abdomen. Storer was hired as a general surgeon to perform mundane procedures such as bonesetting and suturing lacerations. Unlike New York, where J. Marion Sims was performing freewheeling gynecological operations in a crowded amphitheater, the close-knit and conservative physician community in Boston considered these demonstrations to be dangerous quackery. Between 1830 and 1858, six women were operated on for ovarian tumors at Massachusetts General Hospital, and all six died. Afterward, gynecological surgery was not permitted at Massachusetts General until the 1880s, when asepsis, the state of being free from disease-causing microorganisms, was fully established. Surgical asepsis included the use of disposable sterile syringes, needles, and surgical gloves and sterilizable surgical instruments.

Storer, known at Harvard for his rigid and contemptuous behavior toward other professors, was the perfect gentleman with Zakrzewska and the other lady physicians at the New England Hospital. A few months after Storer was hired, Zakrzewska appointed Anita E. Tyng, graduate of the Woman's Medical College of Pennsylvania, as assistant surgeon. Tyng trained with Storer, and he described her as having the demeanor of a surgeon, perfectly fitted to "the nervous strain and shocks of the practice of surgery." Her calm demeanor during surgeries impressed him. In fact, his faith in her abilities was so great, he decided to give her more responsibility. In a letter to the hospital's board of directors, he wrote, "During July and August, I shall be able to visit the Hospital only on Saturdays. During my absence, I wish Dr. Tyng, in accordance with her duties as assistant surgeon, to take my place."

Storer arranged the schedule so that he was the only doctor in the hospital on Saturdays. He told the other doctors that he would take charge and gave them all the day off. He even ran the dispensary. Of course, this goodwill put him in excellent standing with Drs. Zakrzewska, Sewall, and Tyng, at least until they discovered his real motivation.

In all likelihood, Storer's amiable demeanor toward the women doctors was a ruse that hid a tremendous ambition. Working on Saturdays without the prying eyes of the other doctors, Storer was able to schedule the dangerous and experimental surgeries he needed to perform to catch up to his competitor J. Marion Sims.

Women doctors enjoyed a network of support, but males in the medical profession existed in an ecosystem of vicious rivalry. The next best thing to inventing an operative procedure was getting a lucrative patent for surgical instruments and medical devices. Like Sims, surgeons and other physicians learned how to put on a show in order to make money. They read books titled *Dollars to Doctors, Large Fees and How to Get Them,* and *The Physician as Businessman, or How to Obtain the Best Financial Results in the Practice of Medicine.* Universities competed for students, and doctors fought over patients. The more famous a physician became, the more rivals he had to fend off. Yet, paradoxically, doctors were dependent on one another for judgments of success. Women's reproductive organs proved to be the perfect uncharted territory for developing new surgical procedures. In this brutal environment, male doctors came to view women physicians as competitors who threatened their economic survival.

Even though Storer was performing his operations on Saturdays, he was required, like all attendings at the New England Hospital, to report his outcomes. Dr. Lucy Sewall kept diligent records of the hospital's performance each day and wrote the year-end report to board members summarizing every detail. For 1865–1866, Sewall recorded three deaths from surgical procedures, all caused by Storer. These deaths had occurred under circumstances that Sewall described as "hazardous operations," most likely gynecological, including ovariotomies and hysterectomies, and prohibited in Boston. Dr. Mary Putnam, who was an intern at the New England Hospital while Storer was on staff, commented later that the "results of Storer's operations often failed to match the boldness of his plans."

In direct response to these deaths, on August 13, 1866, the board of directors of New England Hospital, which included Ednah Dow Cheney and

Samuel Sewall, voted to approve the following resolution to prevent further deaths:

> WHEREAS: The Confidence of the Public in the Management of the Hospital rests not only on the character of the Medical attendants, having its immediate charge, but also on the high reputation of the consulting physicians and surgeons, and Whereas, we cannot allow them to be responsible for cases over which they have not control—
>
> RESOLVED: That in all unusual or difficult cases in medicine, or where a capital operation in surgery is proposed, the attending and Resident Physicians and Surgeons shall hold mutual consultations, and if any one of them shall doubt as to the propriety of the proposed treatment or operation one or more of the consulting physicians or surgeons shall be invited to examine and decide upon the case.

For Storer, the hospital's requirement that he consult the other physicians before attempting a difficult surgery was the second serious blow that year. Several months earlier, a heated quarrel with senior faculty members had led to Storer's dismissal from his position as assistant in obstetrics at Harvard Medical School. Now, the humiliation he felt at having to clear his surgeries with the women in charge of the New England Hospital stoked his anger to full boil.

Three weeks after the resolution was approved, Storer submitted his six-page letter of resignation to the directors of the New England Hospital. A week later, he shocked everyone at the hospital by publishing his entire letter in the *Boston Medical and Surgical Journal*. It was a full-scale public attack on women doctors.

He began by calling the doctors and board members of the New England Hospital naive and childlike for attempting to oversee a surgeon of his own immense talent and reputation. After condescendingly explaining how a hospital should be run, he blamed the women doctors for his actions: "Having received my resignation, you may consider as gratuitous the remarks I am now to make, and may wish that they had been withheld. The connection that has existed between us has, however, been a public one. It has been severed by your own action, and the changed relation will become a matter of public comment. It is not improper, therefore, for me to say one word more."

Storer then bluntly revealed that he had been lying to them for years, and his tenure with the hospital had all been a deception. The entire time, he claimed, he had been performing an important experiment by "testing the ability of women to become fitted to practice as general physicians."

Overall, his conclusion was dire. "It is sufficient for me to say," he wrote, that because of their reproductive biology, "women can never, as a class, become so competent, safe and reliable medical practitioners as men, no matter what their zeal or opportunities for pupilage." A woman would always be secondary to any man because of her monthly period. He had observed that a woman's nature, far from being an asset, was an insurmountable liability.

He continued with his blaming and patronizing attitude in his final paragraph: "I make these statements deliberately, for they are of public interest. I make them with regret, for to some they will give pain. You yourselves have placed me where I could view the matter in a truer light than might otherwise have been possible."

Zakrzewska, the other physicians, and the board members of her hospital, while shocked and saddened by Storer's scandalous betrayal, refrained from commenting in hopes that the whole episode would quietly disappear. Tyng was appointed as hospital surgeon and took over Storer's cases. Storer had shown himself to be contemptuous and difficult at Harvard, so his criticism of Zakrzewska's hospital did not seem out of character. Eventually, the hospital returned to normal operations. Zakrzewska never hired another male physician.

Still, Storer's argument proved to be very persuasive, and its effects were far reaching. As a leading physician and one who had recently been elected vice president of the AMA, he had supposedly risked his entire reputation to conduct hazardous research in enemy territory. The one thing most physicians agreed on was that women did not belong in the medical profession.

～

According to the AMA president in 1871, "If, then, woman is unfitted by nature to become a physician, we should, when we oppose her pretensions, be acquitted of any malicious or even unkindly spirit." Even though the AMA admitted its first woman before the end of the nineteenth century, the organization did not open its doors to Black physicians for another one hundred years. In 1895, African American physicians formed the National

Medical Association to overcome the AMA's discriminatory policies and improve health outcomes for Black people in a segregated health-care system.

Taking to heart the AMA's opposition to women doctors, Storer never let the medical community forget about his "experiment." In every published article that he wrote afterward that dealt with the topic of female physicians, he footnoted his New England Hospital experience. He always mentioned it when he spoke at medical meetings. The same year that he declared women doctors unfit to serve, he published "The Origins of Insanity in Women." In the paper, Storer claimed that ovariotomies—removal of the ovaries—would cure women who "have become habitually thievish, profane, or obscene, despondent or self-indulgent, shrewish or fatuous."

Five years later, he published a book on the topic titled *The Causation, Course and Treatment of Reflex Insanity in Women.* Ironically, that same year, he institutionalized his wife, Emily Gilmore, for an unspecified mental illness not long after she gave birth to their third child. She died in 1872, and shortly afterward, Storer married her sister Caroline.

While Storer was sterilizing perfectly healthy women in order to demonstrate his surgical prowess, he was also leading the physicians' crusade against abortion. In 1863, he persuaded the AMA to hold a competition for the best essay written by a doctor on the subject of abortion. The prize committee was chaired by his father, David Humphrey Storer, who proceeded to award his son the first prize for his essay "Why Not?" In the essay, Storer argued that abortion was infanticide, that it was epidemic, and that doctors, lawyers, and clergymen must unite to eradicate it. In 1873, the Comstock laws made all forms of birth control illegal, and by 1880, nearly all states had outlawed abortion. None confronted the fact that when embryos and fetuses were protected as fully human, the lives of women became dehumanized and incidental.

Closed Energy System

BY THE END OF 1869, HORATIO STORER HAD OBTAINED A LAW DE-
gree from Harvard and founded the Gynecological Society of Boston. In Paris, Mary Putnam was studying for her final examinations at the
École de Médecine, and despite Storer's crusade against women physicians,
a growing number of young women in America were becoming doctors.

November 6, 1869, was a proud day for fifty-five-year-old Ann Preston,
dean of the Woman's Medical College of Pennsylvania. After petitioning
Philadelphia hospitals the previous thirteen years to allow her students
to attend clinical lectures, she had finally won her battle. In January, her
students had been welcomed to Philadelphia General Hospital's Blockley
Almshouse clinics, and today, Pennsylvania Hospital was opening its doors
to the women.

Preston lifted the hem of her skirt and climbed two flights of stairs to
reach the hospital's brand-new surgical amphitheater. Thirty-four of her
medical students followed. One coughed. Another sneezed. Because they
were women entering a man's domain, hospital managers required them
to take the little-used back staircase, and their long skirts kicked up dust
along the way.

The first thing Preston noticed after entering the amphitheater was the
bright sun pouring through eight double windows and a skylight. The architecture was state-of-the-art. Built like a circus stage to enhance surgical
demonstrations, the octagonal room had rows of tiered seating so that everyone could see. The acoustics were such that any spoken word could be
heard clearly throughout the enormous room. That's why the explosion of
noise that followed the women's entrance into the arena almost knocked
Preston off her feet.

Over two hundred male students from Jefferson Medical College and the University of Pennsylvania stood on the top rows of the tiered seats, most bellowing their disapproval. The men shouted obscenities about the women's looks and clothing. Piercing wolf whistles echoed off the well-built walls. Some read loudly from their medical notes. This spectacle was not some last-minute protest but a planned attack. Warned in secret the day before by disgruntled professors who did not want females violating their sacred space, the young men had passed around a note reading "Go tomorrow to the hospital to see the She Doctors." A record number had shown up, ready to rabble-rouse.

Preston asked her students to halt so that she could assess the situation. Standing there with her head bowed, she looked ethereal. Her petite size and milk-white skin set off by her black silk and velvet dress with its full skirt accentuated her fragility. But her feminine appearance disguised her indomitable spirit. Before the Civil War, her family home in West Grove, Pennsylvania, had been a sanctuary for runaway slaves. The Fugitive Slave Act allowed "slave-catchers" to apprehend runaways in free states like Pennsylvania. Once, when a raiding party approached, she disguised an escaped slave in a Quaker outfit that included thick skirts and a heavy veil, and they both slipped past the raiding party to safety. She was a formidable foe and quite capable of disarming rowdy male medical students.

After a moment, she motioned for her students to take their seats in the first row at the lowest level, below the male students. Seconds later, hospital manager William Biddle burst into the amphitheater. He was wearing a dark, wide-brimmed Quaker hat. His religion required him to keep his head covered at all times, but the boisterous students did not care. "Hat! Hat!" the male students yelled, gesturing for the manager to remove his head covering.

"Boys, we will not have this." Biddle called for quiet and motioned for them to sit down. Filled with anger, he told the unruly mob that the women were there with his blessing and should not be subjected to such insults. "Remember your character as gentlemen," he pleaded. Then he warned them that any student who was found to be insulting the women would have his lecture ticket canceled. At this, the young men hissed.

But Biddle's words had an impact, and the instigators finally lowered themselves into their seats and quieted down. To Preston's satisfaction, the medical demonstrations proceeded normally for the next hour. The first lecturer, Dr. Jacob Da Costa, introduced several patients who were victims of malaria, sunstroke, or dropsy and proceeded to review the diagnoses and cures for these illnesses. After Dr. Da Costa finished his lecture and exited the amphitheater, the surgeon Dr. Hunt swept in, trailed by his assistants bearing a patient on a stretcher.

"Gentlemen," Hunt said, dramatically bowing only to the male students sitting in the upper tiers. He was known for his contemptuous demeanor. Seeing that the esteemed surgeon was ignoring the women sitting in the first row, the young men shouted, clapped, and stomped their approval. Hunt's support of their protest had stirred them up again.

As the noise in the amphitheater grew louder, Dr. Preston touched the knee of the young woman sitting next to her; she then laid her hand on the next woman's knees, and so on. Preston was warning her students to remain calm at all costs. She did not want to give these men the pleasure of evoking an emotional reaction.

Hunt motioned for the men to quiet down, which they did. Then one of his assistants helped the patient out of the stretcher and into a chair. The man's eyes had been severely injured in a mining accident, and ugly scars marked the skin around them.

"What can you see today?" Dr. Hunt asked his patient. Then he pointed toward the lower section where the women were seated and said, "What do you see now?"

A long pause followed as the patient stared in the direction that Hunt pointed. "Patrick," the patient said, indicating the medical assistant standing nearby.

"Look up! Look higher, and tell me what you see," Hunt urged, his voice pitched high for dramatic effect. Male audience members held their breath, waiting for the shocked reaction from the nearly blind man when he saw the females.

The patient squinted. "Light! I see light!" he finally exclaimed.

Someone in the audience laughed. The women strained to keep from smiling. Later, a reporter for the *Philadelphia Evening Bulletin* wrote: "Was there a signification in that blind man's words? Was not *light* dawning upon bigotry and oppression when women were even *thus* allowed to avail themselves of an opportunity for acquiring knowledge that they would dispense for the alleviation of suffering humanity?"

Frustrated by the failure of his stunt, Hunt brought in the next patient; he was placed recumbent on a long and narrow examination table that revolved slowly. The man's broken femur had refused to heal, and he winced with pain when two assistants began pulling off his boots. Another assistant stood at the patient's head, ready to hold an ether-soaked towel to his face until he lost consciousness. This would be a surgical demonstration.

As the two assistants continued to methodically strip off the man's clothing, revealing more and more of his naked body, a low growl of dissent erupted from the male students. In response, Hunt covered the patient's private parts with a blanket, and then the assistants removed his pants.

With the patient lying almost naked on the revolving table, Hunt stepped up next to him and wielded a long measuring stick in dramatic fashion for the audience to see. He proceeded to assess the width of the patient's hips and torso, asking his assistants to write down the numbers. When he got to the patient's thigh measurement, the normally agile doctor made an awkward move with his elbow and briefly exposed the patient's groin. The men shouted with laughter, clapped, stomped, and jeered even louder than before.

Once again, Hunt motioned for them to be quiet, then proceeded with his demonstration. The male students said nothing else, but their abuse of the women continued. Throughout this last hour of the lecture, they rained down on the women wads of tinfoil, paper missiles, and spitballs. Drops of spitted tobacco splattered on skirts. In the silence, there was no peace. But the women did not flinch or retaliate. It appeared to the reporter present that the women stayed calm while the men could not control their emotions.

Seemingly oblivious to the chaos, Dr. Hunt continued with his presentation. Throughout his surgery and lecture, he never once acknowledged Preston and her students.

When the class ended, the turmoil of the clinical lecture spilled outside and onto the walkways near a very busy street. The men lined both sides of the path, forcing the women to run the "gauntlet of their stares" and intimidation.

Upon leaving the building and seeing the mob a few feet away, the women froze, afraid of being attacked. Noticing a different route from the building to the street, Preston called for them to exit in that direction. The men retaliated by singing "The Rogues March," raucously off-key, and following them across the yard. Some gathered up stones along the path and threw them at the women, who put up their arms to protect their faces. When they reached the street, the women separated and hopped into the horsecars traveling in all directions. The men divided into small groups and followed, uttering belching and fart sounds along with swear words and indecent comments.

The news of the episode spread quickly, and it came to be known as the "jeering incident." Newspapers and journals throughout Pennsylvania, Massachusetts, and New York printed articles calling the event disgraceful, blackguardism, and an assault on women. The women had behaved so admirably and the men so badly that those who had hesitated to call on female doctors now felt compelled to do so.

While the public approved of the women's entrance into the hospital clinics, the conservative male physicians did not. A petition against the attendance of women at mixed lectures circulated among physicians in Philadelphia. Its 283 supporters included Charles Meigs, Alfred Stillé (a future president of the American Medical Association), and S. Weir Mitchell, the famous Philadelphia neurologist who was studying the benefits of rest.

In response to the petition, Ann Preston and the faculty of the Women's Medical College said that they would gladly attend separate clinics with only women patients. But the controversy continued until the Pennsylvania Hospital's managers asked the annual meeting of hospital contributors for guidance. The contributors agreed, after discussion, that mixed lectures were unsuitable but urged the hospital to arrange for appropriate and thorough clinical instruction for the women. Separate clinical lectures were scheduled to begin in early 1871.

BOSTON, NOVEMBER 1869

Nine days after Preston and her students were harassed at Pennsylvania Hospital, Edward Hammond Clarke, Harvard professor and one of Boston's favorite medical doctors, wrote a prescription for bromide of potassium and ammonium and explained to his patient how it would ease his epileptic attacks. After expressing his sincere gratitude, the patient called for his servant to get the doctor his coat and have the driver bring the carriage around to take Clarke home. Clarke thanked the man for the offer but declined the ride, saying that a brisk walk would clear his head and improve his appetite.

Because of his reputation as a gentleman with a caring, respectful manner, Clarke treated some of the wealthiest epileptics in Boston. His friend and colleague Oliver Wendell Holmes once described Clarke as "having all the qualities that go to making of a master in the art of healing." Clarke had taken care of illustrious politicians, merchants, industrialists, and poets, including Vice President Wilson, Ralph Waldo Emerson, William Lloyd Garrison, and the entire family of Abbott Lawrence, founder of the textile industry in New England.

Clarke strolled down Berkeley Street, his back straight and the heels of his leather boots clicking rhythmically against the red-brick sidewalks. Many of his patients were from this affluent Back Bay area of Boston. Located near the Charles River on what was once an inland bay, the area had been modeled after Baron Haussmann's Parisian boulevards and it featured acres of connecting neighborhoods and parks. Elegant swan boats drifted along the river. Victorian brownstones four and five stories tall lined the streets like orderly giants. New homes were being constructed every day, and Clarke imagined himself inside one of these, surrounded by servants catering to his every need. More than anything, he wanted to live with the elite in this beautiful neighborhood.

Born February 2, 1820, Clarke was the youngest child of Reverend Pitt Clarke, a Harvard graduate and minister of the first Congregational Society in Norton, Massachusetts. Determined to be like his father, Clarke entered Harvard Divinity School at age seventeen. During his junior year, he became so ill from the stress of his studies that he developed pneumonia and his lungs hemorrhaged. Even though he was first in his class, his poor health forced him to drop out. To regain his strength, he sailed to England, performing common sailor's duties a few hours a day. When the ship reached Southampton, he went ashore and joined the crowd celebrating the coronation of young Queen Victoria.

Despite his sea journey, upon returning home, he remained in poor health for many months and could not attend graduation ceremonies at Harvard. Two years later, he enrolled in medical school at the University of Pennsylvania and studied otology; he graduated in 1846. Although his health had improved, he still felt weak. His physician restricted his studies to three hours per day. To hide his infirmity, he cultivated the demeanor of the perfect Victorian gentleman. During conversations, he showed a devoted and gentle interest in others and never talked about himself. He was always polite to women and had a reputation as a gentleman.

After medical school, he wanted to continue his education by attending the hospital clinics in Europe, but he could not afford passage. By chance, the distinguished businessman and philanthropist Abbott Lawrence approached him about accompanying his two sons, who were both in their twenties like Clarke, on a voyage to Europe. Clarke agreed. He spent the next year traveling and ended up in Berlin, where he hoped to be accepted for clinical training. At the time, Marie Zakrzewska was the head midwife at Berlin's Charité hospital, one of the finest training hospitals in Germany. While touring the Charité, Clarke met Zakrzewska, and they became friends. Impressed by Clarke, the young Zakrzewska used her connections to find him a place in the clinics. Years later, Clarke would repay her generosity by becoming a consultant at her hospital for women and children in Boston.

After returning from Europe, the young ear doctor married Sarah Loud but changed his practice from otology to primary care because he needed a better income. His practice thrived, and in 1855, he became a professor of materia medica at Harvard. Now his students, who admired him for his unassuming yet elegant manner, occupied much of his time. He cared about their futures as if they were the sons he'd never had. Helping them chart their courses through life made him feel like a Christian minister and forthright counselor of men.

Today, though, the closer he got to home, the more depressed he felt. The truth was, Clarke often dreaded seeing his wife, a feeling that caused a surge of guilt. The home was supposed to be the place where a man's emotional needs were satisfied, but since the death of their daughter, Mary, at age three a few years ago, his wife had started attending the popular séances held by spiritualist mediums in hopes of communicating with the beloved toddler.

On impulse, Clarke decided to catch a horsecar headed to the Union Club, one of several gentlemen's clubs in the Boston area. These popular gathering places provided the men with a masculine sanctuary away from their female-run homes. In the middle of the bustling city, clubs afforded private spaces for drinking, smoking, and gambling. The Union Club's many prominent members included Massachusetts governors Alexander Bullock and William Claflin, current and previous presidents of Harvard and MIT, U.S. senator Charles Sumner, Vice President Wilson, Dr. Henry Bowditch, Ralph Waldo Emerson, John Forbes, and Oliver Wendell Holmes.

At the club, Clarke found that his colleagues were not relaxing in the comfortable leather chairs smoking cigars and drinking wine and whiskey but were huddled together in a worried discussion that was growing louder by the minute. The turmoil was over the events that had occurred more than a week earlier at the Pennsylvania Hospital clinic. Clarke had read a small paragraph in the local newspaper about the rowdy young men who had disrupted the amphitheater and embarrassed some women doctors, but he had not given it much thought. He now read the longer articles about the jeering incident, dozens of articles and letters to the editor appearing in newspapers throughout Pennsylvania, New York, and New England. Overwhelmingly, public opinion was in favor of the women doctors. One letter printed in the *Philadelphia Press* read:

"I read with sorrow the disgraceful transaction on the part of the medical students of our city which occurred on Saturday last. . . . I think that the people of Philadelphia will agree with me in censuring the students of the Medical College for their indecent transactions some few days ago." It was signed D.L.S.

A special correspondent to the *New York World* reported, "Philadelphia, the dullest village in America, has undergone a revolution in medical science. The women have triumphed to-day in the most signal manner over the masculines who sought, as it has been understood, to prevent them from attending the clinical lectures at the Pennsylvania Medical Hospital."

Something must be done, the learned men at the Union Club insisted, outraged. Women doctors were ruining the profession.

Clarke disagreed. Even though he was adamantly against admitting women to Harvard and any sort of coeducation for men and women, his friendship with Zakrzewska kept him from arguing publicly against women physicians. In fact, in a speech he had given the previous spring to the graduating class of Harvard Medical School, he said that if they were capable, women had every right to pursue education as doctors. His only stipulation was that it take place separate from men. As he had stated in his speech, a bath was a necessary and purifying process for all, but "it is not wise for the two sexes to bathe at the same time and in the same tub."

And now, reading through the articles describing the appalling behavior of the medical students, he grew angry. The students' actions had betrayed the ideals of their noble profession and Clarke's personal devotion to chivalrous behavior.

But then he came across a letter to the editor of a New Jersey newspaper from a male medical student present at the jeering incident who wanted to set the record straight. He insisted that none of the women had been hissed at or insulted and went on to blame the women for the disturbance. "Who is this shameless herd of sexless beings who dishonor the garb of ladies? This beardless set of non-blushers who infest the rights of four hundred regular medical students who have sustained the clinics from their foundation!"

The words written by this young man must have affected Clarke deeply. He could easily have been one of Clarke's own pupils. Should not those administrators who had invited the women bear some responsibility? Moreover, as the young man pointed out in his letter, the women, simply by learning to be doctors, were themselves being disorderly. They should have known better. What if one day, God forbid, women demanded membership in the Union Club?

Clarke and his colleagues relished their orderly world of manly men and girlish women, and they had good reason to be fearful. The women had surprised them with their persistence over the years and were gaining ground. In 1869, the bright future in medicine that Ann Preston and Elizabeth Blackwell had predicted nearly twenty years earlier was finally arriving. Women were building health-care institutions and forming their own professional organizations. Education standards were improving. Medicine had become a viable part of the separate woman's sphere advocated by Victorian culture. Mary Putnam had been accepted into the École de Médecine, and Elizabeth Garrett had just graduated. In Boston, feminist reformers were petitioning Harvard Medical School to open its lectures to women. At the same time, Marie Zakrzewska was pressuring the Massachusetts Medical Society for membership. In fact, the post–Civil War years saw an astonishing growth of women's organizations of all kinds. Women had taken over the profession of nursing. This feminist challenge brought sweeping changes to education and work, together with legal, political, and social status improvements. Women continued to pour into the workforce. Even those who had to labor in the factories contributed to the perceived threat to the established social order.

For Clarke and his associates at Harvard, these social changes were a growing nightmare. Deep down, they dreaded women as adversaries while simultaneously pitying them for their smaller brains. Something had to be done.

Clarke decided that he would pen a response to the jeering incident for the *Boston Medical and Surgical Journal*. He would calmly state that he agreed with the popular support of the women and would devote all of his free time toward finding a solution to the woman problem in medicine. He owed it to the future of young men. His friendship with Zakrzewska gave him access to some women's organizations, including Julia Ward Howe's influential New England Women's Club. If he was seen as an ally, his opinion about women's place in modern society would seem more credible.

That night, at home in bed, he could not sleep. At four a.m., he arose and started his essay for the medical journal. It began with a warning.

"The recent occurrences in Philadelphia, by which a medical class in that city have acquired an unenviable notoriety, have brought the subject of the medical education of women more prominently before the community than before. Nothing advances any cause so much as the martyrdom or persecution of its disciples. In this way the Philadelphia medical class have given an unexpected impetus to the cause they opposed."

Clarke wrote that a priori a woman had "the same right to every function and opportunity which our planet has to offer, that man has." But, he warned, the real question was not one of right but of capability. If a woman was deemed capable, then no law, argument, or ridicule would prevent her success. Toward the end of his essay, he even stated that he hoped to live to see women get the vote, a declaration he knew would thrill the feminist camp and distract them from thinking too much about what he actually meant by a woman's "capability."

∽

Prior to Darwin's *On the Origin of Species*, published in 1859, the story of Adam and Eve served to keep women in their place. For centuries, the Western world's ideas about what it meant to be man and woman were based on this allegory. In 1833, two paintings by French artist Claude-Marie Dubufe, *Adam and Eve* and *Paradise Lost*, toured the United States under a single billing: *The Temptation and the Expulsion of Adam and Eve*.

The pictures drew greater crowds than any other exhibit in U.S. history. In New York City, over twenty-five thousand people paid to see them. One reviewer observed that Adam and Eve were fascinating because they exposed "the facility of a Temptation to which all the sons of earth fell victims through their beautiful mother."

Men invoked the Bible to assert dominance over their wives. Wives submitted because it was God's will. Then, in the middle of the nineteenth century, women stopped submitting and began moving into the public sphere, and the men in charge, especially physicians, grew fearful.

About the same time that Elizabeth Blackwell graduated from medical school and Harriot Hunt began lobbying to get into Harvard, the AMA started its crusade to control women's bodies by advocating for the outlawing of abortion and birth control. Horatio Storer, in charge of the campaign, used his position to advance the social philosophy of eugenics. He published essays stating that married women, especially those who were Protestant and white, had a moral obligation to reproduce.

"If these wretched women . . . are thus murdering their children by thousands through ignorance, they must be taught the truth," he wrote, "but if . . . they have been influenced to do so by fashion, extravagance of living, or lust, no language of condemnation can be too strong."

But with the advent of science and the writings of Darwin, women activists fought back, reinterpreting the creation story as a feminist allegory. They cheered Darwin for exposing the fraud of Eve and the "rib story."

At an 1869 women's rights convention, Isabella Beecher Hooker, sister of Harriet and Catherine Beecher, reasoned that the parable of Genesis was, in reality, a story about gender equality, and she presented "a number of scientific facts to prove that the highest types of vitality take the female form." Similarly, Illinois lawyer and suffrage advocate Catherine Waugh McCulloch related Genesis to Darwin's evolution. In a leaflet titled "The Bible on Women Voting," McCulloch argued that "the scientists of today quite agree with the Genesis parable concerning the creation, that creation was in the ascending scale, first the lower creatures, then the higher animals, then man, and last at the apex the more complex woman." According to McCulloch, evolution did not support female subordination but "might rather be a reason why men should obey women."

But as Edward Hammond Clarke discovered, medical men no longer needed the myth of Eve to keep women confined. Eager to find a solution to the "woman question," Clarke read the recent books by Charles Darwin, Herbert Spencer, and S. Weir Mitchell. Ideas formed.

Like many other physicians, Clarke subscribed to the belief that the human body was a closed system with a finite source of energy, what he referred to as "nervous force." All bodily functions relied on this metabolic energy. Bodies became battlefields where every organ fought the others for a share of limited energy reserves. Gleaned from the notion of strict determinism, this closed system was also called the "law of the conservation of energy." Herbert Spencer, the English philosopher, biologist, anthropologist, and eugenicist, based his entire philosophic system, later called social Darwinism, on this law.

Also known as the first law of thermodynamics, conservation of energy implied that the energy of a system was always constant, although it diminished over time because energy could not be created or destroyed. Under this law, the human body became an input-output system—food was eaten, energy (which included thought) emerged, and the energy was equal to the amount of food ingested. Thus, bigger was better, and since men had bigger bodies, they had more energy. According to Spencer, individual evolution continued in men "until the physiological cost of self-maintenance very nearly balances what nutrition supplies." At some point, men reached equilibrium, and the white male functioned at the highest level of evolution.

Maturing earlier than boys, adolescent girls skipped the body systems' crucial final evolution. According to Spencer, women's minds had "somewhat less of general power or massiveness." In particular, they lacked "those two faculties, intellectual and emotional, which are the latest products of human evolution—the power of abstract reasoning and that most abstract of emotions, the sentiment of justice."

Thus a grown woman never surpassed the emotional and intellectual development of a teenage boy. In the evolutionary advance of the race, women "lagged behind men much as 'primitive people' lagged behind Europeans." Over the past generations of natural selection, the female had fallen behind the male to such an extent, she was almost a different species. According to these laws of nature, a woman had nothing to offer except for her healthy—and numerous—children. Biology directed that men produced and women reproduced. Any variation would lead to race suicide.

Clarke used his belief in the conservation of energy to build a case against the coeducation of the sexes and, especially, higher education for women. First, he simplified the idea of the competition between organs for functional energy. To reinforce his main point, he claimed that something as common as improper digestion could end in death. "The system," he wrote, "never does two things well at the same time . . . The digestion of a dinner calls force to the stomach, and temporarily slows the brain. The experiment of trying to digest a hearty supper, and to sleep during the process, has sometimes cost the careless experimenter his life."

In this battle for resources within the human body, the struggle between the brain and the female sex organs was particularly dangerous. Somehow, the uterus and a woman's brain were magically linked. In order to grow the proper reproductive system, adolescent girls should use their brains only occasionally. Clarke wrote, "It is . . . obvious that a girl upon whom Nature, for a limited period and for a definite purpose, imposes so great a physiological task, will not have as much power left for the tasks of the school, as the boy of whom Nature requires less at the corresponding epoch."

To further his case, Clarke cited the studies of neurologist and popular physician S. Weir Mitchell from his book *Wear and Tear: Or, Hints for the Overworked.*

According to Mitchell, it was

> better not to educate girls at all between the ages of fourteen and eighteen unless it can be done with careful reference to their bodily health. To-day, the American woman is, to speak plainly, too often physically unfit for her duties as woman, and is perhaps of all civilized females the least qualified to undertake those weightier tasks which tax so heavily the nervous system of man. She is not fairly up to what nature asks from her as wife and mother. How will she sustain herself under the pressure of those yet more exacting duties which nowadays she is eager to share with the man? . . . Our growing girls are endowed with organizations so highly sensitive and impressionable that we expose them to needless dangers when we attempt to over tax them mentally.

Clarke agreed with Mitchell that American white women were a dying species.

> Clinical observation confirms . . . the sad results which modern social customs, modern education, and modern ways of labor, have entailed on

women. Examples of them may be found in every walk of life. . . . Number-
less pale, weak, neuralgic, dyspeptic, hysterical, menorrhagic [abnormally
heavy menstrual bleeding], dysmenorrhoeic [pelvic pain with menstrua-
tion] girls and women, that are living illustrations of the truth of this brief
monograph. . . . The number of these graduates who have been permanently
disabled to a greater or less degree by these causes is so great, as to excite
the gravest alarm, and to demand the serious attention of the community.
If these causes should continue for the next half-century, and increase in
the same ratio as they have for the last fifty years, it requires no prophet to
foretell that the wives who are to be mothers in our republic must be drawn
from trans-atlantic homes.

For confirmation of the debilitating effects of improperly orchestrated
menstruation, Clarke consulted the writings of London obstetrician Charles
West, author of many books, including *Lectures on the Diseases of Women*.
"'It is not enough to take precautions till menstruation has for the first time
occurred,'" Clarke quoted West. "'The period for its return should, even
in the healthiest girl, be watched for, and all previous precautions should
be once more repeated; and this should be done again and again, until at
length the habit of regular, healthy menstruation is established. If this be
not accomplished during the first few years of womanhood, it will, in all
probability, never be attained.'"

For emphasis, Clarke drew from the trauma of his own personal experiences. "There have been instances, and I have seen such, of females
in whom the special mechanism we are speaking of remained germinal—
undeveloped. It seemed to have been aborted. They graduated from school
or college excellent scholars, but with undeveloped ovaries. Later they
married, and were sterile."

Based upon these hypothetical, unscientific interactions with patients,
Clarke endorsed segregated education to accommodate the "periodicity"
of girls, who should study only a few hours per day and rest every fourth
week to accommodate their menstrual cycles. All of this would be overseen, of course, by their physicians.

Along with Mitchell, Clarke adamantly discouraged higher education
for women and cautioned that, if it continued unabated, females would
devolve into a third gender, called "agene," similar to "the sexless class of
termites." For evidence, Clarke told personal stories that linked female

malaise to female accomplishment, sometimes with deadly results. Finally, by relating it all to evolutionary progress, Clarke hoped to influence debates about the science of sex differences for years to come.

As he wrote, he felt like a holy man on a mission. His wife might have called her husband's work "automatic writing," when spirits—perhaps even God—manipulated the author's hand.

Clarke's words were not religious. They were inspired by Darwin. While researching *The Descent of Man*, Darwin had taken a great interest in women's nature. He believed that it was "in the struggle for existence and (especially) for the possession of women that men acquire their vigor and courage." Women's utter dependence on men, along with their desire to be attractive, had to be reinforced or men would not continue to evolve. This belief made Clarke's work more than a doctor's earnest effort to save women's health. It was vital to sustain the natural progression of men. He was writing to keep the white man at the top of the evolutionary mountain.

He gave his work in progress the provocative title of *Sex in Education*. Brief and easy to read, it was more of an extended essay than a book. No scientific work written for a lay audience by a physician had ever discussed women's bodily functions in as great detail.

With encouragement from his colleagues at Harvard, especially Holmes, zoology professor Jean Louis Agassiz, and university president Charles Eliot, Clarke contacted the popular New England Women's Club and got himself an invitation to speak. There, he would present his theory and, perhaps, gain the backing of Boston socialites like Howe. He imagined they would laud him as a savior of women.

Having previously published only a few papers about the ear and a more recent piece titled "The Physiological and Therapeutical Action of the Bromide of Potassium and Bromide of Ammonium," Clarke was not a well-known writer or public speaker. He wanted that to change. In the ensuing days, as he revised his essay on menstruation, Clarke imagined becoming rich enough to purchase the home of his dreams on Arlington Street across from the Public Garden in the prestigious Boston neighborhood of Back Bay.

The Science of Love

DEMONSTRATING FOR HER STUDENTS, PROFESSOR MARY PUTNAM etherized the frog and prepared it for vivisection. Then she made an incision with her surgical knife, removed the skin, and focused the lens of her microscope so that it captured the flowing movement of the amphibian's living bloodstream and organs. She gestured for her students to look through the microscope. One by one they approached, a few with complexions similar to that of the frog.

As a newly hired professor of materia medica at the Woman's Medical College of the New York Infirmary, Putnam was on a mission to use what she had learned at the École de Médecine to create "a scientific spirit . . . among women." Confident that science was the key to women's advancement in American society, she set high expectations for her students. It was a monumental task, especially since "until now, women have not held a normal position as complete human beings, their mental activity, though often considerable has been spontaneous, untrained, unsubjected to systematic educational drill."

When Putnam's students finished looking through the microscope, she helped the frog die peacefully by profound etherization. Then she asked her students to describe what they had seen. Most of their answers seemed generic—it looked like frog's blood or a river back home during a flood. One person might have mentioned the etheric body and God.

Putnam shook her head, mumbling that the women were too lazy, *trop paresseux,* in their assessment. She often vented her frustration by criticizing their work in French so that they would not understand. Nothing galled her more than the fact that young women in America neglected to learn more than one language.

Putnam believed that for young medical students, the view through the microscope should be one of the most remarkable experiences of their lives. It had been for her. Witnessing the real workings of physiology in live animals was both educational and inspirational. For Putnam, "the microscopic shred of tissue from the insignificant animal seemed for the moment to give a glimpse of a mighty vision of endless life, streaming infinite energy into the minutest particles of an infinitive universe. The impression was indescribably powerful." It gave her a sense of being part of something immense, a concrete and objectively proven galaxy of life that was much more comforting for her than any religion. She wanted her students to look at life as she did, like a scientist.

Putnam found herself, ironically, wishing that her students were more like men, who were taught how to study. Women's education seemed to be steeped in the intellectual constraints of religion, but the laboratory was a place of order, logic, and process that required sound reasoning and judgment. It preserved body fluids and pieces of severed bodies. Victorian ideals of femininity were hostile to the gory nature of anatomy and the dissection of live subjects. By doing vivisection in the classroom, Putnam was teaching her students that, as Dr. Marie Zakrzewska liked to say, science had no sex.

Putnam engaged in a broad spectrum of experimental practices that she hoped to include in her teaching. She used vivisection to study the impact of drugs on animals to gauge the corresponding impact on humans. For example, she tested the effects of silver nitrate on the nervous systems of dogs and rabbits, deceased and living. She performed autopsies on the animals, examined the tissue samples under a microscope, and recorded her results. In a lecture that was published in the *Medical Record*, she described investigations on the degree to which the drug atropine accelerated or decelerated the pulses of rabbits and the relationship between pulse rate and arterial tension, a topic of debate. She was developing a whole new curriculum for next semester around the topic of atropine—assuming that her managers, Elizabeth and Emily Blackwell, would not ask for her resignation by then.

After the Blackwells had established, years earlier, the New York Infirmary for Women and Children, they forged ahead with their plans for a medical school. The college finally opened in 1867 after years of fundraising. The beginning of the school, however, marked the end of the Blackwells' partnership. Eight months after delivering the opening address at the

Woman's Medical College, Elizabeth returned to England, her birthplace, permanently.

The Woman's Medical College, reflecting Elizabeth Blackwell's high standards, had a stellar reputation, enrolling almost forty students and graduating five to ten per year. For admission, students had to be at least twenty-one years old with high morals and a good general education. It was one of the first medical schools with a three-year curriculum that offered subjects progressively. In year one, the introductory courses included anatomy, physiology, materia medica, chemistry, and pharmacy along with dissection and other practical work in the anatomical rooms. The second year added instruction in surgery and obstetrics. In the third year, the students learned to evaluate cases and write up clinical reports. The college also required a course in hygiene (preventive medicine), the first offered anywhere in the country. In addition to lectures at the infirmary, students could attend clinical lectures at other New York health-care institutions, such as the Nursery and Child's Hospital, Mount Sinai Hospital, and the New York Eye and Ear Infirmary. Before any student could graduate, she had to pass an oral exam administered by the board of examiners, some of the most notable male doctors in the city.

Even though the college was excellent, Putnam was failing miserably as a professor. Her first few weeks teaching had been riddled with complaints from students about her impatience and contemptuous attitude toward them. Her students, who had looked forward to the arrival of the legendary Mary Putnam, now winced at her unremitting frown and the grim set of her jaw. She was formidable. Students complained that she gave them "malignant criticism," saying that they were unprepared to study medicine and ill-equipped to be doctors. In fact, thirteen of her students, more than a quarter of the entire student body, circulated a petition that they hoped would result in her termination or at least a reprimand. Putnam was distraught and blamed her failure partially on her disagreements with the dean of the school, Emily Blackwell.

During her voyage back to New York from Paris, Putnam had developed a course syllabus based on her studies at the École de Médecine. She wanted to make the study of materia medica (the chemistry of drugs) and therapeutic physiology (assessing patients' symptoms) two separate courses so that students would understand the chemistry involved before prescribing remedies. At most medical schools, the two subjects were taught together, but Putnam was certain that therapeutics required its own course. The treatment of diseases was too difficult for first-year medical students because they did not know any pathology—anything that Putnam told them about the remedial action of a drug would be completely unintelligible—and the second-year students would be bored with the chemical and pharmaceutical history of medicines. She wanted to teach the more knowledgeable advanced students a course on therapeutics. To Emily's dismay, Putnam pursued this change insistently. When consumed by a subject, "there was no limit to her interest in it. It overflowed her mind."

But Emily, who had been left in charge of the college and infirmary when Elizabeth moved back to England in 1869, would not permit Putnam to teach materia medica and therapeutics as two separate subjects, at least not right away. While Emily agreed that Putnam's solution was very innovative, she insisted that the change would be too difficult for the students. Adding another course to their already intensive curriculum might lead them to mutiny or, worse, it could discourage potential students from applying. As administrator, Emily understood the need to attract paying students. She suggested that the course changes be made over a few years and slowly introduced into the curriculum.

Putnam, of course, brushed that argument aside. She was under the impression that Emily wanted to train women to be the best doctors in America, so she ought to welcome these course changes. When Emily refused to yield, Putnam—the young woman who had used her intelligence, charm, and wit to win entry into the world's greatest medical school—felt stymied. Out of desperation, she sat down and wrote a letter to Elizabeth Blackwell begging for advice. After weeks passed and she had not heard back from Elizabeth, she felt abandoned and alone. At least she had her laboratory research and clinical work at the infirmary, now considered to be one of the best hospitals in New York.

⌒

When Mary Putnam returned to America in the fall of 1871, she resided with her family in New York City on East Fifteenth Street near Stuyvesant Park. During the years she spent in Paris, New York had evolved into a modern-day metropolis. In 1870, Long Island City was incorporated as part of Queens. Four years later, New York City annexed the West Bronx, west of the Bronx River. The suspension towers of the Brooklyn Bridge were beginning to rise, tall and gangly, against the horizon. Formed to bring art and education to the masses, the Metropolitan Museum of Art was set to open in early 1872. Mary's father, George Putnam, became the museum's honorary secretary.

The titans of business were busy reshaping America and transforming New York City. Cornelius Vanderbilt, the richest American in history, wanted his newest construction, Grand Central Depot, to be the largest interior space in the nation. The depot would form the nexus for the city's rail lines throughout Manhattan, Harlem, and all the way up to New Haven, Connecticut. John D. Rockefeller had recently incorporated Standard Oil, and Andrew Carnegie would soon begin expanding his steel business.

William "Boss" Tweed was ousted from Tammany Hall in 1871, and the plundering of New York that Tweed and his political cronies had carried out during the 1860s came to an abrupt halt. Immigration spurred the adoption of the Tenement House Act of 1867, which brought housing reform to New York. For the first time, the city established construction regulations, including requiring at least one toilet (or privy) per twenty people. Tens of thousands of tenements would be built in New York City by 1900. They would house a full two-thirds of the city's total population of around 3.4 million. This unprecedented time of far-reaching growth, wealth accumulation, industrialization, and the accompanying corruption was satirized by Mark Twain and Charles Dudley Warner in their 1873 novel *The Gilded Age: A Tale of Today*.

While Mary Putnam felt discouraged and alone at the Woman's Medical College, she experienced the exact opposite living in New York with her large family all under one roof. Her parents' expansive, four-story brick home was brimming with busy young people, from thirty-year-old Mary down to her eleven-year-old brother, Herbert. When she gathered them around to tell her thrilling stories about Paris, their faces glowed with pleasure. Her brother Haven, now part of G. P. Putnam, also lived at the family home with his wife, Rebecca, a schoolteacher. They were looking forward to purchasing a home of their own, but it would have to wait until the family business, experiencing slow book sales since the Civil War, was securely back on its feet.

Her mother, Victorine, kept saying how relieved she was to have her daughter back home and away from those radical Parisians like the Recluses. In fact, Mary kept in close contact with the Reclus family. Tragically, in April

1871 Élisée Reclus had been condemned to the penal colony of New Cale-
donia in the South Pacific for his work with the Paris Commune. His many
supporters from England and America, including Charles Darwin and
Mary herself, attempted to intervene to get his sentence reduced, and Mary
had just received the joyous news that Élisée's sentence had been com-
muted to banishment from France. He would be able to join his brother
Élie, who had also been exiled, and the rest of his family in Switzerland.

Victorine realized that during the years Mary was away, she had grown
even more dedicated to her work. She wished that her eldest daughter
would at least look for a suitable man for marriage. But Mary did not even
try to make herself attractive. Her dresses were all black, and she rarely
shopped for new ones. She refused to wear makeup or even brighten her
cheeks with a touch of the essence of cinnamon. Victorine was thankful for
her daughter's highly active lifestyle because it kept her from becoming too
stout. Mary had explained to her parents that she could never consider becoming attached to a man who was not cleverer than she was, so Victorine
knew she might have to resign herself to having an unmarried daughter.

In the five years since Mary had left for France, Victorine's desire for
her daughter's happiness—which she believed included marriage, children,
and maintaining a certain kind of attractiveness—had not changed. Her
father's attitude, however, had changed almost completely. Putnam's company was building its own book-printing and manufacturing office that
would later be called Knickerbocker Press. Now the man who had once
offered to pay his daughter two hundred fifty dollars *not* to attend pharmacy school had enthusiastically renovated the basement in his home and
offered the space to his daughter for her private practice. He even ceremo-
niously hung a plaque in the window that read DR. MARY PUTNAM. He was
immensely proud of the achievements of his gifted daughter.

Mary was pleased with her office and thankful to her father for his enthusiastic support. If she lost her teaching position, she would have the
income from her medical practice to fall back on. Most of her patients
came from her neighborhood for routine checkups, treatment for minor
ailments and injuries, and some obstetrical and gynecological care. Establishing a new practice was a slow process, especially for a woman. But Mary
counted on her Paris diploma and her seemingly unlimited supply of energy to speed things up.

One of Mary's professional goals was to be the first woman admitted to the New York Academy of Medicine. But even for her, the task would be challenging. The highly conservative institution refused to even acknowledge the existence of qualified women doctors. But in November, she received notice that she had been accepted into other prestigious medical associations: the New York County Medical Society, the New York Pathological Society, and the Therapeutical Society of New York.

She had heard a rumor that Dr. Abraham Jacobi, a very influential pediatric physician as well as the president of the New York County Medical Society, had placed her name in the nominations and then shepherded it through to acceptance. As far as Mary knew, Dr. Jacobi had never overtly supported the cause of women in medicine. Yet Dr. Emily Blackwell had been accepted into the society five months earlier. Perhaps Dr. Jacobi was as fair-minded as this behavior indicated.

Dr. Jacobi's reputation was certainly stellar. In 1860, the New York Medical College had created a new position just for him: professor of infantile pathology and therapeutics. Previously, this subject had been viewed in more general terms: the study of obstetrics and the diseases of women and children. The College of Physicians and Surgeons had then made Dr. Jacobi clinical professor of the diseases of infancy and childhood. From 1868 to 1871, he was joint editor of the *American Journal of Obstetrics and Diseases of Women and Children*. He would later be acknowledged by the AMA as the founder of pediatric medicine.

Born in Prussia in 1830, Abraham was the son of a cattle trader and a shopkeeper. Of Jewish descent, his family was secular and had, like other Jews, assimilated into German society in the early nineteenth century. As a young man, he experienced the vibrant rise of radical politics and the pursuit of unity, justice, and freedom in the Vormärz, a period of political and intellectual unrest beginning in 1840 and culminating in the March revolution of 1848 against autocratic rule in the German Confederation. In March 1848, Abraham started college, where he became part of the underground struggle to overthrow the German aristocracy. He joined the radical pro-democracy and socialist activists and organized students on their behalf. After being prevented from participating in the Baden uprisings of 1849 by the arrival of imperial troops, he moved on to the university in Bonn, where he began his clinical studies. There, he joined the subversive Communist League of Karl Marx and Friedrich Engels and continued to organize students and distribute radical materials until he received his medical degree in 1851. At every turn, he risked capture and imprisonment.

Abraham's escape from political persecution did not last long. In April of 1851, he planned to take his state medical exam in Berlin. While there, he was supposed to meet with a friend and fellow political activist. His friend never arrived. Instead, the police arrested him for distributing revolutionary literature, aiding fellow radicals, and plotting to overthrow the monarchy. He ultimately spent almost two years in prison.

After his release, he fled to England, where he joined other exiles, including Marx and Engels. To make a living, the twenty-three-year-old searched in vain for ways to establish a practice in Manchester. With reluctant financial support from Engels, who called Abraham a "helpless sort of creature," he immigrated to New York along with his childhood sweetheart and fellow activist Fanny Meyer, who was pregnant. They settled in the German district on the Lower East Side of Manhattan known as Kleindeutschland, or "Little Germany." Despite Engels's feelings about Abraham, he and Marx kept in touch with the young German doctor, and in 1857, Jacobi helped form the New York Communist Club. He also began his medical work at the German Dispensary, where he confronted the anguish and suffering of poor immigrant children. At the same time, Abraham faced the greatest loss of his life. Fanny gave birth to a son, who lived for only a few hours, then died of meningitis. The next day, Fanny suffered a blood clot that instantly killed her. Abraham was devastated.

Months later, he married nineteen-year-old Kate Rosalie, the daughter of Irish immigrants. While building his practice, he hoped for a family. Kate gave birth to two babies nine months apart in 1863; both were stillborn. Her next baby lived one day. Almost a year later, she gave birth again, but the tiny newborn was premature and died. She got pregnant for a fifth time but miscarried at seven weeks, and the exhausted and sickly Kate passed away in 1871. Abraham was shattered by the fact that he could not save his wife or his children.

Despite his many losses, he had transformed himself from a struggling immigrant physician to a leading figure in New York. His bereavement moved him to specialize in pediatrics and fight against the staggering rate of child mortality: one out of every four children died before reaching the age of five. He still yearned for a family, but this time, he would find a wife strong enough to survive.

The evening of December 4, 1871, before the start of the meeting of the New York County Medical Society, Mary Putnam scanned the room for Dr. Jacobi. She had the usual trouble seeing over tall men. But when she finally caught a glimpse of the important doctor, she laughed because he was also small. She might not have noticed him if it hadn't been for his impressive head of thick, wavy hair and full, dark, furry beard. His regal air made him look like an elfin monarch. Of course, compared to her, he was a giant.

Mary Putnam was one of twelve new members who would be officially welcomed into the society by President Jacobi. He headed for the podium, walking with fast, elastic steps. Along the way, he greeted colleagues with a series of rapid little nods. He seemed much younger than his age of forty-one.

Speaking with distinctly German r's, Dr. Jacobi paid a gracious tribute to the memory of members who had died that year. Then he greeted the new ones. "It is not a small satisfaction to me," he said, "that in the year of my presidency, one of the most urgent questions of the day should have been quietly answered. The admission of females into the ranks of the medical profession—or, rather, into existing medical societies—had been decided by you by a simple vote." He glanced around the room until he found Putnam. His mouth lifted in a delicate smile when their eyes met. Putnam dipped her chin and looked pleased. "Paris has turned out a woman doctor who will, I hope, prove [beneficial to] . . . this Society, the profession of this city, and our common country."

Putnam was even more pleased when Dr. Jacobi went on to discuss the problem of women in medicine as an educational one, arguing that standards should be raised until there could be no question of their qualifications. Then he tied the acceptance of women doctors to politics by saying that women's lack of equality was an integral part of the challenge to achieving genuine democracy.

"Let it not be forgotten in the history of this Medical Society of the County of New York," he stated in his conclusion, "that we have opened our doors to worthy members of the medical profession, male or female, white or colored, and thus granted reality to the gospel of American citizenship, the Declaration of Independence, according to which we are all created free and equal." Everyone, including Putnam, applauded loudly.

While Putnam was not impressed by any man's good looks, wealth, or status, she did have standards. On occasion, she would repeat this verse, adapted from Tennyson's poem "The Princess," to her family and friends:

The crane, I said, may chatter with the crane,
The dove mate with the dove; but I,
An eagle, clang an eagle in my sphere.

That evening, Putnam identified Dr. Jacobi as her eagle. Would he see her the same way? That same month, at the meeting of the New York Pathological Society, of which Dr. Jacobi was also a member, Putnam demonstrated her current research on an anomalous malformation of the heart. After a meticulous description, she requested comments and questions. Dr. Jacobi jumped to his feet and, with a serious tone in his voice but a twinkle in his eye, asked what, in Dr. Putnam's opinion, was the reason the anomaly had occurred? Mirroring his earnest tone, she gave meticulous and lengthy academic answers. Dr. Jacobi seemed satisfied by her explanations. After the meeting ended, Putnam's own heart thumped rapidly in her chest when he asked if they could continue their conversation while he escorted her home. He also assured the independent Putnam that he knew very well that she was capable of going home unescorted. Of course she said yes.

This back-and-forth flirting continued as the two doctors proceeded to carry out a shockingly public courtship. When Victorine discovered Dr. Jacobi was Jewish, she gulped back her doubts, because at least her daughter was interested in a man. The Putnams were becoming accustomed to Mary's unique attraction to gifted and industrious foreign men. Dr. Jacobi was wealthy and established in his profession; still, Mary's parents feared that life would be more difficult for their daughter with a Jewish husband.

Though New York City had a significant Jewish population, anti-Semitic sentiments were on the rise. Certain private schools, especially those for girls, had begun establishing quotas for or outright rejecting applications from Jewish children. Soon, universities, social clubs, hotels, law offices, hospitals, and other organizations also imposed quotas or banned Jews. Abraham Jacobi did not consider himself to be part of New York's Jewish culture. If asked about his racial background, Dr. Jacobi would admit to being descended from the Jewish race, but he would add that he was not a Jew because he did not attend a synagogue. Like Mary

Putnam, he did not practice any religion. They were interested only in science and each other.

At each meeting of a medical society, Dr. Putnam and Dr. Jacobi would demonstrate and discuss—in detail—their latest scientific experiments. Putnam would sometimes bring her patients along for visual demonstrations. Once, she included a highly detailed report on neurological experimentation and vivisection of a rabbit, which caused a stir, since vivisection, with its carnage, was supposed to be the domain of male scientists only.

The two companions continued to examine pathological specimens, some of which had been removed from patients or cadavers at their individual clinics. When they did not meet professionally in the city, they wrote to each other daily in Jacobi's native German. When Mary told her mother, "My 'Herr Doctor' writes to me every day in German and I reply in the same *Deutsche Sprache*," Victorine shook her head sadly, wondering what other strange kinds of romantic exchanges her daughter might engage in with Herr Doctor. Mary never called him Abraham; she referred to him always as Doctor.

What Victorine did not realize was that Mary had found a soulmate, someone who shared her passion for radical change. As she had fought in the battle for the new republic of France, he had risked his own freedom in Germany's efforts to produce a democracy. Both of them had suffered the disappointment at their defeat, and he had paid a heavy price by going to prison. Now, by fighting together for science and social emancipation, they hoped to engender a greater sense of liberty and freedom in America. Despite Victorine's misgivings, Mary and Abraham were an excellent match.

While Mary Putnam was experiencing the best of times in her personal and home life, her professional life was still miserable. Every day, her medical students disappointed her. After teaching her class, she would be filled with remorse at her own arrogant behavior and surprise at her utter lack of empathy. This inability to find common ground with her students was made even worse by Putnam's frustration with Elizabeth Blackwell. Her mentor still had not responded to the letter Putnam had sent weeks ago. Putnam was at an impasse with Dr. Emily and had nowhere else to turn.

Finally, in January, Elizabeth's reply arrived. Its contents changed her life. By the time she had finished reading, she was in tears.

December 31, 1871

My Dear Mary,

I have just received your letter and am so very sorry for the trouble it indicates. Dr. Emily has not sent me a line since you joined the college, so that I know nothing about the class difficulties. Miss Gould who wrote me some time ago spoke encouragingly of the prospects of the College and thought "Miss Putnam was getting on nicely with the class," so you see I was hardly prepared for the letter which you must have been so unwilling to write and which, indeed, must have been forced out by very severe experience.

But now, my dear Mary, I want you to live down this trouble, and "malignant criticism." You must succeed as teacher and practitioner in New York. I shall care comparatively little for your temporary trials, and the anxiety it gives Dr. Emily can be borne, if only you will be true to yourself and ultimately succeed; but to do this you must be infinitely patient.

There is one sentence in your letter that alarmed me for you, it is where you say, you "now feel thorough contempt for your class." Try and not do this, or you will never get right with them.

It is very difficult, knowing nothing of the details, to write exactly to the point, so I shall say little, but it strikes me that you are making the same mistake that Goldwin Smith did when he settled in America. That clever and learned man, going direct from Oxford, to a raw, manual labor school in Western New York, leaving the most cultivated of cultivated circles for the most imperfectly trained society, saw clearly and only his own superiority in these points where he really was superior, and he began to teach from the height of his superiority, with a certain dogmatism and utter ignorance of the people he proposed to teach, that set him at once in antagonism to the nation!

Now you have lived so long away from America and have become so much of a French woman, that you really must go to school and relearn your own country, before you will be able to teach acceptably; because it is utterly impossible to attempt to teach unless you are thoroughly in accord with your pupils.

It does seem to me, though I speak with diffidence, that it would be a better exercise for yourself (in the study you must make of your present country men and women) to give the short condensed and routine course of materia medica, which all are accustomed to, and see how you can gradually vivify that course, than to proceed at first to enter upon an entirely new road. I am very anxious about the matter. Do, my dear Mary, be very prudent and patient! You are young enough to wait for brilliant success, but you must not fail now.

You kindly ask after me. I am not very strong, but I am happy in my surroundings, and my work. I have finer opportunities for congenial work than ever I enjoyed in my life before. If I could only command the physical vigor of twenty years ago, it seems to me I might be of some use in England, but I distinctly feel the process of growing old, and watch it with curious interest. I am invited to give some rather important Sanitary lectures this spring, which I should like to do, if I feel up to it.

Miss Nightingale has just brought out a little book on lying-in hospitals, which I think an important "study" for the future benefit of those male opprobria. I have, at her request, sent her notes of my ancient experience at "La Maternité" that I hope may be of use. She seems much interested in the training of midwives. I have no interest in such attempt except for a class of nurses. Midwives might be useful in natural labour, but directly you go further you cannot, in justice to women or society stop short of the physician, *accoucheur*. This I have told Miss Nightingale very decidedly, but do not know whether she will accept my statement.

Now, dear child, with sincere hope for your success in the life battle in which you are engaged, of which the class trouble is a little incident,
Believe me, very truly yours,
Elizabeth Blackwell

You must not fail now. Putnam reread the letter many times until she had memorized it. She took Elizabeth's advice to heart, and by the start of the next semester at the Woman's Medical College, she had stopped expecting her students to fail. Instead, she moved forward with her own curriculum despite Elizabeth's plea for patience. By her second year, she ended the "illogical" system of teaching materia medica to students who had no knowledge of pathology or physiology and began working on her course on therapeutics. Putnam was building the reputation she would need, because soon she would risk it all, including her romance with Dr. Jacobi, by defending the future of women.

Battle Lines Are Drawn

O N MONDAY, DECEMBER 16, WHILE MARY PUTNAM WAS WAITING for Elizabeth's letter, the esteemed New England Women's Club in Boston, organized to promote suffrage and other advancements, was holding its weekly education committee meeting. The conference room in its headquarters at 3 Tremont Place hummed with activity. A maid straightened the comfortable chairs arranged in rows for seating; another hastily trimmed dead leaves from the green hanging plants that decorated the parlor. Coffee and tea with milk and sugar in elegant yet practical porcelain teacups were served to arriving guests, who felt properly swept up in the energetic homeyness.

Today, Dr. Edward H. Clarke, a member of Harvard's board of overseers, was scheduled to discuss the important topic of coeducation and higher education for women. Suffragists considered Clarke a powerful ally. In an article published in the *Boston Medical and Surgical Journal* in 1869, he had defended women entering the medical profession. In addition, he was close friends with Zakrzewska, who often spoke about women's health to club members.

Established in 1868, the New England Women's Club held weekly meetings on topics that included history, literature, music, art, and current affairs, such as suffrage and poverty. Men could join as associate members, and Unitarian clergyman and philosopher William Henry Channing, Christian theologian and author James Freeman Clarke, and the essayist, poet, and abolitionist Ralph Waldo Emerson all belonged to the club.

Its founders—Julia Ward Howe, philanthropist Ednah Dow Cheney, suffrage activist Caroline Severance, and Boston's first woman doctor, Harriot Hunt—had declared the club to be a social movement. Among their early projects were the Friendly Evening Association for working women, a horticultural school they supplied with books, microscopes, and specimens, and, in an effort to eliminate the fashionable-but-bone-crushing corset, support for women's dress reform.

The education committee was campaigning to elect the first woman to the Boston county board of education. Even though more women than men were teachers, this was the first time a woman had run for election to a public-school board in the United States.

Club president Howe greeted members and other influential citizens, among them her friend Dr. Oliver Wendell Holmes and his colleagues Professor Jean Louis Agassiz and Harvard president Charles Eliot. Howe raised her eyebrows as they took their seats in the front row. Apparently, the eminent Dr. Clarke had invited his own cheering section.

The legendary suffragist and reformer Lucy Stone and her husband, Henry Blackwell, in their regular seats near the back recorded the names of attendees and got ready to take meeting notes.

Several years earlier, in 1869, Stone, Howe, and Blackwell decided to break away from Susan B. Anthony and Elizabeth Cady Stanton's National Woman Suffrage Association (NWSA) to found the American Woman Suffrage Association (AWSA). Its publication, the *Woman's Journal*, an eight-page weekly newspaper, was fast becoming the national voice of the feminist movement. Unlike the NWSA, the AWSA supported the recently passed Fifteenth Amendment, which gave all men the right to vote, regardless of race or previous enslavement. The amendment did not extend suffrage to women, which made Stanton and Anthony furious. They gave rousing speeches expressing their great disappointment that people whom they saw as inferior had the right to vote and they did not. Taking a more democratic approach, Stone, Howe, and Blackwell viewed Black men's suffrage as an equal priority that would eventually lead to women's suffrage.

Stone was the first Massachusetts woman to earn a bachelor's degree— she graduated with honors from Oberlin College in 1847—and Henry Blackwell's sister Elizabeth was the first woman medical doctor in America. Stone and Blackwell had gained notoriety after their marriage in 1855 when Lucy publicly declared she was keeping her maiden name—with her husband's wholehearted approval.

Howe quieted the room. She was now fifty-three, and her once stunning red hair had turned a delicate strawberry blond. Her sharp intellect, warm heart, and passion for justice gave her a confidence that could be intimidating coming from the famous heiress and lyricist of the "Battle Hymn of the Republic." But her temper rose only when she was defending the human rights of women.

She announced that it was her privilege to introduce the favorite medical doctor of Boston's leading families, Edward Clarke. The women applauded. Women activists depended on the support of influential men who agreed with their causes, and the continued education of girls and women was paramount to them. Public high schools had opened for girls in Boston and New York in 1826, and as more girls received a high-school education, more wanted to attend college. Out of a total of 582 colleges in the United States, twelve were for women only and only twenty-nine were coeducational, but that number was growing. There were hints that Boston College would soon open its doors to women.

Dressed in a dark three-piece suit with a perfectly knotted bow tie and a tailored white silk shirt, the sharp-featured Clarke looked very distinguished. His flinty, Shenandoah-style beard ran the length of his fine-boned jaw, and his thick, dark hair made him look properly stern. As he gazed out at his audience, his face grew solemn.

He informed the ladies present that his lecture would be about more than coeducation. He would address an urgent topic: how the higher education of women influenced their physical conditions. He warned that he would use a stark vocabulary when describing women's biology, and he might reveal information too shocking for some of the gentle ladies in attendance. Yet be assured, he said, that his words were based on the brilliant science of renowned naturalist and biologist Charles Darwin.

The women nodded; they had all read Darwin, of course.

Clarke continued.

There must be discrimination in methods of education between young men and young women, he explained, to attain the highest result; indeed, to attain a healthy development of mind and body for either sex. Once again, Clarke cheerfully conceded that women could pursue every profession that men pursued and could even attain equal eminence among their peers.

"Whatever a woman can do, she has a right to do. The question arises, however: What can she do?" He paused, noting the women's puzzled looks. Then, raising his chin, he continued in his chirpy professor's voice.

It was his unfortunate duty to reveal the truth about the biological devastation being wrought by women's accomplishments. The health of American females today was disastrous, he said. A national tragedy. And it could all be blamed on the current method of educating girls with boys.

"Our present system of instruction for girls is radically wrong," he argued. All coeducation must be fundamentally changed or stopped altogether. Girls were being subjected to a rigid daily routine that was more suited to boys. Because the educators in charge were not considering the menstrual "periodicity" of female students, girls were experiencing a frightful deterioration.

Women's diseases, such as amenorrhea, ovaritis, and hysteria, "are indirectly affected by food, clothing and exercise; they are *directly* and largely affected by the causes that will presently be pointed out and which arise from a neglect of the peculiarities of a woman's organization," Clarke said. These numerous female conditions were not fatal, but they were incurable. And it all started at puberty.

Blank stares turned to quizzical looks on the faces in Clarke's audience.

In his assured bedside manner, Clarke explained that the growth of a girl's "peculiar" menstrual apparatus occurred during the years of her educational life. Think of it, he said. Within her body something extraordinary was taking place: the creation of a delicate "house within a house, an engine within an engine," that had to be well tended or the intricacy would collapse from misuse. In other words, she had only one chance to become fully feminine. This terrible negligence was not only sapping the life and happiness of individuals but also endangering the future of the white race in America.

There was only one solution: less brainwork.

A few women in the audience gasped. One, possibly Lucy Stone, snickered.

The activist women, all educated and healthy and many raising children, could not believe that they were listening to a *male* doctor in public state that women's periods must be appreciated. Howe was deeply offended, but because of the reputation of Clarke and the other men present, she and her fellow club members remained silent.

Oblivious to his audience's mounting frustration, Clarke kept going.

Scientific evidence had proved that if girls studied more than four hours a day, their exhausted bodies could not produce enough energy to grow proper reproductive organs. He gave a basic explanation of a closed energy system where physical, mental, and reproductive expenditures were in competition and could be easily unbalanced, causing illness. Due to her special biology, which included monthly breakdown and bleeding, if a girl put as much power into her brain development as a boy, her intellect—a masculine function—would grow at the expense of her ovaries, he said, which, like the untended rose, would wither and shrink.

He warned that if she kept it up, the female scholar would eventually completely unsex herself, making her incapable of giving birth. As Blackwell wrote, according to Clarke, "The course of education which would make a manly man would kill a woman, and the course of education which would make a womanly woman would emasculate a man."

Clarke explained Darwin's theory of evolutionary biology and emphasized that, according to Darwin, middle- and upper-class Caucasian girls with access to education who studied literature, science, mathematics, and history in the same way as boys did would eventually suffer from incapacitating illnesses that could prevent pregnancy—leading to a complete annihilation of the Anglo-Saxon race. The declining birth rates among white women led academics and politicians to fear being replaced by the invading Mexican, South Asian, Chinese, Jewish, and Irish immigrants. Their beliefs coalesced to form the popular idea of "race suicide"—nonwhite immigrants and lower-class populations becoming the majority.

Finally noticing the stunned disbelief on his audience's faces, Clarke decided to give examples of what would happen if females studied too hard and ignored their periods.

1. Insanity: One of his patients had graduated with honors from the normal school for teachers after several years of studying. Because she worked so hard, she lost all vitality and grew constantly ill. She never attended parties and other social events that all girls lived for. Her illness grew into severe depression, but she was still allowed to marry. Soon after, she had become violently insane and was likely to remain that way for the rest of her life.

2. Sterility: A female bookkeeper who, like the other male clerks, stood at her post all day long making calculations had become ill. Because the female pelvis was wider than that of the male, her body weight while standing pressed on her upper thighs and caused greater fatigue. Moreover, she did not rest but continued to stand during her menstrual period. This woman

believed in doing her work like a man, and she was well rewarded. At about twenty years of age, she asked Clarke for advice about healing her neuralgia, backaches, menorrhagia, leucorrhea, and general weakness. She looked pale, care-worn, and anxious. She tried iron, sitz baths, and other treatments; of course they did not work. To this day, she remained unmarried and sterile, according to Clarke.

3. Death: A young girl worked her way through New England primary, grammar, and high schools, attended college, and graduated first in her class. She worked on her studies continuously from the start of her menstruation without any sort of menstrual considerations. Soon after graduation, she began to weaken, and some years later, she died. A postmortem revealed severe disease, all attributed by Clarke to her unrelenting education.

The club members began to fidget. Several members signaled for Howe to interrupt. It was time to put a stop to this.

Howe rose and suggested that the members present would like some time to discuss Clarke's ideas. The professor, with a patronizing smile, said that of course he would take any questions.

Before any other club member could speak, Oliver Wendell Holmes expressed his hearty concurrence with Clarke's assumptions. President Eliot exclaimed that Clarke had exposed a great evil permeating society. Professor Agassiz said that he would go even further than Clarke and eliminate public education altogether. Holmes nodded and wondered if that should be the ultimate goal.

Discussing Clarke's thesis had gotten the Harvard scholars very excited. In their published research, these three towering academics were at the forefront of the eugenics movement, a thinly veiled pretext for enacting racist, inhumane policies to diminish the so-called unfit in America and Europe. These men considered white women and their wombs critical to their vision of racial supremacy.

When Lucy Stone stood up, the three professors stopped talking.

In her own experience at Oberlin, she said, the lady students not only complied with the normal routine but performed manual labor too—cooking, cleaning, and doing laundry. Yet the health of the young women equaled that of the young men. In fact, when the young men were ill, they too received a special leave of absence.

Lucy's husband, Henry, quoted an old Spanish proverb: "To a man who is well shod, the world is clad in leather." Meaning, he said, that although Dr. Clarke's expert testimony had special weight and value, it might possibly be colored by his constant professional relations with sick women.

Instead of responding to that, Clarke and his colleagues apologized and said that they wished they could stay longer but they had another appointment. Then they hurried out the door. Once they left, the room grew brighter. As Blackwell wrote in his article about Clarke's lecture for the *Woman's Journal*, after the four Harvard men exited, a much more reasonable discussion ensued.

Dr. Mary Safford said loudly that the deterioration of girls' health was attributable more to their unsuitable dress than to any routine of study. Mrs. Abba Woolson agreed and also thought that much of the ill health of girls was due to an attempt to unite the life of a coquette with that of a student. Bad air, improper food, and lack of physical exercise combined with nightly parties had a more injurious effect than studying. Miss Hotchkiss thought that it was high time that women invented a becoming style of dress that didn't suffocate them like those treacherous corsets.

Blackwell added that the sickliest women he had ever seen were in the south and west, where women were not sent to schools at all. Certainly the most educated women he knew, his sisters in particular, were also the healthiest.

The Victorian ideals of purity, chasteness, refinement, and modesty were thoroughly abandoned in this frank discussion of women's bodies. For the rest of the afternoon, the women openly examined a subject that had previously been only whispered about between mother and daughter, sometimes with friends, but never in public. As a poet and essayist, Howe had written about childbirth, breastfeeding, and toilet training. She had published poems about the terrible condition of her marriage's sex life. But like most other Victorian women, she had never openly discussed menstruation or menopause. These subjects held a stigma like no other.

One week later, on December 23, the *Boston Globe* noted in its Personals column that Dr. Edward H. Clarke, Oliver Wendell Holmes, and other prominent gentlemen were wisely against the coeducation of men and women. Other newspapers picked up the notice, and soon word of Clarke's theories spread across America. Satisfied by the overwhelming response to his research, Clarke began writing a book on the subject that he titled *Sex in Education; or, A Fair Chance for Girls*.

In 1872, Horatio Storer began wearing thick rubber gloves during surgery to protect his hands from his patient's infections (not to protect his patients from his germ-ridden hands), but because the heavy gloves hampered his surgical ability, he soon abandoned them and in so doing wrecked his medical career. While operating on a septic patient, he nicked his finger, which became infected. Septicemia followed. He was racked with fever and came close to death. Upon recovery, Storer was so disabled that he abandoned medicine and moved to Italy. Opponents of women in medicine lost their most outspoken champion.

But in 1873, Clarke took up the cause with the publication of *Sex in Education,* so Boston remained the center of the backlash. The book became a bestseller. A Boston bookseller claimed he had sold two hundred copies in one day. At $1.25 each, the first edition sold out in little more than a week, and overnight, Clarke became the world's most renowned expert on women's health.

Reviews across the country praised the book's argument against the higher education of girls. A reviewer for the *Boston Globe* wrote, "Dr. Clarke's book we consider to be the most important contribution to the cause of female education which has, as yet, been made." Editors at the *Chicago Tribune* claimed, "It is an earnest, honest, and competent exposition of the manifold and increasing evils which the established system of sustained and exacting study during the critical years between 14 and 18, inflicts upon the health and constitution of the women of our country." On the West Coast, the writer for the *Sacramento Union* hoped that the book would be a "snag" on which the cause of women's rights would be shipwrecked. He called Clarke "one of our most eminent physicians; one who is a very oracle in all matters pertaining to his profession."

Zakrzewska was notably quiet about Clarke's book. In fact, the year it was published, Clarke joined the consulting staff of the New England Hospital. Clarke viewed his friend as an exception to her sex. And Zakrzewska was careful not to do anything that would risk her hospital's closing, including challenging Clarke. Their continued association required deft handling.

But for Zakrzewska's good friend and benefactor Julia Ward Howe, her colleagues at the New England Women's Club, and women activists throughout the United States, *Sex in Education* was devastating. Girls and women would now be evaluated according to Clarke's standards. Public discussions on the controversies outlined in his book were organized across the country. At the annual convention of the American Social Science Association, held mid-May in Boston, the session on Clarke's book featured a formidable panel of speakers that included Julia Ward Howe, Harvard professor Jean Louis Agassiz, Harvard's president Charles Eliot, Vassar's president John Raymond, and Thomas Wentworth Higginson, a Unitarian minister, author, militant abolitionist, and Civil War hero.

Every member on the panel held fervent opinions about Clarke's theory, and audience members were riveted by the war of words. Along with Howe, Higginson was an editor of the *Woman's Journal*. He had been part of the Secret Six, the group of men who secretly funded abolitionist John Brown during the Civil War, and he had served as colonel of the First South Carolina Volunteers, the first federally authorized Black regiment. Following the war, he famously corresponded with the poet Emily Dickinson, becoming her devoted mentor. First to speak, Higginson read his essay titled "The Higher Education of Woman." In it, he argued that all women should have the opportunity to go to college and that men and women should be educated together. His firm minister's voice carried across the room, attracting devoted attention from the crowd.

In St. Giles, London, "there is or was a sign inscribed, 'The Good Woman,' with a painting of a woman without a head," he began. "It seems a simple and rudimentary joke enough, but it condenses in a few square feet of space the opinions of many of the greatest men. When Lessing said, 'The woman who thinks is like the man who puts on rouge—ridiculous;' when Voltaire said, 'Ideas are like beards—women and very young men have none;' when Niebuhr thought he should not have educated a girl well, for he should have made her know too much, these eminent men simply painted, each in his own way, the sign of the Good Woman."

Higginson then dismantled what he called the fallacies about the "Good Woman" preventing women from pursuing higher learning. For instance, Clarke, in his book, wrote that girls' education should be different from boys because girls menstruate and boys don't. Higginson looked at the audience and shrugged. "Why so, if they do not need different physical diet?" If girls are so physically different from boys, why not different foods along with education?

A good question, the audience responded.

The second fallacy Higginson outlined was "the assumption of the hopeless intellectual inferiority in the case of women." Only the records kept by public schools could reveal the true intellectual accomplishments of girls, and these were ignored completely.

The third fallacy was that of hopeless physical inferiority. In that case, Higginson said, "If every woman is a life-long invalid, then it would mean that the Lord did not know how to create a woman." When Higginson finished, the audience stood and applauded.

Now Professor Agassiz stood up hesitantly and faced the crowd. Seeing that they overwhelmingly agreed with Higginson's opinion, the portly Agassiz, in a ham-fisted bid to win over the room, boasted that it was he who had thrown open the doors of the Harvard Museum of Comparative Zoology to women. He also intended to open the Anderson School of Natural History to young women. In fact, he had received this year an equal number of applications for admission from both sexes. He neglected to say that neither of these institutions were directly connected to Harvard University.

Next, Vassar president John Raymond proclaimed that his school had long since stopped questioning whether girls could keep up with boys. He had spent seventeen years as a professor at a men's college before Vassar, yet he had never been as challenged to keep up with his classes as he was at Vassar. As to the effect of higher education upon the health of young women, he stated that he knew of no healthier occupation than study correctly pursued. Then he attacked Harvard directly. Why was it necessary for women in the nineteenth century to plead that the "mother University of the land" (Harvard) merely open a side door and let the girls in? In fact, he hoped that the esteemed institution would open the front doors.

Harvard president Charles Eliot stepped up on the platform to speak. Not yet forty, he was the youngest president Harvard had ever had. A handsome man who never smiled, he had furry sideburns that reached below his jaw. His stern demeanor telegraphed his thoughts. While Eliot alleged that Harvard had a diversity of male students, including Jews, Catholics, and Italians (Harvard had not admitted any Black men), he enthusiastically supported the maintenance of racial purity through segregation. (Unsurprisingly, in 1912, he would serve as vice president of the First International Eugenics Congress in London.)

Today, Eliot told the crowd that he adamantly opposed the education of women. He said that, unlike Colonel Higginson, he was absolutely against the education of boys with girls. In fact, he claimed that the experimental system of coeducation that had been tried in the West was now being abandoned.

At this statement, those in the audience looked at one another and shrugged. These educated members of the American Social Science Association knew Eliot's words were not true. Most had read the articles, and some had even traveled west themselves, and they knew that those youngsters being schooled in the western territories had to be taught with both sexes together in one-room schoolhouses because of the lack of teachers in those vast areas. This system saved time and was, so far, a great success.

Spurred on by the sour looks from his audience, Eliot continued. From the time of the Egyptians to the present, he proclaimed, education had existed only for men. Why change now? He insisted that women's colleges should become day schools of manners that offered basic reading and writing courses that would not injure women's "bodily powers and functions." Male and female minds were essentially not the same, he continued, his eyes narrowing. Furthermore, housing women together at colleges led to abuse. Dark things happened when large groups of girls got together, he warned.

Just then, as if he were shocked by the thought of those "dark things," Eliot lost his balance and had to grip the podium to right himself. "It requires special care to prevent evil in the contact of large numbers of girls," he warned after regaining his balance. To protect young women from themselves, he recommended that any higher education should take place only in day schools where the women could be closely watched.

During Eliot's speech, loud gasps and statements of shock came from the audience. They knew what he meant. He was insinuating that young women living together in college dormitories, away from the supervision of fathers or husbands, would become lesbians, nymphomaniacs, and prostitutes. Eliot had turned the whole thing into a sex talk.

Julia Ward Howe, who had been sitting straight as a beam while listening to Eliot, had finally had enough. Throughout her life, she had advocated for young women, and she felt each insult from Eliot jab at her own heart. In her personal life, she had put up with a philandering husband who gaslighted her for his own amusement. She jumped to her feet in furious anger and shouted that she would not tolerate his contempt for the morals of young women. He was projecting his own fantasies on young women. She was insulted by his very presence.

"You are the enemy of humankind," Howe thundered at Eliot. "Privileged men like you have a responsibility to others," she said. She heartily advocated for his abdication as the conservative leader of educated men. "If, like the Bourbons, [you] can neither learn anything nor forget anything, [you] must give place to a wiser dynasty." She criticized the "*a priori* ignorance" in all of his assertions. They were his own fabrications and had no resemblance to facts. Why could he not contain himself? She finished with a warning. She told Eliot that she knew some of the dark things and moral delinquencies among the young men at Harvard College that were never spoken of, things that would be "scared away like nightmares and dreams" in the presence of women students and their shining morality.

Howe finally had to stop speaking because the audience's boisterous cheering and clapping drowned out her words. Eliot looked like he had been physically struck. Most likely, he had never encountered a woman's unchecked anger. After grabbing his hat, he exited the conference without saying another word. Agassiz jumped to his feet, huffed and puffed at Howe, then followed Eliot. Higginson, Howe's friend and coworker, stood calmly and waited for the audience to grow quiet. When he spoke, he pointed out the falsehood the deluded Eliot had tried to sell when he said that the coeducation taking place in the western territories had failed. In fact, it was ongoing and gaining strength.

Then he spoke the final words of the session in defense of Howe. The unfortunate accusations of President Eliot regarding the general morality of young women were particularly dire, he said. He could not expect any woman, solicitous for the character of her sex, to hear such a statement without indignation.

Despite Higginson's defense of Howe, scandalized reporters throughout the country detailed her "ghastly" unladylike behavior. Conversely, newspapers characterized Eliot as the wounded gentleman, insinuating that the crazed Howe had "verbally castrated" the earnest college president. "It is on this account, however, that Social Science Conventions have a value for the community," the *Chicago Tribune* stated, "and it was particularly unfortunate for the cause of woman in this particular discussion that Mrs. Julia Ward Howe lost her temper, and thereby furnished the scoffers with material for maintaining that women are not adapted for deliberative discussions."

Howe never regretted her attack on Eliot. In fact, she decided that the assault on women coming from Harvard and echoed in the newspapers deserved her full attention. She worried about the life-and-death urgency underlying the reaction to Clarke's *Sex in Education*. This was a terrible escalation in the battle for women's rights. She, along with Lucy Stone and other suffragists, realized that if science supposedly proved women were too feeble to be educated, they could not possibly be trusted to vote. Women's suffrage would die.

Howe and other prominent activists clearly needed the expertise of intellectuals, scientists, and physicians on their side to launch a full-scale retaliation against Clarke's popular thesis. The number of qualified women scholars was infinitesimal, but there was one woman in America who had obtained three medical degrees, published numerous clinical studies in prestigious journals, and been accepted into the Medical Society of the County of New York: thirty-year-old Dr. Mary Putnam. Only she could lead them into battle.

But first, she would have to be convinced to join the fight.

Counterattack

I N A DINGY ROOM AT CITY HALL WITH COLD GRANITE FLOORS AND A sign above the door that read MARRIAGE BUREAU, Mary Putnam and Abraham Jacobi stood together before New York City mayor William Havemeyer as he pronounced them man and wife. The ceremony was a formality, witnessed by strangers. To Mary, it felt surreal yet perfect. The marriage announcement published in local newspapers described it as an "exhibition of eccentricity," noting that if "it was intended as a defiance to the conventionalities of fashion . . . to make 'the judicious grieve,' it was an unquestionable success."

Mary remembered her friend Élisée Reclus's diatribes against the "barbarous" rites of matrimony, though she did not go so far as to agree that marriage itself should be eliminated. More than anything, she wanted to have a family with Abraham. Élisée would have been proud of her for wearing a black dress, but she was not in mourning for the loss of her freedom as a single woman. On this Tuesday, July 22, cloudy and unseasonably cool for midsummer in New York, Mary and her entire family were mourning the death of her father.

The previous October, a few days before Halloween, Abraham and Mary had announced their engagement at a family dinner party held in Abraham's enormous home at 110 West Thirty-fourth Street. Its imposing entryway, with its ornate ceilings, marble floors, and walnut staircase that led up to the spacious parlor, drew gasps of delight from her youngest sibling, twelve-year-old Herbert, who raced up the staircase and then slid down the long banister. An impressive library, waiting room, and doctor's office occupied most of the first floor. It was clear that Abraham, one of the most respected physicians in New York, was a wealthy man. He had invented the field of pediatric medicine and was consulted by doctors from all over the world. His many books and essays always sold well. His expansive home delighted her family.

Mary's brother Haven heartily approved of Abraham and for some reason nicknamed him "Hugo." Her father, George Putnam, who was by nature slow to warm up to anyone, considered Abraham worthy of his eldest child. The two men were alike in many ways; they had both worked hard for success, and they were both unassuming yet charming enough to get what they wanted.

Sadly, Abraham and George never got the chance to become great friends and laugh over the antics of their children and grandchildren. In mid-December, Haven noticed that his father was looking older than his sixty years, more tired, and graying. After attending the funeral of an old friend, George Putnam had trouble climbing up the steps to his home. Even so, he insisted on finishing some contract business in his bookshop. Haven offered to help. Suddenly, in the middle of a sentence, George slumped forward. Haven caught his father in his arms and knew immediately that the family's beloved patriarch was dead. He called for help, and he and a servant carried George's body to his bedroom, laid him on the bed, and closed his eyes. Someone went for the doctor while Haven notified family members.

At the news of her father's sudden death, Mary felt her legs go numb. She worked to catch her breath amid her tears as she tried to imagine her life without him. The doctor eventually diagnosed the cause of death as stroke. George's widow, Victorine, had many children to comfort her, but it was almost entirely up to Haven to handle the affairs of what became G. P. Putnam's Sons.

Notice of the publishing magnate's unexpected death appeared in newspapers across the country. In her grief, Mary wrote a lengthy, unsigned obituary titled "Appreciation." George Palmer Putnam was an unworldly man, she wrote, not "by virtue of a profound reflection" but "by the same instinctive purity and naivete of feeling that we fancy we detect in a child who prefers flowers to diamonds. . . . When he was young he looked persistently on the bright side of things because it attracted him; when he was older he kept his eyes fixed steadily in the same direction because he would have esteemed it a wicked unthankfulness to have done otherwise. He was looking forward, I think, to a quiet old age, to an afternoon of beneficent leisure, filled with social plannings such as becomes the legitimate reward of a broad and sympathetic and reverent life. It seems hard that this should have been denied him."

Mary and Abraham postponed their wedding until they could not wait anymore. It felt wrong to have a festive ceremony, and by July, the family was scattered about New England. No one felt like celebrating, so they married in city hall.

Immediately after the formalities in front of Mayor Havemeyer, they left for their honeymoon at Lake George. They would stay in a cottage on a little island that Abraham owned. Mary was looking forward to seeing the island, but Abraham expressed concern about the two-hundred-mile journey north, teasing her that she hated traveling. Mary assured him that she loved to travel. "It's only sightseeing I object to," she said. "Rushing about from one place to another and staring at things so you can check them off your list."

They packed only a couple of suitcases of clothes, but they brought a heavy trunk full of books, journals, and writing paper. For the first leg of the journey, they took the train to Glen Falls, passing through the Hudson River Valley with its picturesque rolling hills and the flinty cliffs. When the tracks ended, they climbed on top of a glittering red stagecoach that flew along behind six strong horses galloping down the newly built wooden-plank road. The initiated, Abraham explained, always reserved seats outside the coach and near the driver in order to watch for the Hudson River Falls, Cooper's Cave, and a good view of Bloody Pond, where the corpses of two hundred soldiers had stained the waters red during the French and Indian War.

Heavy forests bordered the road, and the scent of balsam and pine whipped through the air. Wind swept the dust into Mary's hair and clothes, but she did not care. The journey was thrilling. She loved the idea of exploring the land that as a young girl she had read about in *The Last of the Mohicans* and the tales of Ethan Allen.

Soon, turquoise gleamed through breaks in the dense forest. Lake George, beautiful and isolated among the vast Adirondack Mountains, revealed its clear waters sparkling in the sun. The lake attracted artists and the wealthy, including the Roosevelt, Vanderbilt, and Rockefeller families, who would build mansions along Millionaires' Row in the first decade of the twentieth century.

Their stagecoach did not go beyond Caldwell, one of the few sites along the mountainside that could be cleared for a town. This was the end of the journey for most of their fellow passengers, who were planning to stay at the elegant Fort William Henry Hotel.

The Jacobis still had ten miles to go to reach their destination near the lumber town of Bolton. Even that small village was beginning to attract those who wanted to experience a vanishing wilderness. The Mohican House, built in the 1790s, had expanded to accommodate vacationers as well as woodsmen and lumber buyers. Bolton Landing could be reached by carriage over a rough country road, but the two doctors preferred to go by steamboat.

As the *Minnehaha* churned through the calm waters, Abraham pointed out the sights: Tea Island, one of over 170 islands scattered throughout the lake, was named for the teahouse that had burned down in 1828; Dome Island, which looked like a big "knob of moss"; Diamond Island, where pieces of quartz sparkled in the sand; and many other fir-plumed islands—some no bigger than their living room—the best of which, he assured her, was their own. The region reminded him of the Black Forest in southwestern Germany where he had played as a child. Finally, after reaching Bolton Landing and acquiring supplies, they made the last leg of their journey by rowboat.

Covered in tall white pine, elm, and cedar, Hiawatha Island, tucked into Huddle Bay on the western shore of Lake George, was perfectly secluded. Abraham had purchased the island in 1867 for fifty dollars. Their cottage sat at the very edge of water that was so clear, Mary could see darting trout, pickerel, and bass. Having lived near a lake during her childhood, she felt instantly at home and soon fell in love with the cottage. An early riser, she delighted in the mountain ridges that looked like the backs of dinosaurs emerging from the mists. During rough weather, the whitecaps rode high and lashed the island. Mary loved the stormy days even more than the sunny ones because then they could stay inside and write, a joy for them both.

They were both *working*. They had planned it that way. This was a time to assemble notes, put papers into final form, search the literature, and outline projects for the future. In addition, Mary prepared her lectures for the upcoming fall semester at medical school.

Ensconced in their comfortable cottage, the Jacobis collaborated on a second edition of Abraham's book *Infant Diet*. To address the issue of poor nutrition among newborns, part of the cause of high infant and childhood mortality, Abraham had given the New York Board of Health recommendations for the systematic improvement of infant health, a paper titled "Rules for Feeding Babies." These guidelines were also meant to help solve the child health crises in the tenements. He went on to publish these rules under the title *Infant Diet*. It was the first book of its kind and led to a vital improvement in public health.

For the second edition, Mary adapted the content for a new audience: mothers. The mother would become "the intelligent passenger on a vessel, who learns how to read the chart . . . so the mother may learn the general plan of her child's life, its future course, and the accidents that beset it." Mary chose to write for mothers as a way to introduce basic science into raising families. She described how the health of the mother affected infant feeding and warned that diseases such as consumption, syphilis, and epilepsy could alter a mother's ability to feed her child naturally. She explained the chemical composition of breast milk, talked about why it was better for babies than cow's milk, and recommended proper exercise for all mothers.

Mary viewed her coauthored book with Abraham as a translation for the general population. Published in 1875, the new edition was advertised as "revised, enlarged, and adapted to popular use" by Mary Putnam Jacobi and was part of the popular Putnam's Handy Book Series of Things Worth Knowing.

Mary and Abraham believed that science and medicine should be used to improve the lives of all people, especially the poor and laboring class. They both worked for "the humane evolution of society" and criticized the doctors who pandered to the rich. They believed that birth control and family planning were essential to health care and the economic stability of middle-class families. Because Abraham spoke out against the Comstock laws of 1873 that made promoting and practicing birth control illegal, he was labeled "a revolutionist against the government of God" by reactionary conservatives.

By the time they left Lake George for New York City, Mary Putnam Jacobi was eight weeks pregnant. Since she believed that pregnancy was a nutritional process beneficial for women's bodies, she did not see any reason to lighten her workload. Jacobi kept regular office hours and paid home visits to her patients. She continued to lecture, wearing maternity skirts and dresses with boxy jackets. She never worried about hiding her pregnancy. Her father, whom she missed every day, would have laughed at her insistence that being pregnant gave her *more* energy, not less.

In fact, her life was busier than ever. Out of concern for the dire lack of proper clinical training for women physicians, Jacobi organized the Association for the Advancement of the Medical Education of Women (later the Women's Medical Association of New York City) and would serve as its president from its inception in 1874 until 1903. Her public promotion of higher education for women catapulted her into the circle of professional women educators that included the renowned philosopher, writer, and feminist Anna C. Brackett.

Brackett had grown up in Boston and graduated from the state teaching school in Framingham. At the start of the Civil War, she left for a teaching job in New Orleans and then St. Louis, where she published the first English translation of several German works on the philosophy of education. In 1863, she became the first woman in America to be appointed as principal of a secondary school: the St. Louis Normal School, primarily focused on preparing students for careers in education. Brackett negotiated with the board of education to allow young women who were training to be teachers access to the same higher education as young men had. In 1872, Brackett moved to New York City with her domestic partner, Ida M. Eliot, the daughter of U.S. congressman Thomas D. Eliot, and opened the Brackett School for Girls, a college preparatory school located at 9 West Thirty-ninth Street. She wrote essays about the philosophy of education for *Harper's Magazine* and other well-known publications and served as an editor of the *New England Journal of Education*. She was a force to be reckoned with when it came to educating women.

The enthusiastic response to Clarke's book *Sex in Education* from the men in science and education stunned Brackett and spurred her into action. In 1874, she wrote "The Education of American Girls," an essay stating that a young woman must be guided carefully through two steps of the learning process, the "perceptive stage" and the "conceptual stage." No girl could develop fully and excel in life without achieving both of these steps. According to Brackett, an education such as the one that Clarke recommended, confined to the conceptual stage, would result in girls who were undereducated and untrained in abstract thinking. She pointed out that women who were confined to the family circle would not be able to fully mature into moral and intellectual beings. They faced two dangers. First, they would fail to be capable adults out in public and thus prove the stereotype of the "incompetent woman." Second, they risked being exploited by men. Brackett believed that coeducation was vital for the advancement of women.

Jacobi's brother Haven and the editors at G. P. Putnam's Sons were impressed by Brackett's essay. As a response to Clarke's book, they wanted to publish "The Education of American Girls" and several other essays in book form; Brackett would be the editor. Prominent educators and activists, including Ednah Cheney, Caroline Dall, and Lucinda Stone, would contribute pieces, and Brackett encouraged Jacobi to write a response to Clarke for the book too. Jacobi enthusiastically accepted. She had returned home from her honeymoon excited to share the news of her pregnancy only to find an army of feminists whose sole purpose seemed to be to refute Clarke's essay. Books were being planned and speeches were being given.

Jacobi was not shocked or angry at Clarke the way Julia Ward Howe and Brackett were. Her feeling about *Sex in Education* was more like what she experienced when she encountered the lazy, self-important male medical students in Paris—utter disdain. Responding to the male physicians who believed that there were "in the woman's physiological life disqualifications for such continuous labor of mind as is easy and natural to man" seemed like an ideal research project.

As she nourished herself, caring for her unborn child by eating nutritious food and taking long walks for exercise, she began forming her theories about female physiology and women's educational rights. The essay that she wrote for Brackett's book, "Mental Action and Physical Health," was a coolheaded, sharply drawn, and exacting refutation of Clarke's major claims. In her distinctive voice—dry, self-aware, analytic yet passionate— she tore his arguments to pieces. As she had done when revising *Infant Diet*, she used language that communicated complex physiological and scientific information to a lay audience.

Calling Clarke out by name, Jacobi accused him of exaggerating the incapacities of menstruating girls and falsely attributing menstrual issues (amenorrhea and menorrhagia) to excessive studying. Her reasoning was brutal. For example, she wrote that Clarke "relates a certain number of cases, interesting in themselves, but whose histories are lacking in many important details" in which healthy girls, after two or three years of study at school, began experiencing monthly "hemorrhages" so excessive that their health was compromised. Clarke had found no organic cause for these disorders but noted that when the girls stopped studying and doing all other activities, their health improved, and when they resumed their usual activities, including studying, their symptoms returned. Clarke wrote that these cases proved his theory that the intellectual demands of studying incapacitated young females.

Jacobi, using her acerbic wit, wrote that "this argument might be exactly paralleled by the following, which should prove whisky-drinking to be an efficient cause of yellow fever. A physician might select twenty cases of men, personally known to him, who had lived twenty and thirty years in New York or Boston, and never had yellow fever. During this time they had taken little or no whisky, but afterwards, removing to New Orleans, they fell into the habit of drinking, and, at varying intervals from that date, caught the fever, and in many instances, died. Therefore, fever was due . . . to the newly contracted habit of drinking whisky."

Next, she made fun of Clarke's theory that the brain and the uterus were intimately connected by some invisible force. Clarke's contention that studying "is capable of affecting an apparatus apparently so remote from the organ of the intelligence as is the vascular system of the uterus, certainly implies some most interesting physiological facts." His explanations of women's physiology were, at best, vastly oversimplified. Jacobi then described the human nervous system for her lay readers. She explained that nerve force in humans was communicated from the brain and spinal cord through an extensive nervous system via fibers with tiny brain-like structures. While boa constrictors, for instance, fell into a state of torpor while digesting food, humans could easily converse over dinner due to this powerfully independent nervous system.

The human nervous system was complicated; it was nothing like, for example, the simple ganglionic structure of crustacea and mollusks. These creatures "possess neither brain nor spinal cord; their nerve-centers, instead of being concentrated in a cranium and vertebral canal," were in sections throughout the trunk. In fact, Clarke and others who insisted on the incompatibility between cerebral action and the process of ovulation "have thus, perhaps unconsciously, reduced [women] to the anatomical level of the crustacea."

In his book, Clarke had prescribed a week of rest during menstruation. But in reality, Jacobi wrote, menstrual discomfort experienced by most girls and women usually lasted hours, not days. In fact, Jacobi asserted that his overprescription of rest would greatly increase pathologies in women because illnesses did not result from too much studying—rather, they arose from too much sitting on the couch and eating pastries.

She listed the factors that might cause uterine hemorrhage; none were related to studying. She described the power of thought and the stimulation of the intellectual functions of the brain, the radical difference between emotion and thought, and the causes of exhaustion. She took the reader on a tour of the brain, detailing its physiology, function, and possible location of the emotion center. She destroyed the idea that a bigger brain meant higher intelligence. She spent the last few pages drawing conclusions as to why and how coeducation, especially for higher learning, was healthy for both sexes. Finally, she compared Clarke to the French writer Jules Michelet, who claimed that women were not only sick but wounded: *La femme est une malade.* In other words, Clarke's theories about women's health were literary and romantic, full of passionate feelings, and completely unscientific.

G. P. Putnam's Sons was set to publish *The Education of American Girls* with Jacobi's essay in March of 1874, right when her baby was due. Since her brother Haven and his wife, Rebecca, had recently become the parents of a second little girl, the Putnam family thought it would be nice if she had a boy. She and Abraham simply hoped for a strong and healthy baby.

But this time, hope did not bring happiness. Mary went into labor on March 17 and gave birth to a baby girl. At once, everyone could see that something was wrong. The pale and listless infant did not cry but only whimpered. Mary's tears were lost in the sweat that covered her exhausted body. Taking the child in his arms, Abraham wished for a miracle. But his examination revealed that his daughter would not survive.

Their baby lived one day before she died from what doctors at the time termed "atelectasis pulmonum," a lung disease found in infants and newborns. For those few hours that the baby lived, her parents held her close. Losing the child was the worst thing that had ever happened to Mary, and she could not begin to imagine her husband's grief. For the sixth time, Abraham buried a child at Green-Wood Cemetery. Though devastated, Mary was determined to try again. She told her brother Bishop, "I always felt that my first baby would not live—I can scarcely know why, except that a great misfortune so often precedes a great happiness."

Her premonition about success after great misfortune would come true sooner than she anticipated. "Mental Action and Physical Health" was seen as a tour de force and catapulted Mary Putnam Jacobi into the public eye in the battle against Edward Clarke. Her essay received glowing reviews in newspapers, magazines, and journals across America and Europe. The *Westminster Review*, a British quarterly that published works by John Stuart Mill, George Eliot, and T. H. Huxley, was deeply impressed by "Doctress" Putnam Jacobi's essay and wrote that it "possessed merits far beyond this of the great majority of medical essays by her male contemporaries." American newspapers agreed. Admiration for Jacobi's intellect and scientific abilities grew. Soon, she would be asked to risk her reputation to help save the lives of American women.

Jacobi's essay became part of the contentious public response to Clarke's book; numerous articles appeared, and four books rebutting his arguments were published in 1874. The books, titled *The Education of American Girls*, *Sex and Education*, *No Sex in Education*, and *Woman's Education and Woman's Health*, contained essays written by leading educators, philosophers, and activists and were reviewed in major newspapers and journals. The authors recognized the threat of leaving Clarke's theories unchallenged. Using fiery rhetoric and passionate appeals to sanity, they denounced Clarke's attempt to enforce moral discipline on women through an alleged expertise over their bodies.

Clarke's covert plan "has been a crafty one and his line of attack masterly," wrote Eliza Bisbee Duffey, the well-known painter, poet, newspaper editor, and printer who was also the author of *No Sex in Education, or An Equal Chance for Both Boys and Girls*. "He knows if he succeeds ... and convinces the world that woman is a 'sexual' creature alone, subject to and ruled by 'periodic tides,' the battle is won for those who oppose the advancement of women."

Like Jacobi, most of the authors agreed that Clarke's theories would fail any scientific test. In *Sex and Education: A Reply to Dr. E. H. Clarke's "Sex in Education,"* edited by Julia Ward Howe, Thomas Wentworth Higginson accused Clarke of indiscretion, pointing out that the seven cases that he presented with only his "assurances" that there were more where those came from was simply not enough for anyone to accept his assertions as facts. Furthermore, Clarke had not presented any "representative males" for comparison but assumed that boys could automatically withstand the pressures of education.

In the same book, the resident physician at Vassar, Alida C. Avery, called Clarke a liar for the example he used of a girl who had supposedly attended Vassar. In a defiant tone, Avery noted that the case of Miss D—, described on page 79 of Clarke's book, was not even possible, since the college had never admitted anyone as young as fourteen. Next, she wondered why he had chosen a case from a women's college when he was supposed to be denouncing the evils of coeducation. Avery defended Vassar as a well-managed, respectable college. "I regret that you should have taken as your most elaborately discussed and aggravated case one which so misrepresents the college that any person who is at all acquainted with its rules and management can hardly help having his confidence in the book shaken," she wrote.

In her own essay, Howe called Clarke's assertions pure fiction: "That women in America particularly neglect their health, that women violate the laws of their constitution as men cannot violate theirs, and that the love of intellectual pursuits causes them to do so,—this is the fable out of which Dr. Clarke draws the moral that women must not go to college with men."

Howe asserted that he deliberately ignored any other facts—poor diet, restrictive clothing, lack of sleep—that might challenge his original theory. Rather than suffering from the pressures to keep up with the male students, women were, Howe wrote, victimized by Clarke's constant reminder that for them education did not matter.

Educator Anna Brackett also asked why Clarke had not considered other factors when drawing his conclusions about women's health: "We want to know also the kind of food she eats, and how cooked, and the regularity of her meals. We want to know the state of ventilation of the school room and her home; we want to know how many hours of sleep she has, how many parties she has attended, what underclothing she wears. . . . We want also to know what proportion of cases come from pampered, half-educated devotees of fashion, and what proportion from well-educated, hard-working women."

Caroline Dall, a prominent author and famed champion of women's rights, expressed great pain at the harm done by Clarke to those women who followed his disastrous recommendations. She accused him of wanting to humiliate women, most egregiously after having pretended to be their friend. She also condemned Clarke for ignoring other factors that might be at fault. "In all books that concern the education of women, one very important fact is continually overlooked. Women, and even young girls at school, take their studies in addition to their home-cares. If boys are preparing for college, they do not have to take care of the baby, make the beds, or help to serve the meals. . . . Women have [studied] in the nursery or the dining-room often with one foot on the cradle." God forbid that a community "undertook to train young men to the functions and duties of fathers," she wrote sarcastically.

The authors firmly rejected Clarke's vague proposal of a special education program for women that stipulated a week of rest during their menstrual periods. Duffey asserted that Clarke's plan would work only if students all menstruated at the same time. And what of the teacher, who was also likely a woman? "She too requires her regular furlough." Duffey wondered if Clarke would extend his argument to the home so that wives could leave their families for a week out of every month and take a break. "I think a concerted action among women in this direction," she wrote, "would bring men who are inclined to agree with the doctor to their senses sooner than anything else."

In an article for *Sex and Education* that voiced similar concerns, Mary Peabody wrote, "One would think, judging by Dr. Clarke's 'dreadful little book' . . . that women had generally been educated to death, while the deplorable fact is that she has only been half educated at the best."

These four books excoriating Clarke and his theories were published in March of 1874, a year after Clarke's book. By August, Clarke was ready with a backhanded response. He refused to name his critics or answer them directly because the thoughts of women, even brilliant women, were not supposed to be taken seriously. But the nature of Clarke's reaction made it clear that he and his allies were furious.

The executive committee of the National Education Association asked him to prepare a paper to present at their next meeting on the subject of the education of girls. Clarke wrote back that he had not intended to publish anything more on that subject and that, like the godly force of nature itself, he preferred to remain silent and let the seed that was sown "germinate and grow without my interference. On the other hand," he wrote, "I am not insensible to the obligation which rests upon every one to render whatever service he can, however little, to any good cause that is brought to his notice."

Clarke turned his thirty-minute presentation to the NEA into a 153-page book titled *The Building of a Brain,* published in the fall of 1874. Divided into three sections—"Nature's Working-Plans," "An Error in Female Building," and "A Glimpse at English Brain-Building"—it was a camouflaged reply to all his critics but especially to Jacobi's "Mental Action and Physical Health."

He began his treatise by stating that two duties were imposed on human civilization and, thus, on educators. "The duties are, first, to secure the perpetuation of the [Caucasian] race in America; and, secondly, to provide also for the survival of the fittest." It was a difficult but crucial task for civilization to evolve in the *right* way, but fortunately, educated white men like Clarke were there to guide the whole complicated process. The stakes were high: Unless white men and women both had "normally-developed" brains, the entire nation would crumble.

"The best brains, the only sort the world needs, are built by education, in accordance with working-plans that Nature furnishes. . . . Build the brain aright, and the Divine Spirit will inhabit and use it. Build it wrongly, and the Devil will employ it."

Clarke was again employing a popular, as opposed to academic, style of writing, but this time, he had made himself the purveyor of God's will. Once again, Clarke preferred salaciousness over science. And his use of pious rhetoric was strategic. His book ended up being reviewed in hundreds of newspapers. In fact, the entire piece was reproduced in full in *The New York Times*, in tiny print stretching across three wide columns.

The most powerful review, however, came from his friend Oliver Wendell Holmes. In the *Atlantic Monthly*, Holmes wrote that Clarke had gathered a large mass of information that proved that "the health of our women demands a more careful management of our girls with regard to special physiological conditions, which have been commonly enough winked wholly out of sight by our educators."

Holmes then introduced his own brutal rhetoric by comparing the process of educating girls to warfare: "Many young women may pass through the dangerous ordeal of forced education without manifest injury, as many soldiers go through a campaign unhurt. . . . But the fact remains that flying bullets and habitual neglect of physiological laws are always dangerous, and sometimes fatal." According to Holmes, women and girls were "forced" into education like young men were conscripted into the army. With the trauma of fighting the Civil War fewer than ten years past, Holmes had set out to shock his readers.

Then he made an accounting of the white races breeding in America and how "there is a prejudice against this continent as a home for white men." He reported that European experts in biology, natural history, botany, and other sciences found Americans to have feeble bodies and minds that "mature earlier and decay sooner. . . . Children born to [Europeans] in America are less hardy than those born and bred in Europe. Women cease bearing children after thirty."

Holmes, who had coined the expression *Boston Brahmin* in 1860 to describe his social class as the physical and mental elite, identifiable by its noble, inherited physique and aptitude for learning, refuted these European observations with statistics from the U.S. Army and American life insurance actuary tables that showed the opposite: Americans were living long, healthy lives. This evidence led him to conclude that "the imported American race, properly cared for and with fortunate crosses of blood, can not only continue itself, but can also develop exceptionally fine types of manhood and womanhood."

But only if properly managed.

Holmes's account then turned into a longing for eugenics: "If we could only bespeak a brain for one of the freshman class of 1890 as we lay out for an unborn colt to run for a cup in two or three years! But we have to take the brains as they come." Holmes expressed regret that S. Weir Mitchell, his colleague in Philadelphia, had not been given the time to carry out his own history of the white race in America.

Because America represented the commingling of the white races of Europe, scholarly men like Holmes were salivating at the opportunity to breed the Caucasian superman. Yet women were not cooperating. While they fought for better education, birth rates were plummeting, and the white race, especially in the South, according to Holmes, seemed to be declining.

"Dr. Clarke startles us at the outset by saying that no human race has kept a permanent foothold on this continent, and that the Anglo-Saxon race will die out here like those which have preceded it, unless it can develop an organization and a brain equal to the demands made upon it by its conditions. To keep up the race is not enough; the individual must also be developed to the highest point."

People had heard a great deal lately about the rights of women, Holmes wrote. "It may be very desirable that she should vote, but it is not essential to the tolerably comfortable existence of society. It is essential that she should be the mother of healthy children, well developed in body and mind. It is not essential that she should know as much as man knows, or produce as much by her ordinary labor of mind or body as he does. It is essential that she should save her strength for the exhausting labors which fall to her lot as woman."

According to Holmes, in this fight to pacify the females so that they would calmly and happily get married and reproduce, Clarke was akin to Lincoln, leading the learned white men into a battle that they must win.

～

In 1871, Harvard president Charles Eliot, a chemist, brought controversial changes to the medical school. In addition to a new three-year curriculum, he emphasized clinical training and evidence-based research. Plainly stated, Eliot brought science to Harvard's medical school. After implementing these transformations, he was called a pioneer and the greatest of Harvard's leaders. Of course, the same pioneering changes had been initiated several years earlier by Elizabeth Blackwell and Ann Preston at their own colleges. The scientific curriculum at women's medical schools grew even stronger with the arrival of Mary Putnam Jacobi. Yet none had the reputation or resources of Harvard, and women physicians, including Jacobi, still fought for that school to admit qualified women.

Naturally, important Harvard physicians like Holmes and Clarke, who wanted to eradicate coeducation, abhorred the idea of any woman attending their alma mater. When Harriot Hunt applied to Harvard's medical school, she was given permission to attend lectures. But after the all-male students protested, the faculty convinced her to bow out. Sixteen years later, in 1866, Lucy Sewall, M.D., and Anita Tyng, M.D., physicians at the New England Hospital for Women and Children, applied for admission to Harvard. Sewall had graduated from New England Female Medical College and Tyng was a graduate of Philadelphia's Women's Medical College. Harvard quickly rejected their applications. When Susan Dimock and Sophia Jex-Blake, both excellent students at New England Hospital, took up the gauntlet in 1867, their joint letter of application was reprinted in newspapers and widely read. These same newspapers also printed Harvard's wishy-washy rejection: "Neither the corporation nor the faculty wish to express any opinion as to the right or expediency of the medical education of women, but simply to state the fact that in our school no provision for that purpose has been made, or is at present contemplated."

Unwilling to accept Harvard's dismissal, Jex-Blake scheduled interviews with every faculty member and recorded each professor's attitude toward the admission of women. Mary Putnam had employed her personal charm and intellect to gain admittance to the Paris medical school, and Jex-Blake used the same approach. She obtained expressions of support from four faculty members, including Dr. Oliver Wendell Holmes. Perhaps he was merely placating her, but he did note that, while women's sole purpose *was* reproduction, a few exceptions should be made. However, those instructors who were willing to admit women warned that they would vote for it only if the rest of the faculty did as well. At the faculty meeting held in November 1867, members voted anonymously, and only one ballot was cast for admission.

The barricade against women at Harvard seemed insurmountable.

The Boylston Medical Society was part of Harvard's medical elite and represented the best of Boston's physicians. The society's founders, James Jackson and John Collins Warren, also established Massachusetts General Hospital and the *New England Journal of Medicine* and oversaw relocating Harvard Medical School from Cambridge to Boston. Each year, a prestigious committee in the society devised special essay topics for the annual Boylston Medical Prize. The competition was meant to encourage research into little-known areas of medicine. All essays were submitted and judged anonymously.

At the close of 1874, the committee, whose members included Boston's most important medical men, among them surgeon Henry Jacob Bigelow, obstetrician David Humphreys Storer (Horatio's father), and surgeon Morrill Wyman, decided to add fuel to the fire raging over women's health and higher education. They proposed the following question for 1876 two years in advance to allow enough time for research: "Do women require mental and bodily rest during menstruation; and to what extent?"

The Boylston committee's topic shocked and excited leading activists like Julia Ward Howe, Caroline Dall, and Anna Brackett. Since the competition was judged anonymously, these women begged thirty-three-year-old Jacobi to compose an essay for submission. Even though no woman had ever been allowed to participate in the competition, they were hopeful. Their champion had proven herself to be smarter than most men. She could win. But they were disappointed. Jacobi, who was pregnant again and optimistic this time for a healthy birth, reluctantly turned them down.

Fighting Back with Science

JACOBI YEARNED TO INVESTIGATE THE EFFECTS OF MENSTRUATION and submit an essay to the Boylston committee. She could think of no subject more relevant to her life. Yet she hesitated. The judging was anonymous, but she believed that if she won, they would disqualify her. Given her pregnancy and current workload, she did not want to put her heart and soul into a competition that she had absolutely no chance of winning because she was a woman. For now, she would continue with her own experiments.

Working in her lab, Jacobi made last-minute adjustments to the sphygmograph, a mechanical device that resembled a small metronome. Made of levers hooked to a scalepan with weights, the machine measured blood pressure and pulse rate. It was meant to be attached to the underside of a wrist, but for her experiment, Jacobi used a different site. An otherwise healthy boy had fractured his skull eighteen months earlier, and although the wound had healed, the bones had not fused closed. Jacobi carefully placed the lever pad of the sphygmograph into the two-and-a-half-inch-wide crack and rested it against the thin, pulsing membranes covering his brain.

Jacobi occasionally asked her patients to take part in her research studies to test drug hypotheses or merely to observe specific chemical changes or physiological responses. She measured patients' arterial tension and pulse rates after giving them alcohol, caffeine, or medications. She and her assistants, advanced students from her classes, meticulously documented her findings because she intended to publish the results in the *American Journal of Medical Sciences*.

Nineteenth-century medical journals often published studies that included experiments, surveys, and results from pathological examinations. With the explosion of public interest in science, medical writing took many forms: clinical studies, case histories, arguments for new forms of treatment, public lectures, memoirs, and scientific papers about puzzling anomalies. As a skilled author, Jacobi wrote unpretentious prose that, depending on the purpose of her scientific investigation, employed most of these formats.

～

While Jacobi continued with her experiments, activists promoting higher education for women confronted a turning point in the fight for equality. Their future success hinged on a woman winning the Boylston essay contest. They needed Jacobi to participate, so they set out to convince her that she could win even after the judges discovered that she was a woman. Since the contest was judged by Harvard professors, Cambridge feminists volunteered for the job.

One person was already acting on Jacobi's behalf. Esteemed teacher C. Alice Baker had sent a copy of *The Education of American Girls* to her friend Dr. Morrill Wyman, a prominent physician and Harvard Medical School faculty member who served on the Boylston committee. She included a note encouraging him to read Jacobi's article in Anna Brackett's book. The doctor followed her advice, read "Mental Action and Physical Health," and responded that, although he was no supporter of women's higher education, he was very impressed by Jacobi's work.

Baker owned and operated a successful private girls' school in Boston with her partner and housemate, Susan Minot Lane, an artist born in Cambridge. As a friend later wrote about the two women, "In course of time there came a day, when the Cambridge lady, Susan Minot Lane, calm, self-poised, strong, with keen but quiet and kindly wit, met Charlotte Alice Baker, all on fire with generous impulses, warm sympathies and ardent longings. The two came together, and it was not long before the union was complete, as each chose the other for a life companion."

A writer and historian, Baker had recently been elected honorary and corresponding member of the New-York Historical Society. Her father had attended Harvard Medical School at about the same time as Morrill Wyman had. Her father died when she was six, but the influence he had over her life was enormous. In "The Doctor's Little Girl," she wrote about the wonders of her youthful adventures with the man who raised her to be as independent as any boy. The story was published in 1870 in ten parts by *Robert Merry's Museum,* a children's magazine.

Baker had important connections to needed resources. After receiving Wyman's enthusiastic response, she invited him to dinner so that she could find out more. She and her partner, Susan, were charming conversationalists who could make anyone feel at home. Wyman had a kind face, a long nose, and white hair that curled around his ears. He was the favorite doctor of Harvard president Charles Eliot, but unlike Eliot, Wyman genuinely liked the company of women. It was a good thing, because all they talked about at dinner was Mary Putnam Jacobi.

That night, Baker struck gold. Wyman revealed that he did not consider Clarke's book *Sex in Education* "a dignified or trustworthy exposition of the subject." In fact, he harbored some resentment toward his colleague. Clarke had brought an enormous amount of attention to Harvard, not all of it welcome. His book was popular because it told salacious stories about female patients; it was an embarrassment.

Wyman praised Jacobi's work and spoke of her writing "with great respect." Baker learned that Wyman had encouraged a few other members of the Boylston prize committee to read Jacobi's essay, and they found her work to be "strong and sound in its physiology."

Finally, she asked Wyman the most important question: Would an essay submitted by a woman physician be eligible to win the Boylston Medical Prize? To her delight, he said yes. If she won, Jacobi would not be disqualified from the anonymous competition after her name was revealed. Each entry was to be submitted in plain and distinct handwriting, and when Baker suggested to Wyman that Jacobi should write "in a masculine handwriting," he strongly agreed.

Official rules required essays to be bound in book form and sent to Dr. J. B. S. Jackson, Boston, on or before the first Wednesday in April 1876. Revealing any clue that identified the author to the judges would result in automatic disqualification. The essay should be accompanied by a sealed envelope containing a note with the author's name and address. In addition to recognition, the winner of the Boylston prize would receive two hundred dollars.

The next day, Baker wrote Jacobi about her interesting conversation with Wyman and said that she hoped this would encourage her to compete for the Boylston Medical Prize. She reported that the Harvard physician spoke of Jacobi with great admiration, expressing an earnest desire that she should expand the discussion about menstruation that she had begun with her piece in Brackett's book. Baker believed that Wyman and his colleagues felt "that the honor of the profession required a more careful consideration and handling than [Clarke] had given the subject." If Jacobi did submit an essay, copied in a masculine handwriting, she would have a good chance of winning. Boston feminists crossed their fingers and prayed that Jacobi would accept the challenge.

～

For Jacobi, Baker's letter was a delightful surprise; it changed everything. She loved Baker's description of her secret meeting with Wyman and how she calmly finagled vital information from the staid Harvard physician. Jacobi must have felt like General George Washington receiving top secret intelligence from his network of spies. With growing excitement about the competition, she sat down and wrote to Baker that she was thankful for the news and ready to get started.

Jacobi began her research for the essay nearly a year after the Boylston committee's announcement about the menstruation topic, and she needed help gathering the evidence for her study so she would have enough time to interpret the data and write her essay. Inspired, she decided to join forces with the vast network of the women's rights movement. She devised an innovative technique for gathering information that had never been used in scientific research but would allow women to speak for themselves: She would send out a questionnaire. For the statistical analysis to be sound, it was vital that she reached women from a variety of occupations and backgrounds with a wide range of educational experiences. Baker volunteered to help copy and distribute the survey and then gather responses.

Eventually, they sent out a thousand of the following questionnaires:

The undersigned, desirous of collecting reliable statistics in regard to the menstruation of women in America, would feel indebted to all who would answer accurately, the following questions. No signature is necessary.

1. Age of going to and of leaving school.
2. Health under 13. Specify any disease of parents or sisters.
3. Number of hours a day spent in study at school.
4. Hours spent in exercise every day during the same period.
5. Studies pursued between ages 13 and leaving school.
6. Occupation (if any) since leaving school, and hours of work.

7. Health, general, since leaving school. Specify date of any illness. Do you have headaches or neuralgia?

8. Date of first menstruation.

9. Pain at menstruation, while at school and since leaving.

10. Does pain occur before, during, or after flow? Spasmodic, cramp-like, or steady and burning?

11. Does pain exist between menstrual periods?

12. What is duration of flow? Has it ever been excessive or too scanty?

13. Has it been necessary to rest during period? If so, how long? When did this first become necessary?

14. Strength, as measured by capacity for exercise. How far can you walk?

15. Have you ever been treated for uterine disease?

16. Are you thin or stout, rosy or pale, tall or short? Has any change taken place since twenty in color, flesh, or strength?

Next, Jacobi formulated a series of experiments to be carried out with the help of her colleagues Dr. Victoria White, Dr. Mary Baldwin, "and other ladies connected with" the New York Infirmary. They set out to do something unheard of in medical research. Using the most current experimental technologies, they intended to map the physiological and chemical signs of menstruation related to muscular strength. They would gather information to measure the levels of nutrition in a small number of subjects over a period of three months. Jacobi wished she could do more, but it was all they had time for.

She immediately set up her laboratory at the hospital and began her experiment. For each participant, she measured pulse rates with the sphygmograph, which created a visual graphic: small wave lines recorded on a rectangular board that illustrated the rise and fall of arterial tension throughout the women's menstrual cycles.

Next, Jacobi and her assistants tested urine samples for urea, a substance excreted by the kidneys. They used Liebig's volumetric method to estimate the depletion and replacement of the substances in muscular tissue. At the same time, she evaluated physical strength with a dynamometer. It was possible to gauge the tractive or compressive strength of all of the body's major muscle systems up to 175 pounds by pressing or pulling correctly on the straight or inverted handles. Finally, each participant recorded her own temperature by mouth, armpit, and rectum at hourly intervals during her monthly cycle. She noted that their body temperatures changed through-out the cycle. Her breakthrough would lead to the discovery that these temperature changes indicated ovulation. Eventually, other doctors would use her evidence to conduct their own studies, and in the 1930s, a Chi-cago physician, Leo J. Latz, published *The Rhythm of Sterility and Fertility in Women*, advising a form of natural family planning and birth control known as the rhythm method.

~

Through her years as a student, scientist, and doctor studying cellular nu-trition, treating patients, and teaching medicine to young women, Mary Putnam Jacobi had come to understand that the notion of female inferior-ity was a fiction, propaganda devised to keep women isolated and bound to a domestic sphere of existence. Even though this truth was obvious to her and those who fought for women's rights, telling stories about strong women would not suffice as evidence. She had less than a year to prove it scientifically.

But first, she had to give birth.

In the early summer of 1875, before she could conduct her experiments, Mary found herself in the middle of a disagreement about her own health-care choices that involved her coworkers at the infirmary and her family at home. She and Abraham wanted to take their annual summer leave to Lake George for the delivery of their child. Despite the island's remote location, Mary considered it an ideal spot for the last weeks of her pregnancy. How-ever, Dr. Emily Blackwell, consulting physician Isaac Adler, and her brother Haven all urged her to remain in the city.

She insisted that she had nothing to fear. There was no doctor in Man-hattan who knew more about obstetrics than Mary and Abraham Jacobi did. In addition, a number of excellent physicians summered at Lake George and would be on call if needed.

Once again, the long, picturesque journey to the lake was wondrous but exhausting. Mary, in her last weeks of pregnancy, carried thirty extra pounds that made her shed clothing to stay cool. When they boarded the *Minnehaha* for the last leg up the lake to Bolton Landing, she could fi-nally relax and enjoy herself. As always, she had brought more books and research than clothing. But this time, she had packed extra for the baby. Despite her professional self-confidence, she was tearful when she thought about having the baby. She and Abraham were filled with anxiety. She worried about the pressure on Abraham to attend the birth, telling her mother, "My Doctor is in a most exalted state of mind. If everything goes right, he will be in 7th heaven. But, what an *if*." That's why the couple decided he would not attend the birth but would go for the doctor in town when her labor started.

On the evening of August 3, Mary's water broke. Abraham helped her into her loose-fitting birthing gown, and they both took deep breaths to calm his nerves and her labor pains. Just as the sun went down, Abraham left to fetch the doctor from Bolton Landing. Mary remained on her own with only a servant for help. But she, the physician who had delivered scores of women and attended to countless infants, realized her labor was progressing quickly and was shocked to find she was ready to deliver. Easy as that, she reached for her son, and he took his first breaths that soon became a crying wail. Abraham had just pushed the boat away from the island when he heard the newborn's cry, and he came scrambling back home. Mary had given birth on her own to a healthy boy.

They named him Ernst, after their late friend, fellow physician, and Forty-Eighter Ernst Krackowizer. After experiencing so many losses, Abraham expressed his joy by waltzing around the house with his son in his arms. Mary told her mother that Abraham's delight "is so intense as to be touching and almost awful." Undoubtedly, Ernst was Abraham's greatest joy. In a letter to her brother, she wrote, "The loss of our first baby, last year, makes this one, if possible, all the more precious. . . . But now, the doctor at least, has had so many misfortunes that it seems as if the time had come for him to be perfectly happy,—or rather to stay as happy as he is at present." Mary herself cared for the boy with the ease of having grown up the eldest child of a very large family. Having a baby around felt perfectly normal.

While still at the lake, with the help of a nanny caring for Ernst, Mary Putnam Jacobi, the scientist, continued to interpret her Boylston research. She ordered and reordered the survey responses that Alice Baker had sent in the mail, putting them in piles and imagining the lives of the women who had made the effort to answer honestly. Her demeanor epitomized the detached objectivity necessary for laboratory work, yet in a way, the essay would be entirely self-referential; one of the most highly skilled and educated women of her time was researching and drawing conclusions about her own anatomy. It had never been done.

Being immersed in reproductive physiology while nursing her own baby led her to reflect on the unique characteristics of a newborn in a letter to her mother: "A baby is not even a boy or a girl but just a baby, and that is really something wonderful." Yet the further along she got in her research, the more frustrated she became. While organizing her thoughts about how to write her essay, Jacobi sat on her hands, leaned back in her chair, and tried to suppress her anger. The existing research on menstruation seemed utterly ridiculous! Most of these men of science who were celebrated for solving the riddle of life had never once asked a woman about her own body. Were they too afraid or utterly repulsed? She could not decide. It took all of her will-power to squeeze the irritation out of her writing and keep it objective. That meant that she had to overcome her own secret fear: that she would end up proving Clarke's theory correct.

But when she started combing through her piles of completed questionnaires, her worries subsided. Even at first glance, it was plain that most women did not give their periods much thought, and when they did, it was only when their menstrual flow stopped for pregnancy. They all had hopes and dreams beyond motherhood. Besides, Jacobi herself was living proof that Clarke was wrong. She took a deep breath and began to write.

Jacobi set out to efficiently reject the premise of Clarke's *Sex in Education* by drawing on her expert knowledge. In addition to proving that women should not be sequestered during menstruation, she wanted to subvert the ideas of female passivity and frailty and show that men and women had equal capacities. She intended to do this by applying her own extensive research on cellular nutrition, but first she had to address the existing theories about women's reproductive physiology.

She began her essay with a broad statement about the idea of limitations. Throughout history, she explained, men had found ways around anything that constrained their progress. For example, "knowledge of the limits of muscular strength stimulates the invention of machines many times man power." Similarly, men of science never regarded their own reproductive organs as debilitating or " 'limiting' in its nature," she wrote. Quite the opposite. The effects of the male ability to procreate "have been portrayed in brilliant colors by even sober pens."

This was not the case, however, when male physicians turned their sights on women's reproductive organs: "Such indeed is the audacity of the human intellect; that the discovery of limits usually proves hopeless in only one case, namely, when they are perceived to apply to a different race, class, or sex, from that to which the investigator himself belongs. . . . As soon as there is question of the other, the fundamental conception of the subject seems to be changed." Indeed, with women, "the sex itself seems to be regarded as a pathological fact, constantly detracting from the sum total of health, and of healthful activities."

Next, Jacobi reviewed the research history of women's reproductive biology. It was very brief. For over two thousand years, from the time of Hippocrates (around 400 BC) up to 1845, "Menstruation in women, muscular force in man, growth in children, were held to be more or less exact equivalents to one another." Women's physiology was simply a man turned inside out, making her a lesser version of the masculine.

At the beginning of the nineteenth century, physicians and scientists still had no concrete notion of how women's reproductive systems actually worked. They left it up to midwives or used the bits and pieces of knowledge gained over the centuries to build odd theories, often drawn from their basest fears about women's sexuality. A woman's reproductive physiology was hidden deep in her body and remained a complicated secret. Except for the assumption that men created life and women provided the home (womb) for it, nothing stuck as a theory of reproduction until the middle of the nineteenth century. This "breakthrough" idea about women's physiology began with a doctor's experiment on his female dog.

In December 1843, Theodor von Bischoff, a German physician and biologist, noted that a large female dog in his possession was going into heat. He immediately tried to breed her with a male dog, but she refused. After keeping her caged for two days, he allowed her contact with the male dog again, and this time she was interested. Before they could mate, Bischoff separated the animals and removed one of the female dog's ovaries. He found the ovary swollen and ready but not yet burst. Five days later, he killed the dog and observed the remaining ovary and fallopian tube. He was surprised to discover four eggs. He concluded that the dog ovulated during heat whether or not she mated. She did not require a sex act to become fertile. This piece of information was seen as revolutionary.

The world of science was elated to hear of his findings. Physicians took this discovery and applied it to women even though the doctor who had sacrificed his dog to perform his surgical inspection admitted that there was absolutely no proof that his theory extended to women. It just seemed logical. After all those years, Hippocrates was proved wrong. Women were not lesser versions of men. They were something else altogether, sexual machines whose stunted bodies were caught up in an evolutionary melee that even Darwin regarded as wholly dangerous.

By the mid-nineteenth century, even though no other mammal menstruated monthly and scientists had never seen a human egg outside of the uterus, it was "common knowledge" that menstruation corresponded with the sexual excitement known as the rut in dogs, pigs, cats, horses, and so on. This "rutting" theory was referred to as spontaneous ovulation. As the eminent New York gynecologist Augustus Gardner wrote: "The bitch in heat has the genitals tumefied and reddened, and a bloody discharge. The human female has nearly the same." In 1843, the *Lancet* pronounced that the swelling and rupture of the reproductive organs "occurring in the human female at the menstrual period [occur also] in animals during their rutting season." It was also assumed that, just like dogs, women ovulated during menstruation (heat). As a result, doctors recommended coitus occur at no more than eight days after the onset of menses to ensure conception. No wonder birth rates were plummeting.

In her essay, Jacobi fiercely opposed this ovulation theory because it "isolated menstruation from all other physiological processes" in women and turned a natural bodily function into a pathology. She noted that the theory of spontaneous ovulation was presented as a brutal progression similar to a death march into battle:

"The congestion of the ovary, ripening of the ovule, effusion of the serum and blood into the Graafian follicle; its rupture; the escape of the reproductive cell; its seizure by the fimbriae of the fallopian tube; its journey along the oviduct and descent into the uterus; the hyperannia of the latter, the turgesence of its mucous membrane, the rupture of its blood vessels, and local hemorrhage. . . . For the first time the periodicity of menstruation began to be considered as a morbid circumstance."

In other words, simple ovulation began with a time bomb of sexuality called the rut and ended with a ruptured ovary that expelled eggs, wounded the uterus, and caused a monthly outpouring of blood and gore. A woman's entire body suffered in sympathy with her reproductive organs. In that way, the ovulation theory kept women shackled to their bodies in fear of being consumed by both illness and their animal natures. As Jacobi wrote: "Thus one of the most essential apparent peculiarities of the menstrual process, its periodicity . . . has come to be considered as a mark of constantly recurring debility, a means of constantly recurring exhaustion demanding rest as decidedly as a fracture or a paralysis."

According to some doctors, to overcome this monthly "curse," women should simply stay pregnant. Jacobi quoted a prominent professor of obstetrics in Washington, DC, Dr. A. F. A. King. According to King, gestation was the proper function of the adult uterus, while menstruation was "fraught with danger . . . proof of functional inactivity on the part of the uterus, which becomes therefore liable to atrophy by sclerosis." King advised girls to marry at puberty in order to cure the morbid state of menstruation with pregnancy.

And the rut—the recurring heat that caused female dogs and cats to change from delightful pets to frenzied devils—attributed to menstruating women perfectly explained the fear that arose in men at the idea of attending classes or performing jobs with females who could, at any time, become fiendish, uncontrollable sexual sirens. It also provided a convenient excuse for men to behave violently toward women.

Women had absorbed the widespread cultural view that their bodies were sick, wrote Jacobi. She was determined to replace this cult of weakness with her theory of strength.

To refute the brutal theory of the rut and its exploding ovary, Jacobi supplanted it with a picture of serenity. She reconceptualized menstruation as a nutritional process, not a sexual one, by referring back to another idea that originated under Hippocrates, the plethoric theory of menstruation. This ancient concept described menstruation not as physical depletion but as the simple evacuation of a plethora of leftover nutrition. In her essay, Jacobi proposed a modern interpretation of women's reproductive physiology based on the theory that menstruation was simply the body's evacuation of nutritional surplus.

Jacobi had studied the process of cellular nutrition for years, beginning with her introduction to cellular theory at pharmacy school. Throughout her career, she used the concept of nutrition to explain health and the manifestation of illnesses. In this case, *nutrition* did not mean simply the dietary consumption of food. Rather, it described the continuous regeneration of cells and tissues to preserve life. The circulation of blood through bodily "force" delivered the chemical substances that nourished the cells and promoted growth. Other physicians also believed illness resulted from the body's general failure to build and break down tissues properly. For example, the famous neurologist S. Weir Mitchell, in what would become known as the "rest cure," related female emotional instability, or hysteria, to nutritive deficiencies. But while Jacobi and Mitchell agreed on the scientific fundamentals of nutrition, they disagreed completely on how to apply them to women.

With her essay, Jacobi guided the study of women's health away from ovarian and uterine diseases and their connection to mental illness and toward the simple process of cellular nutrition. In this framework, the menstruating woman was undergoing not a crisis of sexual stimulation but a normal event in the growth and death of tissues. Menstruation was not a violent congestion of the uterus, not an erection of the female organs, and certainly not a brutal hemorrhage. It was not equal to heat or rut in other mammals. It was simply part of the process of forming nutritional reserves.

Menstruation was a recurring bodily function that had distracted male scientists from understanding the true difference between men and women: cellular nutrition. For example, girls did not develop muscles like boys because nutrients in girls were naturally diverted away from muscles, and an "afflux of blood to the uterus" occurred to increase the functional capacity of the uterus and prepare the body for menstruation or pregnancy. The process of ovulation and menstruation had no connection to a sexual act. Women's bodies stored nutrition for pregnancy and, when conception did not occur, shed that overproduction through menstrual blood. Men and women were different, Jacobi argued, because of these varying nutritional requirements.

She also rejected the theory that ovulation and menstruation occurred simultaneously. Neither menstruation nor pregnancy, she reasoned, was tied to the time of ovulation. In fact, hundreds of cases presented in the most recent research indicated that ovulation actually occurred about two weeks after the onset of menstruation. The amount of blood flowing to the uterus was far less than the amount of blood transported to the stomach and intestines during the digestive process. She pointed out that there was no evidence that the uterus or ovaries became aroused during menstruation and no chemical evidence linking ovulation to the supposed excitement of "heat."

This process of nutrition that Jacobi described was neither momentary nor sporadic, but continuous and reoccurring, like waves in an ocean. She argued that women experienced "rhythmic wave[s] of nutrition" or "rising levels of vital force" throughout their monthly cycle. Using the evidence provided in her surveys and experiments, she proceeded to demonstrate how the wave of vitality and nutrition increased in her subjects before and during menstruation, which served as a powerful argument against rest.

∾

Jacobi then analyzed the results of her questionnaire. Of the thousand distributed by Baker and others, 268 were returned, an acceptable number. They came from a varied cross-section of American women. Performing extensive statistical calculations using simple averages, Jacobi evaluated the relationships among her questions, divided respondents into categories, and standardized their responses. Then she took these self-reports from women and inserted them into her report, thus adding, for the first time, women's stories to the medical record.

In one table, Jacobi correlated the respondents' general health with the number of miles that they walked daily. Answers to the question about general health included "Very fine," "Mens. this morning. Some pain of steady character," "Good. Sick headache," and "Good until child bearing." They reported miles walked daily as "Long dist.," "2–3," "Four miles till after 2nd child," "All day," and "20 miles."

Next, she reported facts about menstruation and menstrual pain. While 65 percent of respondents suffered varying degrees of menstrual pain, from almost nothing to fairly severe, a full 35 percent reported suffering no pain at all. She correlated these answers with amount of exercise, family history, education, and occupation. Jacobi found that immunity from menstrual suffering did not depend on rest but on a healthy childhood, proper exercise, a sound education, marriage at a "suitable" time (when she was old enough to make her own decisions), and a steady occupation.

Overall, the survey portrayed American women as active, healthy, and industrious; women with "excellent" health who walked five to twenty miles a day were not likely to be incapacitated by menstruation. They were the opposite of fragile. She used their voices to counteract Clarke's paternal and condescending style of reporting so-called true stories about his unstable, sickly, and feminine patients. Jacobi's firsthand reports were more authoritative than Clarke's personal stories about his handful of patients could ever be.

She concluded this section by stating, "Rest during menstruation cannot be shown, from our present statistics, to exert any influence in preventing pain, since, when no pain existed, [rest] was rarely taken." She noted one exception: working-class women, those who labored in the fields or factories and were on their feet for hours. Depending on the job conditions, these women might require extra rest during menstruation, but for the most part, too much rest was injurious. In fact, because women experienced a buildup of nutritional reserves during menstruation, Jacobi argued that it was actually a time of "increased vital energy," not sickness.

To prove this assertion and demonstrate the wave theory of women's reproduction, Jacobi did further research on a small number of subjects at the New York Infirmary. In a section titled "Experimental," she tracked their cycles, measured pulse rates, took their temperatures, and determined their strength.

She began the section by stating her premise: "On the hypothesis that the menstrual period represents the climax in the development of a surplus of nutritive force and material, we should expect to find a rhythmic wave of nutrition gradually rising from a minimum point just after menstruation, to a maximum just before the next flow."

After tracking her subjects' physiological signs for ninety days, Jacobi concluded that menstruation was like any other bodily function: "Reproduction in the human female is not intermittent, but incessant, not periodical, but rhythmic, not dependent on the volitions of animal life, but as involuntary and inevitable as are all the phenomena of nutritive life." Any pain or disability related to menstruation was relieved not by rest but by action. "Practically," Jacobi explained, "we find that the habit of disordered and painful menstruation is more frequently associated with habits of feeble muscular exercise than with any other one circumstance." As a result, Jacobi advised physical activity, calisthenics, sports, and even exercise machines to build women's health.

In "Conclusions," Jacobi summarized her findings and made recommendations using the precise and formidable language of science. She also mocked Clarke and other physicians who prescribed rest: "The menstrual flow is the least important part of the menstrual process, and arguments for rest drawn from the complexity of the physiological phenomena involved in this, should logically demand rest for women during at least twenty days out of the twenty-eight or thirty. In other words, should consign them to the inactivity of a Turkish harem, where indeed, anemia, if not dysmenorrhea is said to be extremely frequent."

Last, she wrote that her findings "do not in the least show that menstruation, *per se*, constitutes any temporary predisposition to either hysteria or insanity." Just as food digested, hair grew longer, and hearts beat rhythmically, women menstruated.

⤳

She signed the last page with the Latin phrase *Veritas poemate verior* ("A truth truer than a poem") and mailed it in according to the instructions for anonymity.

While Jacobi knew that she could win, she understood that there were many reasons for the judges to shun her once they discovered her sex. The menstruation question, in many instances, was the only excuse for keeping women out of Harvard University.

It took some time for the committee to choose a winner because the members had to read over three hundred submissions. Finally, a few weeks after mailing in her essay, Jacobi received a letter from the committee. When she slit open the envelope, she felt more nervous than the day she had given birth to Ernst. A slip of paper floated out of the envelope and onto her desk. When she turned it over, she discovered that it was a bank check containing the Harvard insignia and made payable to Mary Putnam Jacobi for the amount of two hundred dollars. She leaned back in her chair, closed her eyes, and laughed. She had won.

For a moment, she wondered if Professor Wyman had shepherded her essay through the committee, gently revealing her gender to his associates to soften the blow. Perhaps, once they uncovered her name, there had been a great debate about giving her the award. Or maybe, for once, she had been granted the prize simply because her essay was the best. In any case, she was grateful. She responded by showing appreciation for the Boylston committee. She wrote that she was greatly honored that they "willingly conferred their prize upon a woman." She noted, modestly, that the piece was but "an imperfect beginning of labor" and conveyed plans to expand her experimental observations in her published work.

Nationwide, newspapers reported that a woman had competed with hundreds of men and won Harvard's Boylston Medical Prize. The fact that she was Mary Putnam Jacobi, the Parisian scholar and famous woman doctor, made the news less shocking. In any case, Jacobi's essay was probably the most scientific of any submitted. She had not only invented a new form of medical research by including data from surveys but also performed unprecedented experiments to determine the effect of menstruation on women.

While Harvard sponsored the Boylston committee and announced the winners' names, the university did not publish the actual winning essays. Those remained the property of the Boylston committee. Jacobi decided to present her argument to the public. She simplified her narrative, expanded her research, and rewrote the content to make it a more overt attack on Clarke's *Sex in Education*. G. P. Putnam's Sons published her book *The Question of Rest for Women During Menstruation* in 1877.

Months later, after her book had been delivered to bookstores, Jacobi received a letter from Richard M. Hodges, a member of the Boylston committee, alerting her to the fact that she had neglected to include the required disclaimer in her book stating that the committee did not "approv[e] the doctrines contained in any of the dissertations." As it stood, it looked like Harvard endorsed her attack on Clarke. Not wanting to stir up conflict, Hodges politely asked Jacobi to correct the error, "not because there is any expressed dissent on the part of the committee from your doctrines," he said, "but simply because the rule is deemed an important one to be followed."

Jacobi wrote back and apologized, claiming that she was absolutely "mortified" by her error and would add the disclaimer in future printings. Secretly, though, she might have been smiling. Neglecting to include the disclaimer worked in her favor. From then on, her book and professional standing would be attached to the Harvard award.

The medical community praised Jacobi's book. The *Medical Record* called *The Question of Rest* "masterly" and wrote that "every page in the book gives evidence of great erudition." The *Philadelphia Medical and Surgical Reporter* admired the book's "wide range of observation, experiment, and new statistics." In *The Nation*, Dr. Henry Bowditch of Harvard Medical School said that "her successful competition for the Boylston prize, rendered her sex a far more important service than if she had directly advocated their claims." Agreeing with Bowditch, the editors of the *Woman's*

Journal, including Julia Ward Howe, Lucy Stone, and Henry Blackwell, wrote: "The friends of the higher education of women are to be congratulated upon this result of the patient, candid and exhaustive research, which Mrs. Jacobi has given to this important subject. It is one of vital interest to all women. . . . This result is itself a final and conclusive practical refutation of the theory of Woman's physical disability for the highest professional attainments."

Surprisingly, many other physicians approved of her dismantling of the ovulation theory, because, from practical experience, they had begun to question the supposition that ovulation and menstruation occurred simultaneously. Continuing to say that women went through "heat" every month made them look silly. Jacobi's work on the menstrual wave was cited by colleagues, and in some instances, her laboratory experiments were duplicated and expanded.

Of course, many physicians dismissed her conclusions about rest and the ability of women to enter the public sphere of higher education, professions, and politics. A woman's biology would continue to be used as an excuse to keep her out of certain fields, such as engineering and mathematics, many leadership positions, and even the American presidency. Edward Hammond Clarke died in 1877 from heart ailments, but his book, though much diminished, lived on.

Jacobi's battle for equality had just begun. She vowed to lead the fight for the acceptance of women into the nation's finest medical schools, including Harvard. Her research into women's health care turned to neurology and hysteria, which seemed to plague so many women. Jacobi would challenge the findings of America's famed expert on women's mental pathologies, the formidable S. Weir Mitchell, who had invented the wildly popular rest cure.

12

God's Gift to Women

LIKE MARY PUTNAM JACOBI, S. WEIR MITCHELL LIVED AN EXPERI-mental life. Tall and slender with a Vandyke beard and piercing blue eyes, the distinguished Philadelphia doctor was known as a pioneer of the female nervous system. His powerful charisma attracted fawning attention from both women and men, who referred to him as the Benjamin Franklin of his time.

His writings had been cited by luminaries such as Charles Darwin and William James. One admiring journalist described him as "God's gift to women."

His typical patient was frail and thin with sallow skin and dark circles beneath her eyes that looked like bruises. Overwhelming fatigue had weakened her muscles, and she could not stand erect because of the aching in her spine. She did not remember the last time she had menstruated. In her late twenties or early thirties, she was an aging shadow where a full-blooded human had once existed. Whether caused by brain trouble, selfishness, exhaustion, an abusive husband, the death of a child, nursing, dyspepsia, or low fevers, the illness had taken control of her life.

To soothe her deepening melancholy, she drank anesthetizing tonics made of bromides, opium, chloral, and brandy. As the weeks passed, her nervous instability led to hysteria. An endless string of nerve doctors and gynecologists prescribed plaster jackets, braces, and water treatments, but nothing made her feel better. When every action had failed and nothing else could be done, the family found the money to call in Dr. Mitchell for his miracle rest cure.

Mitchell's self-assuredness was immense. A Renaissance man, he wrote extensively, penning case studies, children's books, and long narrative poems. Brave young heroes, dark villains, and ultrafeminine women with small hands and delicate feet populated his romance novels. On darker days, he liked to experiment on himself with hallucinatory drugs like mescal and peyote and then write stories. Throughout his life, the only person he ever looked up to was his father. As a result, he had acquired an almost pathological obstinacy that led to nervous breakdowns and required long camping trips to restore his vigor.

Now forty-eight, he had started out in his chosen profession decades earlier and claimed to be a devoted practitioner of scientific medicine. His first taste of fame came with his research on the effects of poisonous-snake bites.

∽

During his childhood, young Mitchell had, according to his father, indulged in his emotions and lacked discipline. A prominent Philadelphia physician, John Mitchell was the chair of the obstetrics department at Jefferson Medical College. Professor Charles Meigs was a colleague and a good friend. Young Weir upset his father because, though bright, instead of studying, he devoured books like *Robinson Crusoe* and *The Arabian Nights*. He wrote flowery-sounding poetry and had started several stories about true love.

At age fifteen, Weir entered the University of Pennsylvania and spent his time drinking and playing billiards. He never received his undergraduate degree. Two years later, when he finally decided to study medicine, his father reacted with disgust: "You have no appreciation of the life. You are wanting in nearly all the qualities that go to make success in medicine."

Despite his father's misgivings and his lack of a college degree, Weir entered medical school at Jefferson Medical College in 1848. John Mitchell insisted that his son take up the manly pursuit of surgery. But the gore, the screams, and the flying jets of blood horrified Mitchell and he always fainted at operations, so instead, he focused on anatomy and physiology, chemistry, physics, and obstetrics. His favorite professor was Charles Meigs, who had recently published *Females and Their Diseases*.

Mitchell observed Meigs's upbeat, gossipy lectures with fascination. His sympathetic style won over Mitchell, especially when Meigs disagreed with his father. For example, the popular obstetrician refused to administer the chloroform anesthesia that the elder Mitchell always used on his patients to ease the pain of childbirth. Meigs's reasoning was that "the female, at the most interesting period of her life, the time of labor, should, all other things being equal, have her mind unclouded, her intellect undisturbed, her judgment fully adequate to realize and appreciate the advent of a new and important era in her existence—the birth of her child." Even if she begged for anesthesia, he refused to administer it. According to Meigs, labor pain was God's curse upon women, and her suffering was necessary to induce maternal love.

Pain and suffering that ultimately led to pleasure made perfect sense to Mitchell. He stopped fainting at the sight of blood but still rejected surgery. Instead, he chose neurology and physiology. After graduating, he traveled to England and France for further medical training. In his letters home, he commented on the uncouth women who traveled alone. He found the English women ugly. French women, on the other hand, were willowy, trim, and petite with "the neat foot in the neater shoe," the "tasteful costume, and the modest down looking eyes."

While in Paris, Mitchell fell in love with the Latin Quarter. During the day, he pursued his studies. Even though he hated the process of writing letters to gain introductions for clinical instruction, he managed to get himself invited to attend rounds at prominent hospitals. As his French improved, he learned about diagnoses and operative surgery in hospital clinics, watched innovative cataract surgery, and found out how to use a catheter. At night, he visited lively cafés and attended the theater.

After spending several months in the clinics, he received a letter from home asking him to return because his father had fallen ill. In 1851, he cut short his European medical education to return to Philadelphia and join his father's practice. Seven years later, his beloved father, after suffering numerous strokes, died of typhoid pneumonia. Mitchell found solace by working in his laboratory and soon began experimenting on animals. During the next two years, he presented papers at the Academy of Natural Science on topics such as the blood of the sturgeon, reflex and conscious action, and vivisections of opossums, muskrats, frogs, and fish, all of which he had injected with various poisons.

When he discovered that very little was known about snake venom, he began collecting all kinds of poisonous snakes, especially rattlesnakes. He found the reaction of a large rattlesnake when surprised on a remote footpath to be "one of the finest things to be seen in our forests. The vibrating tail" projected from the coils and "the head perfectly steady, the eyes dull and leaden, the whole posture bold and defiant, and expressive of alertness and inborn courage." It took practice, the help of knowledgeable lab assistants, and numerous snakes, but soon he had learned the proper way to safely handle rattlesnakes.

His elaborate laboratory was lined with wooden boxes containing snakes. Every morning, he and his assistant would spend an hour subduing each one, forcing a large glass tube into its stomach, and feeding it milk and finely chopped flies, grasshoppers, and raw beef. He hoped to increase the potency of their venom. Because snakes ate very little in captivity, Mitchell had invented a whole set of tools and contraptions to manipulate and control the snakes' bodies during force-feeding and venom extraction.

Mitchell spent his afternoons exposing his research animals—dogs, cats, rabbits, pigeons, and frogs—to snakebites and recording the animals' subsequent acute and chronic stages of poisoning. Because of their larger size, dogs lived longer after being bitten, and when the venom was slow in killing the animal, Mitchell had more time to watch and record the toxicological effects. On one occasion, Mitchell placed a white mongrel weighing seventeen pounds in a cage with a large snake that struck twice. The dog "suffered terribly, and during two hours whined and yelled incessantly." A dog's death could take from twelve minutes to nine hours of suffering.

Bunnies and birds were much more susceptible to venom, and birds sometimes died in seconds. Mitchell wrote that so minute "was the quantity required to kill a small bird, such as the reed-bird, that under certain circumstances these little creatures became very delicate tests of the presence or relative activity of the venom."

In 1860, Mitchell performed experiments that resulted in the deaths of over 150 animals, including one hundred pigeons and reed birds and twenty dogs. Anti-vivisectionists, aware of his experiments from his publications, strongly objected to Mitchell allowing animals to die long and painful deaths. But no laws existed to prevent animal suffering, and he could proceed as he pleased without consequence.

That same year, he published the results of his experiments in *Researches upon the Venom of the Rattlesnake*. Mitchell's ornate, almost romantic, style and startlingly sexual language cloaked the reality of his torturous research and kept his readers—all educated white men—turning the pages to see what happened next.

For example, he wrote that the rattlesnake fang must be "fully erected" in order for the duct to work properly, and that the poison gland was so constructed that it "resembles very strikingly, in section, the appearance of a small testicle." When the snake's deadly blow occurred, the fang "ejaculated" the poison, and in snakes that were "perfectly fresh, healthy, and undisturbed for some weeks in summer, the first gush of their venom was sometimes astonishingly large."

Soon after this book was published, Oliver Wendell Holmes, a close friend of Mitchell's father, wrote him to say how impressed he was with *Researches*. Holmes expressed a camaraderie with Mitchell because, coincidentally, he was writing a novel about rattlesnakes.

Elsie Venner: A Romance of Destiny told the story of a girl whose pregnant mother was bitten by a rattlesnake just before her birth. The venom gushed into Elsie's blood, engulfing her nervous system and making her personality seem more snakelike than human. Those who cared for her feared her stony eyes, wild beauty, and sensual but menacing reptilian behavior. The novel explored themes of original sin, hereditary influences, and human nature. Both Holmes and Mitchell had studied what they believed were inherited characteristics, such as the differences between common country boys who had been bred to bodily labor and those elite young men from the "Brahmin caste of New England" who were "commonly slender," with delicate features, bright eyes, and supreme intelligence—men like Holmes and Mitchell. Mitchell told Holmes that he was planning to scientifically investigate the "physical statistics of our native-born white race."

With the publication of *Researches*, Mitchell gained prominent admirers and an international reputation. In 1861, he was elected a member of the Boston Society of Natural History, and that same year, Darwin, who was researching his tome *The Descent of Man, and Selection in Relation to Sex*, requested a copy of Mitchell's book. Mitchell, who had also inherited his father's medical practice, experienced great success, but that was put on hold with the eruption of the Civil War.

In October 1862, he became a contract surgeon for the U.S. Army, working in Philadelphia. He was particularly interested in gunshot wounds and injuries to the nerves, and soon he was getting all the severely wounded soldiers from around the city referred to him by other surgeons.

Mitchell found the bloody cases in this "hell of pain . . . of amazing interest." Over the next two years, he saw hundreds of patients in such agonizing pain that they were being driven mad. He treated them with a mixture of opiates and an extreme form of rest that he described as the "absence of all possible use of brain and body." Some survived, but most did not. In 1864, ill and exhausted from war, he resigned his position and suffered a complete breakdown. As a result, he turned his research toward hysteria and resolving the plague of "American nervousness."

After fully recovering, Mitchell joined the staff of the Orthopedic Hospital and Infirmary for Nervous Diseases in Philadelphia. Patients suffering from the most hopeless, pathetic, and disturbing cases traveled great distances to seek his help, especially after reading his book of lectures titled *Rest in the Treatment of Nervous Disease*, published in 1875 by G. P. Putnam's Sons. In it, he outlined case after case of patients who had suffered for years from pain caused by broken bones, sciatica, writer's cramp, and injuries and who were cured by a treatment of rest and dietary therapeutics.

In 1877, he began to call his treatment the rest cure. Most of his patients were women whose health had been gradually deteriorating despite seeking advice from many doctors. The affluent women who could afford Mitchell's fees spent their lives indoors sewing, sketching, reading romances, planning meals, supervising the household, and having children. The more wealth a man accumulated, the more leisure time his wife had—the icon of status in the industrial age. The boredom and confinement among the genteel ladies led to a popular trend of "female invalidism." A pale and worn-out appearance and a wardrobe of airy white gowns were all the rage, and popular women's magazines featured stories about "The Grave of My Friend" and the "Song of Dying." Women avoided sexual relations, housework, and other unwanted tasks by retiring to bed with "sick headaches" and a host of other illnesses. The waiting rooms of prominent physicians grew crowded with ladies of fashion, and physicians made a fine income off these "sickly" females.

This pervading view of upper- and middle-class women as inherently sick provided a compelling argument against allowing women to be healthy. A whole industry that depended on her invalidism had risen up. Sometimes, a woman confined to a life without any other options would erupt in fits of screaming, laughing, and crying. She might exhibit explosions of rage, chronic fainting, violent contortions, hair tearing, and attempts to bite herself. These frenzies became known as "hysteria," and if they lasted long enough, the family's last resort would be to call in Mitchell.

When he appeared at the home of a new patient, a frail young woman with sallow skin, she was too far gone to be enraptured by his enigmatic presence. She noticed the doctor and his devoted nurse only when they forced her to leave the familiar confines of her bedroom and move out of her home and into his clinic. Mitchell demanded seclusion away from family and friends for all of his rest-cure patients.

Mitchell ran several tests to make sure the new patient's illness was not biological; cancer often caused some of these symptoms, and tuberculosis was epidemic among American women. If Mitchell found nothing chemically wrong, he diagnosed her with neurasthenia—a vague medical condition with symptoms of lassitude, fatigue, headache, and irritability associated primarily with emotional disturbance—and began his rest-cure treatment. A patient's stay at his clinic could range from six weeks to two months.

First, the patient was put in a room with a chair, a daybed, and a door that the hospital staff kept locked. Enjoyable pastimes like reading, writing, and sewing were strictly forbidden. She could not do anything but lie there. According to Mitchell, "To lie abed half the day, and sew a little and read a little, and be interesting as invalids and excite sympathy" was not his intent for his patients. In other words, if she wanted to shirk her duties and retire to the fainting couch, then he would keep her there for a very long time. Mitchell removed her daily family life and replaced it with himself. He made all of her decisions for her.

In addition to seclusion and rest, the patient received massage, electrotherapy applied to all areas of the body, and forced feedings called "dietetics and therapeutics." Many of his patients were anorexic and had to be fattened up. The crux of the rest cure was forced feeding. If she proved to be constipated, Mitchell would insert an electrode into her anus and administer a brief shock to stimulate bowel movements. If that didn't work, he prescribed enemas. Each day until she produced sufficient stool, the doctor would force a long tube at least six inches up the rectum and inject a cup of olive oil through the tube followed by a quart or more of flaxseed tea. For the worst cases, an assistant would help the enema treatment along by compressing the anal opening to keep the fluid from leaking out. This treatment took two to four hours. If the patient had not been hysterical at the start, she would be shrieking with pain by the end.

When her bowels were emptied, she was ready to proceed with her feedings. During the first week, she was, like a newborn, restricted to a milk-only diet. After that, her day began at seven thirty a.m. with cocoa, coffee, hot milk, beef broth, or hot water (the doctor's choice, not hers). At eight thirty, she ate breakfast in bed. At first, she was given only toast and juice, but later she was allowed fruit, steak or mutton, potatoes, coffee, and a goblet of milk. She was required to clean her plate.

From ten to eleven, she received a Swedish massage. For the first week, the masseuse used a gentle touch for a half hour. Gradually, the bodywork became more intense, to stimulate blood flow, and lasted for an hour. After the massage, patients received another thirty minutes of electrotherapy with currents strong enough to contract the muscles. Massage and electrotherapy compensated for the muscle atrophy that naturally occurred as a result of complete bed rest for weeks or months.

At noon, she was allowed to rise and slowly dress. Toward the end of her stay, if she behaved properly and was getting better, she could see visitors or read her mail. Letter-writing was forbidden. Lunch, the chief meal of the day, was served at one thirty. Afterward, she could move to the daybed for more rest. At three o'clock, she received a snack of milk or soup. Supper was served at seven. She drank hot milk at bedtime, ten p.m.

After weeks of a specialized diet, massage, and electric shocks, when she had grown fat enough to be of some value to her family, she would be returned to the exact home-life situation that had caused the hysterical symptoms in the first place. In his reports, Mitchell always claimed victory over the poor woman's wild hysteria and rarely followed up on cases. Full of rosy-cheeked health, she was now, as Mitchell liked to say, as he had made her.

A demure patient who acquiesced to Mitchell, cleaned her plate at every meal, and never complained was normally treated well. If a patient became obstinate, Mitchell did not hesitate to threaten or inflict physical pain through a whipping or even a strong shock. Making quick, creative decisions about what kind of punishment to employ seemed to energize Mitchell. When he was a visiting physician at the Providence Hospital in Washington, DC, a woman claiming to be paralyzed had baffled several doctors; they sent for Mitchell to help solve the perplexing case. After examining the patient, he asked the other doctors to step out of the room. A few minutes later, he rejoined them. They asked, "Will she ever be able to walk?" He answered, "Yes, in a moment." Soon, the door flew open and the woman rushed out and down the hallway, followed by billows of smoke. Mitchell had set her bed on fire.

In the fall of 1877, the same year that Mary Putnam Jacobi won the Boylston Medical Prize, Mitchell published his rest cure in *Fat and Blood: And How to Make Them*. The book received rave reviews, and Mitchell's practice exploded. Doctors added the rest cure to their repertoire of wonder treatments for hysterical girls and women.

The one essential ingredient in all rest cures was the dominant *male* physician who could ensure "belief in his opinions and obedience to his decrees" and who could entice "childlike acquiescence" from his patients, especially if they had strong wills that needed breaking. Even the most capable women doctors would fail because they could not "obtain the needed control over those of their own sex." Mitchell hated the idea of women attending regular medical schools. In fact, he was vehemently opposed to all higher education for women. The very thought of it sent him into a rage. Like Edward Hammond Clarke, Mitchell believed that educating women was of absolutely no use because of their innate biological weakness. Nature's laws were unalterable, he often said. A woman was born into her profession; a man was not. It was as simple as that.

～

While Mitchell was still reveling in the success of *Fat and Blood* in Philadelphia, Mary Putnam Jacobi was holding a fundraising event in New York to benefit the Association for the Advancement of the Medical Education of Women. On the evening of March 26, 1878, the lecture room at the Union League, located on Madison Avenue, was filled with wealthy New Yorkers interested in improving the quality of education for American women doctors. Tonight, Jacobi, Emily Blackwell, and the women doctors of the New York Infirmary sat listening to U.S. congressman Robert B. Roosevelt speak to their cause.

A renowned citizen of New York, Roosevelt had been instrumental in establishing paid fire and health departments in the city. He avidly supported his nephew Teddy's campaign to be elected to the New York State Assembly. Speaking with sincere concern on "the Social Influence of Women Physicians," he stated that one of the reasons that the medical profession and the public discriminated against women physicians was the perception that they were not as well educated as male physicians. He congratulated women doctors for their tenement work and for caring for the "pale, delicate and always suffering and thoroughly shattered and broken-down young woman who needed proper medical advice and treatment."

He stated that it was his belief that most of women's ill health could be blamed on a lack of women physicians. That evening, Roosevelt showed himself to be an important ally and advocate for women's higher education.

Next, Dr. Emily Blackwell took the stage to talk about the medical education that she and her sister Elizabeth had received as well as the history of women physicians in the United States. It was a long and thorough chronicle meant to convince her audience that women were making vital contributions to medicine. Since arguments against women doctors included the belief that they stopped practicing after marriage, Blackwell finished her speech by sharing impressive data about the work history of alumnae from her medical school. Of the forty-six graduates, most were still working, and many were excelling. Six were wives of physicians and in practice with their husbands; four were in practice with their fathers; five were missionaries, one of whom had established a hospital for women in East Asia; seven were studying at universities in Europe; two had passed examinations for hospital appointment; and one was a member of Mount Sinai's medical staff. Blackwell finished by inviting all those present to visit the infirmary for a tour.

Jacobi then delivered a speech titled "Our Future Aims." She described the infirmary's plans for providing education equal to or better than the best medical schools in the world. The college would need funds for cutting-edge laboratory equipment and excellent instructors. She closed the meeting by asking attendees for donations. Afterward, Jacobi and Blackwell mingled with the wealthy visitors, thanking them for their support. Several congratulated Jacobi on winning the Boylston prize and publishing her book on the question of rest for women.

A few weeks after this meeting, Jacobi discovered that she was pregnant again. This time, her family, including Abraham, celebrated the news without any panic. Their toddler, Ernst, was a constant source of joy for the couple; his lively presence brightened each day.

During her pregnancy, Jacobi remained busy teaching classes, seeing patients, and working on a study of anemia, a condition believed to be closely related to hysteria, with her friend and associate at the New York Infirmary Victoria A. White. Over the past two years, they had published the results of their research in several medical journals. When Jacobi discovered Mitchell's book *Fat and Blood*, describing his "rest cure" for hysteria, she became curious about his findings. Each night, she settled in bed next to Abraham and read a few pages. By chapter 2, she began to feel uncomfortable. When she was about halfway through, she was fuming with anger and wanted to fling the good doctor's treatise across the room.

It was not just that he described his patients in a condescending and churlish manner; it was that, like Clarke in his *Sex in Education*, Mitchell projected his own feelings and emotions onto them. He wrote about his cases using overly dramatic language that turned patients into characters similar to those populating his fiction. She could only ask: Where is the science?

Jacobi openly scoffed at literary physicians like Mitchell who lived for good reviews and compliments from admirers. These men played at being physicians. Their passionate rhetorical style turned the results of their research into publicity that sold books rather than elevated science. But for Jacobi, it was not just Mitchell's writing style. She realized that, in the cases he presented, he had failed to properly monitor his patients. He did not report taking temperatures, blood samples, or urine, and Jacobi was concerned for his patients' well-being. She rejected his old-fashioned explanations for hysteria that attributed the condition to female biology and mental decline resulting from overactivity. Jacobi's own studies revealed that hysteria was caused by physiological and nutritional deficiencies that resulted from the unlivable constraints on women's lives. While a time of rest could be very important for overworked women, most needed stimulus rather than sedation to free themselves of hysterical symptoms. Scientifically speaking, in Jacobi's view, Mitchell's rest cure did not work.

Once again, Jacobi thought, a man had achieved wide public recognition for inadequate work. But his exaggerated prose and incompetent science were not the only reasons she was upset. Apparently, he had read her previous studies on anemia, because certain prescriptions for his patients were identical to the ones she and Dr. White had published a few years ago. Jacobi was convinced that Mitchell had claimed her work as his own.

Jacobi's clinical studies focused on how to diagnose and cure anemia. Similar to Mitchell's, the first step of her cure was to relieve constipation. However, she used simple cold-water enemas. She did not isolate her patients or keep them from reading or sewing. To calm their stomachs and provide nourishment, Jacobi prescribed a milk diet and soups for the first few days, but she never forced anyone to eat.

Within a week, Jacobi's patients improved. Since they were sleeping much better at night, Jacobi increased their daily food intake and pre-scribed a few days of bed rest followed by regular activities. But unlike Mitchell, Jacobi limited the amount of rest and preferred to stimulate her patients with the use of cold packs. To apply the treatment, Jacobi's assis-tant enveloped them in a wet sheet surrounded by a dry one and then six blankets drawn tightly around each patient's body. While the patients were wrapped in sheets and blankets, Jacobi traced their heartbeats with the sphygmograph and recorded their body temperatures. She applied mas-sage therapy to stimulate circulation following the cold packs.

After the massage, Jacobi or her assistant took urine and blood samples to measure urea and hemoglobin levels. Unlike Mitchell, she constantly monitored her patients. Laboratory analyses showed that the therapy pro-duced higher levels of urea and rising levels of hemoglobin, both demon-strating that increased stimulation of body tissues resulted in more cellular nutrition and better health. Jacobi's data revealed that as long as her pa-tients obtained proper sleep at night, any additional rest was of the least consequence to their health.

⤻

Mary Putnam Jacobi gave birth to a plump, healthy girl, Marjorie, in De-cember 1878, and the entire Putnam family gathered to celebrate. Her mother, Victorine, had watched how Abraham grew fearful every time Ernst came down with the sniffles while Mary never worried until it was absolutely necessary. The couple's temperaments were completely at odds these days. Victorine realized that the little boy now constituted the bond between Abraham and Mary. "Ernst is a darling child," she told Haven. "I tremble to think how much they depend upon him for their happiness. . . . One child is a terrible anxiety."

Whether or not she consulted Abraham on the matter, with the arrival of her baby daughter, thirty-six-year-old Jacobi put childbearing behind her and entered one of the most productive periods of her life.

Spurred on by her antagonism toward Mitchell, Jacobi and her part-ner Dr. White continued their research. Two years later, *On the Use of the Cold Pack Followed by Massage in the Treatment of Anaemia* was published by G. P. Putnam's Sons. The book contained eleven case studies. The first described their successful treatment of a patient who had previously un-dergone Mitchell's rest cure and had gotten worse, not better. In her book,

Jacobi attacked Mitchell's findings, launching a professional debate between the two that would last for decades.

Jacobi had published more than a dozen papers in medical journals on a wide range of topics emphasizing diseases of women and children and research in neuropathology. And yet, like all women physicians of the time, she was barred from working as a physician in the major New York hospitals. But as a wealthy New Yorker, she often benefited from her elite connections, especially in publishing.

Nonetheless, her wealth could not protect her from public expressions of bigotry.

In 1877, Henry Hilton barred wealthy financier Joseph Seligman, founder of J. and W. Seligman and Company, from his swank Grand Union Hotel in Saratoga Springs, New York. This incident became one of the most publicized anti-Semitic occurrences in America up to that point and inspired other hotels to put up placards that read NO JEWS OR DOGS ADMITTED.

In 1880, when Marjorie was two and Ernst was five, Jacobi and her children traveled to Staten Island for a holiday at the shore. When she tried to register for a room at the St. Mark's Hotel, the owner turned her away, saying that his establishment did not cater to her people. While she wasn't Jewish, her name was, and she and her children were forced to find other lodging. Days later, the hotel found its name mentioned quite disparagingly in several newspapers, including Jewish publications; they reported that the eminent Jacobi, a Protestant descended from Revolutionary War generals, and her children had been turned away due to "the shameful prejudice which certainly does exist, and whose manifestations should be deemed disgraceful and humiliating by all true Americans."

Abraham Jacobi was outraged by the hotel's rejection of his wife and children. When a reporter asked him what he thought of the matter, he called the incident "perfectly ludicrous. . . . I consider [the hotel manager's] scheme simply an advertising dodge. Dr. Adler, who was formerly an assistant of mine, was treated in the same way at the hotel this week." When asked to respond, the hotel manager said that he did not want his establishment to be known as a "Jew House."

During the 1880s, anti-Semitism spread like wildfire through the vacation grounds of New York State. Ten years after the Seligman incident, the Catskills resorts were equally divided between those with an all-Jewish clientele and those that accepted only Protestants. The swank clubs that sprang up along Millionaires' Row at Lake George restricted Jewish membership too.

Eventually, Jacobi forgot about the hotel incident because, months later, she achieved another high point in her medical career. When the New York Post-Graduate Medical School was opened, Jacobi joined the faculty, lecturing to both male and female physicians on children's diseases. She received no pay, but her opening session was a remarkable event, with diagrams and case histories of children's physiology and pathology.

Jacobi's growing success may have sparked a rivalry between husband and wife. After Marjorie was born, Abraham Jacobi changed. He began to make requests of Mary that she considered unreasonable. Perhaps he wanted another child; she did not. Although they employed a nurse and other household servants, Abraham expected his wife to make the professional and personal sacrifices needed to raise a family. He began asking her to stay at home. Mary brushed off her husband's growing dissatisfaction as stress from overwork. He was tired, that was all. And of course she did not ignore their children. She loved to romp about the house with them and often took them on adventures around the city. Life with Mary Putnam Jacobi was never boring.

Jacobi idealized Abraham, and for as long as she could, she held on to the idea that their marriage was a union of equal partners. She had seen such a marriage in France between Élie Reclus and his remarkable wife, Noémi, who worked outside the home as a schoolteacher and activist. Using the Recluses as her guiding star, Jacobi believed herself to be a pioneer in matrimony as well as medicine. She intended to live the fullest life possible with her medical career growing right along with her children. But while her career continued to soar, the idyllic image she held about her life with Abraham would be shattered.

Part Three

Breakthrough

[Women should unite] as the bees work,
without any special reference to individual
advancement, but the intention of
contributing to the upbuilding of the hive.

—MARY C. PUTNAM JACOBI, "ADDRESS BEFORE
THE WOMEN'S MEDICAL ASSOCIATION"

Success, but at What Cost?

AFTER WINNING THE BOYLSTON MEDICAL PRIZE, JACOBI CONTINUED to expand her pioneering inquiry into women's reproductive health and publish her findings in medical journals. The president of the American Society of Gynecologists, George J. Engelmann, cited her study of menstrual waves in his own published research. Even after duplicating Jacobi's experiments, Engelmann still concluded that during the premenstrual period at the height of the wave, American girls exhibited "morbid nervous symptoms as characterized by the hystero-neuroses" that indicated pathology, not, as Jacobi had concluded, vitality.

Other physicians failed to reference her at all. Even worse, some, like Mitchell, appropriated her research without giving her credit. When scientists did cite her study, they snubbed her achievement. In 1882, William Stephenson, professor of midwifery at the University of Aberdeen in Scotland, published a medical paper discussing nutritional waves in which he *did* reference Jacobi's work, although he rejected her conclusions about increased vitality during menstruation. In a tragic but predictable turn of events, the menstrual wave became known as "Stephenson's Wave."

As time passed, Jacobi grew resentful and angry. It was a bitter realization that, because she was a woman, her work would never be fully recognized by the medical community. She had always assumed that because of her sharp intellect, she would eventually break down every barrier to her success. But now she realized that the overarching cultural belief that women were not supposed to achieve anything also applied to her.

Still, she found solace in hard work and her practice. The greater the difficulty she had in diagnosing a patient's disorder, the stronger her determination to discover the cause and bring it to light. She used her imagination to visualize the possible physical causes of her patients' illnesses, conceptualize an accurate diagnosis, and develop cures for the most puzzling cases. As a teacher, she gave her soul to her students, finding as much pleasure in their accomplishments as she did in her own. More than anything, she wanted bright women to be given the chance to learn and excel. If she could not get the recognition she deserved, she resolved to change things so that they would.

In the early 1880s, pressure to accept women into regular medical schools was growing. In Boston, Dr. Henry Bowditch, a supporter of Dr. Marie Zakrzewska and the New England Hospital for Women and Children, kept proposing that qualified women be admitted to the Massachusetts Medical Society. He reminded his colleagues that Harvard Medical School's continued refusal to accept women forced prospective students to search elsewhere for medical training; they either traveled to Europe, attended the (so-called) inferior women's medical schools in the United States, or learned what he considered to be the medical quackery of water cures and homeopathy.

At the annual meeting, Bowditch and his associates were ready with the following arguments advocating for the admission of women. First, the society had an obligation to protect the community from improperly educated or incompetent physicians. Second, it was important for other physicians to know which female practitioners were competent. Third, admitting women would automatically reduce the number of those practicing irregular medicine like homeopathy.

The large faction opposing Bowditch insisted that the society was as much a social organization as a licensing agency, and therefore its members could determine with whom they would socialize. One physician, in an obvious misunderstanding of Bowditch's proposal, was upset at the possibility of having to admit "such nuisances" as Julia Ward Howe. Another quoted Joseph Lister, who had told the British Medical Association "that he could not consent to be a member of an association [with] the unseemly practice of discussing medical topics in a mixed company." Yet another faction presented the clichéd yet popular argument that women were incapable, by their very nature, of being qualified practitioners. Women should not undertake a profession that God would not allow, blah-blah-blah.

At a meeting of the Association for the Advancement of the Medical Education of Women in 1881, the members began by lamenting the fact that women were still barred from attending the best medical schools in America.

Jacobi interrupted. She said that, as a student in Paris, she had used her wits and charm to convince professors and administrators to allow her into their clinics and seminars; however, if she thought that her request was taking too long, she tried something even more persuasive. She purchased access to facilities normally open only to male students. Flashing a *chez mon banquier* had, unsurprisingly, opened doors more quickly.

Admission to medical schools in America could be similarly acquired, she told them. "It is astonishing," she asserted, "how many invincible objections on the score of feasibility, modesty, propriety, and prejudice will melt away before the charmed touch of a few thousand dollars." Several members laughed, but Jacobi was deadly serious.

In the fall of 1881, Emily Blackwell, Marie Zakrzewska, and Jacobi decided to put her theory to the test. They joined forces to spearhead a very public attempt to purchase admittance to one of the larger medical colleges in the country. Calling these funds an "endowment," they would be used to "purchase direct partnership rights." Ready to push forward, they decided that Harvard, because of its status in the world of medicine, was the most logical choice. Even though in the past, Harvard president Charles Eliot had proved to be an immovable force against women's higher education, things had changed since his confrontation with Julia Ward Howe: Harvard desperately needed the money.

In 1874, Eliot had launched a drive to secure $200,000 for a new building, but only half the funds had been raised. Upon receiving notice of the women's endowment, Eliot put aside his own great prejudices against women's higher education and suggested that $100,000 would be a "good sum" to start with, exactly the amount to finish the building. Perhaps he thought that such a large amount would dissuade any further inquiries.

Moving quickly, the New England Hospital Society formed a committee and organized the fund drive. The committee, led by Dr. Emma Call, contacted women's medical colleges for help in raising the necessary funds. Eager students and their professors went to work asking for money. Although the Woman's Medical College in Philadelphia did not participate, a substantial amount was raised in Boston and New York; not $100,000, but enough to make a solid impact. In September 1881, the committee sent the following letter along with a check to the president and overseers of Harvard University:

Gentlemen:

Would you accept the sum of fifty thousand dollars for the purpose of providing such medical education for women as will entitle them to the degree
of Doctor of Medicine from your University?

This sum to be held by you in trust, and the interest of the same to be
added to the principal, until the income of the fund can be used for such
medical education of women.

If such an arrangement cannot be made within ten years, the fund to be
returned to the donors.

Sincerely,

Marie Zakrzewska, Emily Blackwell, Lucy Sewall, Helen
Morton, Elizabeth M. Cushier, Alice Bennett, Eliza Mosher,
and Mary Putnam Jacobi

The committee waited patiently for an answer. Month after month, there
was no reply. But the lack of response did not mean a lack of interest on the
part of Harvard. In fact, the impact of the letter resembled that of a bomb
tossed into a whirlwind. The blast spread to all corners of the hallowed
institution. Jacobi had been correct; money did speak loudly.

Because even President Eliot had voiced a desire to accept women if
the price was right, there was a real chance that petticoats and perfume
would invade the sacred lecture rooms and marble halls of Harvard Medical School. The male students warned that if Harvard stooped to accepting
women, attending the prestigious university would stop being an honor.
Enraged faculty members threatened to sabotage the project from within.
Professors from other departments joined with the medical faculty to
spread ugly rumors of mass resignations. Fear and chaos ran amok.

During this time, the editors of the *Boston Medical and Surgical Journal* published a series of articles that also argued against the admission of
women to Harvard, but their reasoning was unexpected. They wrote that,
because women had their own accredited medical schools in Philadelphia
and New York that were "as good as the best colleges," they did not need to
be admitted to Harvard or any other regular medical school. Thus, one of
the most prestigious medical journals in the United States acknowledged
that women physicians were as well trained and as competent as men. This
development would help Bowditch finally win the admission of women to
the Boston Medical Society in 1884.

Jacobi, who had lambasted the Woman's Medical College of Pennsylvania fifteen years earlier for its poorly trained faculty and appalling curriculum, would now agree wholeheartedly with the Boston journal editors' upbeat assessment. In the eighteen years since she had attended the college, the quality of education offered there had risen sharply. For example, Ann Preston had, before her death in 1872, "utilized its legacy of $100,000 to fully equip its beautiful college building with amphitheaters, lecture rooms, and even embryo laboratories, museums, and libraries." Jacobi had stated in a recent journal article that she was very satisfied that its graduates were "quite as carefully trained as those in any other medical school."

In New York, Jacobi and Emily Blackwell worked endlessly to make the infirmary's medical school one of the best in the country. In 1881, out of a desire to increase the competency of its students, they upset some feminists by requiring entrance exams. As Jacobi explained, "When people first began to think of educating women in medicine, a general dread seemed to exist that, if any tests of capacity were applied, all women would be excluded." But by 1881, those who were proponents of higher education for women understood that the highest possible standard for their medical education must be enforced.

Jacobi attributed the success of women's medical training to the rise in power of those pioneering women. Not only did they open schools, they created a thriving network of hospitals for women and children run by women doctors who, in turn, offered clinical training to women medical students. In addition to the New York Infirmary and Boston's New England Hospital for Women and Children, women's hospitals had opened in Philadelphia, Chicago, San Francisco, and Minneapolis. A total of ninety-four women physicians worked at these hospitals, which treated 18,600 patients per year, not including the patients treated in private practice by the hospitals' physicians.

In the late 1860s, Freedmen's Hospital in Washington, DC, partnered with Howard University College of Medicine to train African American medical professionals, including women. In 1877, Canadian Eunice P. Shadd was the first Black woman to graduate from the program. By 1900, twenty-five Black women (out of 552 graduates) had received their MDs from Howard University's medical school. Dr. Sarah Garland Jones, class of 1893, was the first African American and the first woman certified to practice medicine by the Virginia board of medicine. She later founded the

Richmond Hospital and Training School for Nurses, renamed the Sarah G. Jones Memorial Hospital in 1902.

But the fact was, keeping separate but equal colleges of medicine for men and women required an extraordinary amount of money, often paid by taxpayers and donations from wealthy citizens. A community might not be willing or able to fund both a men's and a women's institution if they were both providing the same first-rate education. In the end, during economic downturns, the women's smaller institution would always suffer. Men would continue to benefit from the best teachers, the best laboratories, the best libraries, the best facilities for training, the best hospitals, and the best clinical opportunities.

"There is no manner of doubt," Jacobi wrote, "that coeducation in medicine is essential to the real and permanent success of women in medicine. Isolated groups of women cannot maintain the same intellectual standards as are established and maintained by men."

In her inaugural address at the opening of the Woman's Medical College of the New York Infirmary on October 1, 1880, Jacobi explained to her students what it took to be a practicing physician. She vividly described an individual case of a fractured skull from beginning to end to illustrate her point about the strength of education needed to be a doctor. She knew her audience well and used precise yet dramatic language to tell a thrilling story. Each student could imagine herself as the doctor tending the patient.

"The physician is summoned in haste, and learns that an hour previously the patient had fallen from a scaffolding to the street; had been picked up unconscious, and brought home in the same state, that shortly after reaching home he had vomited. . . . The physician finds the patient in bed, motionless and insensible. His eyes are closed, but if the lids be raised the pupils will be found to contract, perhaps sluggishly, to the light, and the lids quiver more or less if the conjunctiva is tickled. The breathing is slow and rather labored, and at each respiration the cheeks puff out as if the man were forcibly smoking a pipe. Perhaps from time to time one of the arms is raised and moved convulsively backwards and forwards, then falls again. The face is pale, but when the doctor lays his finger on the pulse he finds no sign of exhaustion, the pulse is full and hard, and rather slow. He will notice that the clothes are wet with urine."

Jacobi described the head wound and how to examine it and how the physician was not required to make a diagnosis because it was a clear case of a fractured skull. Even so, the amount of expert knowledge required to care for the patient was breathtaking.

"But, before the physician can understand either the extent or the consequence of this injury, he must be extremely familiar with the anatomy of the injured region." She listed every detail the doctor must know in order to perform a complete examination. In addition to anatomy, the doctor must understand physiology, the science of the functions of the body's organs.

"I have spoken of the clear fluid running from the patient's ear. To the uninitiated this would seem to be of much less importance than the blood which matted his hair. But the physician sees in it a symptom of very serious import, he knows that it is a sign of the fracture of a certain portion of the base of the skull, and foretells almost certain death."

After demonstrating the complex process of patient care, Jacobi encouraged her students to gain a foothold on the "broad, intellectual basis of general medicine." She asked them to look at themselves "as a colony just landed in a new country; compelled to found a state in spite of hardship, and peril, and danger, and isolation, by means of the vigorous and intelligent co-operation of each of its members. . . . This is the austere, self-denying, intelligent heroism, which is needed for our enterprise—for this also still deserves to be called heroic."

Six months after the women submitted their proposal, in April 1882, each of them received a letter with Harvard's spineless reply.

Dear Madam:
I have the honor to enclose a copy of a vote recently passed by the President and Fellows of Harvard College, in relation to the Medical Education of Women in Harvard University.
Yours very respectfully,
E. W. Hooper, Secy.

At a meeting of the President and Fellows of Harvard College in Boston, April 24, 1882.
Upon the question of accepting the proposal contained in the communication received by this Board on September 26, 1881 . . . in relation to the medical education of women in Harvard University.
Voted, that while the President and Fellows of Harvard College recognize the importance of thorough medical education for women they do not

find themselves able to accept the proposal contained in the communication above referred to.

A true copy of Record

Attest: E. W. Hooper, Secy.

Jacobi and her colleagues felt betrayed by Eliot's shallow promises. Yet Eliot himself was in trouble. Rumors spread that Harvard's governing board was looking for his replacement. Intent on protecting his own position, Eliot had decided to jettison the hated woman's issue. Even so, a final, desperate effort was made the following year when Henry Bowditch, himself a Harvard graduate, approached the faculty with a plan to use the recently vacated old medical building as a separate women's medical college with a separate faculty that would provide an identical education so that women could be awarded a Harvard medical degree.

Bowditch's proposal was rejected. This would be the last time for decades that the esteemed university considered admitting women to its medical school.

～

After losing the Harvard proposal, Jacobi turned to her thriving career, choosing to ignore the growing turbulence between herself and her husband. She and Abraham were raising a charming son and an adorable daughter who spent glorious days playing with their growing tribe of cousins supplied by Jacobi's numerous younger brothers and sisters. The family also spent long summers on the island at Lake George and busy working months in their big house in the city, where Abraham's monthly medical association meetings were attended by New York's leading physicians.

Both doctors had a tremendous capacity for work. Together, they campaigned for raising the standards of medical education, including postgraduate study. In 1882, the New York University Medical College founded the New York Post-Graduate Medical School, where Jacobi lectured on children's diseases. This teaching job was in addition to her regular duties at the New York Infirmary and its college and her private practice. She was quickly becoming one of the most popular physicians in New York.

Abraham remained at the forefront of pediatric medicine. He was famous for his achievements in infant nutrition, which included advocating for breastfeeding and nontoxic breast-milk substitutes. After Louis Pasteur had established a way to safely pasteurize milk in 1865, Abraham told parents to boil milk until bubbles appeared. Raw milk was dangerous. His recommendation to boil milk probably saved more lives than any measure at the time besides antibiotics. In 1880, he founded the pediatric division of the American Medical Association, cementing his reputation as the father of children's medicine.

The tributes Abraham received delighted Jacobi and brought recognition to her family. She and Abraham were known as the "first family of medicine." Jacobi began making plans for their time away at the lake in July and August, where they would celebrate their tenth anniversary and her forty-first birthday.

Immersing herself in the happiness she had found, she called the previous ten years of her life the "Golden Decade." According to Jacobi, "the prize of life" was not the constant striving for heaven but the development of her earthly intellect to the greatest extent possible. When declaring what she wanted from life, she wrote, "Everything that the experience of thousands of years shows that it has in store for us."

But during the past months, her dreams had been threatened by a more mundane reality. Jacobi loved having an equal partner in Abraham, someone she could go to for advice and sympathy who also valued being part of a thriving community of professionals. Their collaboration on *Infant Diet* had proved stimulating as well as lucrative.

Yet he was older and taciturn; she had an ebullient personality. She thrived on making connections with sympathetic friends and sharing her ideas with them. This ability was her superpower. Attending dinner parties and festive celebrations made her feel more enthusiastic about life, especially when she met interesting new people to connect with. Abraham, at age fifty-three, liked the familiarity of his study. After hours alone, he would emerge fully charged and ready to accompany Jacobi to medical events or family gatherings. Their complementary personalities had been the basis for their strong attraction and successful marriage. But now it was causing them to grow apart.

Abraham's best friend since childhood, Carl Schurz, a German statesman and journalist, had recently moved to New York. Like Abraham, Schurz was a revolutionary who had jumped into politics soon after immigrating to America in 1852. He campaigned forcefully for Abraham Lincoln, who subsequently appointed him minister to Spain in 1861. After the Civil War broke out, Schurz resigned his post and returned home to serve in the Union army. Even though Schurz was not a trained military man, Lincoln appointed him brigadier general and later major general. After the war, Schurz was hired as an editor at the *New-York Tribune*, then the *Detroit Post*, and, finally, the *St. Louis Post*. In 1869, Missouri elected him to the U.S. Senate, the first German immigrant to attain that position. After Rutherford B. Hayes won the 1876 presidential election, he appointed Schurz secretary of the interior.

Schurz and Abraham kept in touch, seeing each other occasionally when Schurz visited New York. After Hayes left office, in 1881, Schurz moved to New York permanently and became part of the management team of the *New York Evening Post* and *The Nation*. Abraham celebrated his good fortune when he heard that his best friend was coming to live in New York. They soon became inseparable, fighting for civil rights and political reform, writing drafts together, attending the same political meetings, and eventually becoming summertime neighbors after Abraham built Schurz a house at Lake George.

In the meantime, Mary and Abraham stopped collaborating and drifted apart. She adapted to the situation, of course, because it was in her nature. But something was lost between the two that could not be regained. Perhaps she was jealous. Schurz, who had impressed Abraham Lincoln enough to be put in charge of an army, was so much like Mary Putnam Jacobi in temperament—outgoing, charming, and full of optimistic energy—that people began to gossip about their similarities. But what disappointed her most was her realization that Abraham, like so many husbands, preferred his male companions to his wife.

On the night of Carl Schurz's fifty-fourth birthday celebration, Mary arrived home after work elated that she and Abraham were invited to mingle with Schurz's well-known associates. Abraham was working late, so she changed her clothes, organized their gifts, then waited for him to get home. After a few minutes, she could not wait any longer. She instructed the children's nurse to tell Abraham that she would meet him at the party. When Abraham got home and found that Mary had left, he became angry and refused to go himself. He ate supper with the children and went to bed.

The next day, Mary and Abraham left for work without seeing each other. At supper that evening, when Mary sat down to eat with her family and asked Abraham about his day, he pressed his lips together and refused to speak. Perturbed, Mary asked him what was wrong. Abraham looked at her as if she were one of the children. You should not have gone last night, he told her. Mary stopped eating and put down her fork. Why not? she asked. Carl is my oldest friend, he told Mary. Someone needed to stay with the children. It should have been you.

Mary pointed out that their full-time nurse could have taken care of the children. Abraham said that Mary was the mother, and it was her job to care for the children. She was the one being unreasonable.

He might as well have said that he was sending her to prison. Her face turned red with anger. She rose from the table and, without saying a word, packed a bag and marched out the front door. A few days later, Abraham received a letter saying that she was staying with a friend, most likely Victoria White, her colleague and collaborator. He immediately returned the letter to her, saying that she could "speak but not write." After describing his own account of the quarrel, he said he wished that they could find some way to work out a peaceful coexistence or, as Abraham described it, "a quiet and rational *modus vivendi*." He told her that if she had more patience and less arrogance, she would remember everything that he had done for her career. That alone should have caused her to give in to his wishes and show him the appreciation he deserved. He complained that Mary stubbornly lived by her own decisions, and her actions only made him angry. When it sounded like he would never give in, he finally gave her an out.

"You will find that I shall not show you by sign or word that I bear you a grudge for this hasty step of yours," he wrote. If she came home, he would not "mention it at all and the children will be glad to see you though childlike they do not miss you."

Shortly after receiving his letter, Mary went home, and Abraham kept his word and said nothing more about her behavior. Yet the essence of their quarrel continued to haunt their marriage. It was always there in the background. Abraham expected her to be more attentive to their children. Mary, a scientist at the forefront of medical research, could not abandon her vision. What Abraham saw as a peaceful coexistence, Mary saw as utter confinement.

Toward the end of May in 1883, Mary and her two children went to the dock to bid farewell to her mother, Victorine, who was sailing to Europe for the summer. On the way, Ernst complained about the terrible heat and wished he could sail his own boat on the cool waters of Lake George. He was looking forward to their annual visit, when his family would celebrate his eighth birthday, making him three years older than little Marjorie. Hurrying to keep up, Marjorie kept asking Ernst if they would see any trains.

Trains were not important today, he informed his sister, reminding her that they were going to see a boat that carried hundreds of people across the ocean for days and days with no land in sight. Then Marjorie complained that she was tired and needed to rest.

The next morning, both children had fevers and sore throats. Mary kept them in bed, and Abraham took their temperatures. The thermometer read 102 degrees. They had runny noses and swollen glands. Mary and Abraham grew sick with worry.

Abraham soon diagnosed both Ernst and Marjorie with diphtheria, an acute bacterial infection spread by personal contact. It was the most feared of all childhood diseases, especially for children under five, like Marjorie. Ernst's parents thought that he was past the danger because of his age. They were wrong.

All patients with diphtheria were cared for in their homes. No hospital on Manhattan Island would admit anyone with an infectious disease like diphtheria, scarlet fever, or even measles. In fact, if a case arose in a patient already admitted to one of the large hospitals, the patient was removed and the entire hospital was thoroughly scrubbed and disinfected.

Diphtheria puzzled physicians. Considered to be a poor person's disease because experts argued it was caused by unsanitary conditions in the homes, treatments included broths, gruels, warm baths, and willow bark for the fever. There was no cure. As the disease progressed, patients developed pasty-white membranes in their throats that could grow large enough to constrict their breathing and suffocate them. Abraham treated diphtheric croup with intubation—the passage of a tube down the throat to help the patient breathe. One of the nation's leading experts on the disease, Abraham had published *Treatise on Diphtheria* in 1880, which explained how to prevent, identify, and treat the disease. Because of Abraham's expertise, Mary let him take the lead in caring for their children.

Both Ernst and Marjorie became very ill, but Mary worried more about her son. She saw his pallor, debilitating weakness, rising fever, and worsening cough. In her view, a more intensive course of action was needed to increase the boy's power of resistance. Her recommendations might have included applying glycerin and salicylic acid to disinfect the upper respiratory tract and using calomel or boric and phenolic acid added to water to dislodge the membrane. Perhaps she wanted to intubate Ernst right away. When she approached Abraham with her counsel, he would not listen. Even though Mary believed that he was making his decision based on emotion and outdated science, she followed his instructions for care.

While Mary and Abraham agreed that science was the foundation of medicine, because of the timing of their training and experience, they meant different things by *science*. Abraham was a member of the group of European physicians influenced by the physiological and pathological studies conducted at midcentury. They valued physician assessment over laboratory research and believed that knowledge of pathology and proper application of therapeutic principles would cure patients, not experiments in laboratories. The human organism "is not a test tube," Abraham wrote.

Mary thought differently. Trained almost two decades later, she had complete faith in laboratory data. She was a leading proponent of vivisection and evidence-based practice and would often bring the results she found experimenting on animals in her laboratory to therapeutic use. She also fully believed in the new science of bacteriology recently popularized when Louis Pasteur succeeded in immunizing sheep and cows against anthrax.

At the forefront of laboratory science, Mary was well on her way to being publicly recognized as a pioneer in applying microscopic and chemical analysis to the treatment of patients. While she never pursued significant bacterial research herself, she urged one of her brightest postdoctoral students, Anna Wessel Williams, to obtain a position with William Park, the bacteriologist and director of the New York City public-health laboratory who made bacteriology an important aspect of diagnostic and preventive medicine in America. A decade later, Williams would discover what became known as the Park-Williams strain of diphtheria bacteria, from which a much more effective antitoxin was derived.

Unlike Mary, Abraham believed that new claims about bacterial agents symbolized an ominous new trend in scientific inquiry; he called it "bacteriomania."

"Any young man can look through a microscope," he said. While Abraham understood that diphtheria was highly contagious, he did not accept that a simple bacterium was its sole cause. He focused on the pathology—how the symptoms developed—and rejected the "no bacteria, no diphtheria" dictum. Mary strongly disagreed, which caused an even greater rift between the two physicians and explained why Abraham would not listen to her words of apprehension about Ernst.

Abraham thought that his only son would naturally weather the storm. But soon, Ernst developed a barking, croupy cough and struggled even harder to breathe. Abraham then performed the necessary intubation. But nothing could save the child. In his final hours, his heart beat too fast, then sporadically, and finally, it just stopped.

On June 12, 1883, the following notice appeared in *The New York Times*:

Died: Jacobi, Ernst, of number 110 West 34 Street, on Sunday June 10, age 7 years 10 months and 7 days.

Little Marjorie, however, recovered fully. When she discovered her brother was gone, she asked for him over and over, tears streaming down her face, until her grieving mother silenced her: "Do not ask for him anymore, he has left us and will not return." It was heartbreaking.

Abraham was so devastated that he could hardly put one foot in front of the other. He could not accept that his beloved son had died from a disease that he had spent years fighting. While Mary cared for Marjorie during her recovery, she also cared for Abraham. His tremendous grief overshadowed hers, as she later told close friends: "The loss of this darling boy has been so overwhelmingly terrible to the doctor, that I have scarcely dared to think of myself. You could imagine what the loss of any son must be to him—after he had waited so long for one."

The Jacobis buried Ernst with Abraham's other wives and children at Green-Wood Cemetery in Brooklyn, near a large gravestone marked THE BABIES. On Hiawatha Island, where Ernst was born, close to the shore on the north end of the island, Abraham erected a five-ton granite monument to his son that read:

ERNST JACOBI.
BORN ON HIAWATHA ISLAND. AUGUST 3rd, 1875.
DIED IN NEW YORK. JUNE 10th, 1883.

Abraham continued to suffer in silence. But Mary brandished her grief for all to see. Each day, every hour, she relived the decision she had made about his care, punishing herself for not being able to save him. "This rooted feeling of self contempt . . . helps me to bear this terrible grief, though in other ways it makes it worse," she wrote to a friend.

Mary had come to firmly believe that her recommendations would have saved her son's life. Thinking about it made her sick. She wished that she had more strongly questioned her husband's authority and now blamed herself for Ernst's death. Because of her understanding of bacteriology, she also lamented that she and Abraham had not taken more protective measures in the first place, recognizing that their wealth and status did not make their children immune from disease.

In 1883, just months after Ernst's death, Friedrich Loeffler, a German bacteriologist, discovered the bacteria that caused diphtheria. He was able to grow the microbe in his laboratory and subsequently infect guinea pigs, rabbits, and other test animals with his lab-grown cultures. Five years later, other German scientists developed an antitoxin from the bacteria that was used to alleviate symptoms and reduce deaths from the disease. These discoveries about the etiology and transmission of diphtheria worsened the fault line between Mary and Abraham that would, ultimately, never heal. They blamed each other for their son's death, Mary because Abraham would not listen to her therapeutic recommendations, and Abraham because Mary, the famous doctor, was too busy to protect her son. He continued to resist universal bacteriological explanations and named the real "scourge of the community" to be those with mild cases of diphtheria who ignored their symptoms and continued to move about the city. Several years later, he wrote a paper titled "Diphtheria Spread by Adults" in which he stated that "spontaneous" cases of diphtheria were due not to unsanitary conditions like moist walls or faulty drains but to sore throats in adults not sufficiently ill to be confined to bed yet ill enough to spread contagion.

Abraham's contagion theory certainly partially explained the spread of diphtheria. But he used this explanation to exonerate himself and other wealthy parents from bearing any responsibility for their children's deaths. Despite his Marxist beliefs, Abraham was a member of the city's professional class and educated elite, so he accused domestic servants, who happened to be mostly women, of posing the greatest threat. Poor and working-class women's bodies could not be trusted. To save face, he publicly blamed his children's favorite nurse for spreading the disease and sent her back to Germany.

But the reality behind Ernst's death might have been much darker. When Abraham performed the intubations or tracheotomies to save other children, their fluids would spatter onto him, and, like the ignorant surgeons carrying disease from patient to patient in operating rooms, Abraham did not change his clothes or make any extra effort to clean himself afterward. He made the old-fashioned assumption that physicians had "a certain degree of both active and passive immunity." Throughout his life, he would never admit that he could have been the cause of his son's demise.

Abraham never recovered. After losing a promising boy like Ernst, he did not *want* to recover, turning away from his wife and family and suffering alone. Only his good friend Schurz could help him find the hope and humor in life again. Mary, however, faced her pain openly so that, eventually, she could salvage her capacity for happiness, for Marjorie's sake. The child emerged from the trauma of her own illness to a world without her big brother and her beloved nurse and with a father whom she was a little afraid of. For that reason, Mary kept her daughter close. When she was not in school, Marjorie accompanied Mary to work, association meetings, and other public gatherings, including meetings about the fight for a woman's right to vote.

As tensions strained her partnership at home, Mary Putnam Jacobi turned to women's suffrage and found a family of activists waiting. Ironically, she had been indifferent about suffrage for years, not publicly denouncing it but not endorsing it either. Women's education and work in the professions were bigger priorities for her because she believed that they could provide the true means for gender equality. But at this stage, science and suffrage became inseparable. She now considered "the real basis of democracy, republicanism and justice" equality among human beings. When women were denied the vote and full political participation, they were also prevented from being fulfilled and complete human beings. Jacobi believed this denial explained a "large share of . . . the physical ill health of women, not to speak of [their] moral unhappiness."

In 1885, in an article in the *Woman's Journal*, she vowed her support for women's enfranchisement: "Please count me henceforth among those who believe in woman suffrage." Besides the idea that women's full participation in society led to a healthier democracy, she was forging a life without her husband at her side. A year later, Jacobi achieved one of her highest goals: she became the first woman to enter the New York Academy of Medicine.

The Agony of Her Mind

DESPITE JACOBI'S CRUSADE EXPOSING MITCHELL'S REST CURE AS ineffectual and potentially harmful, patients continued to flock to his clinic, making him rich and famous. The honors he won in toxicology, neurology, and biology were too numerous to count. Throughout Europe, his cure was gaining in popularity. His peers had elected him president of the College of Physicians of Philadelphia. A top-rated literary physician, Mitchell wrote poetry and novels that were bestsellers because of their "wholesomeness." Newspaper editors, biographers, and historians referred to him as a First Citizen of America.

Of course, Mitchell had been catapulted forward in life by his marriage to the heiress Mary Cadwalader, a member of one of Philadelphia's oldest and wealthiest families. Her fortune was the reason they could afford their mansion on Walnut Street. Still, he owed his celebrity to the lives of sick women, and many of them certainly admired his work and were grateful. But as he would soon learn, not all women would succumb to his powers of healing.

Each morning when he arrived at the Philadelphia Orthopedic Hospital, the nurses lined up to greet him and, after he had passed, quietly gushed over his lordly manner and handsome face. Predictably, his vanity and arrogance had grown with his fame. Since Mitchell had taken over running the hospital in 1871, it had expanded from a two-room clinic to a sprawling health-care facility with wards, thirty-six private rooms, and modern facilities located at the corner of Seventeenth and Summer Streets in Philadelphia.

Hanging on the wall outside his office were several before-and-after portraits of some of his patients, women who, upon arrival at the clinic, looked skeletal and appeared to be approaching death but who, after weeks of his rest cure, were fattened up with rosy cheeks and sparkling eyes. The differences between the before photographs and the after photographs were so startling that visitors sometimes gaped at them for several minutes.

In his practice, Mitchell treated patients who were in the worst health. One young girl vomited all her food and had bowel movements only once every ten days. The "wretched, wilted, starved creature" followed his movements with attentive eyes, "although she never turned her head." Another young girl kept her eyes constantly closed and could not eat before nine p.m. She was "a queer little shriveled creature, tawny of tint, and the skin covered with bran-like scales, washing being a rare ceremony." Her thin legs and arms were drawn up and hid her "cunning little visage, which seemed so blind with its closed but quivering lids, and yet so unnaturally astute in its intentness of attention when her own case was mentioned or discussed." These women seemed barely human, and Mitchell had made some of them whole again.

These success stories helped him attract a cult of followers. Former patients, aspiring patients, and their husbands plied Mitchell with gifts and admiring letters. His name had become legendary among the wealthy and middle class. Blessed with a never-ending supply of anxious women, Mitchell had perfected his brand of authoritative healing.

In his office, Mitchell displayed his medical degree plus an honorary law doctorate that he had lately received from Harvard. In fact, he had gotten so many honorary degrees from universities around the world that he had no room to display them all. His secretary had organized file cabinets that were filled with these honors plus thick folders full of the fan mail and small gifts he received from hundreds of patients and admirers.

His office at the hospital, however, was Spartan compared to the large, elegant study at home. Family portraits by famous artists lined the walls. All of his important papers, coins, and some extra cash were stored in a tasteful safe. Along a mantelpiece and on the tops of bookshelves were items from his large collection of antique porcelain and glass vases. But the room's centerpiece was a striking chandelier with twelve arms made from cut crystal that hung over his ornate claw-foot Chippendale desk and reflected like glowing icicles in the enormous mirror over the fireplace across the room. Finely crafted chairs and recliners that he had collected on his many European adventures were arranged strategically throughout the room. The bookshelves contained his medical books, novels, and poetry.

The most prominent of his books was *The Hill of Stones*, a volume of poetry recently published by Houghton, Mifflin and Company featuring his
famous poem of the same name. Written in blank verse and eleven pages
long, it told the metaphorical origin story of the rocky formations around
Fontainebleau Forest near Paris. The poem described the outward world
of the heroic king and his court and the hidden realm of the forest maid-
ens, who were happy to live in nature with their "Diana-like queen." Even
though the self-sufficient forest women kept to themselves and harmed no
one, the king, his masculinity threatened, ordered his knights to capture
them. Just by existing, these independent, natural, and smart women who
held festive celebrations threatened the social order. The queen was the only
spirited and fearless character in the entire poem. She turned each knight
who attacked her women into stone. But eventually, one brave knight, clad
in white robes, subdued them all, and the queen and her women were
transformed into a "tumbled heap of dreary rocks." Subconsciously, Mitchell had written the perfect allegory for his rest cure and its intended effect
upon women.

On a day in late April 1887, he was waiting in his office for the arrival of
his next patient, twenty-six-year-old Charlotte Perkins Stetson, remarkable
only because her great-aunt was Harriet Beecher Stowe. At this point in his
career, Mitchell had seen hundreds of young women, but he always organized their problems under one of two categories:

1. selfishness and disobedience that led to malingering and hysteria
2. mental and physical overwork followed by exhaustion, breakdown, and
   finally hysteria

He had already placed Charlotte in the first group: a young, frivolous
woman who had flouted the rules of her sex and must now pay the price.
She was one of those Beecher women, after all, and since he had treated
two of them, he knew for a fact that they were overly arrogant and spoiled.
He was sure that Charlotte would prove to be an aggressive, dominating,
and manipulative woman who sought independence and self-fulfillment
over marriage and family. She deserved little sympathy. In fact, she was one
of the lucky ones. Mitchell was the only doctor in the world who could help
her. This knowledge always left him calm and self-assured.

Preparing for Charlotte's initial physiological assessment, he set out his stethoscope, thermometer, and stopwatch for recording her pulse. Then he straightened his broad shoulders, sat tall in his chair, and waited.

Charlotte Perkins Stetson always felt better when she traveled away from her husband and child, and riding the train from Providence to Philadelphia had lifted her spirits. But now, entering Mitchell's five-story hospital and being directed to the private wing for rest-cure patients, she felt the shadows coming back. Somehow, the place seemed eerily confining. A stout nurse and a young orderly were helping with her things. As they walked along, the nurse explained that Charlotte would not need many day clothes, only those for a long stay in bed.

The nurse, who irritatingly reminded Charlotte of her mother, assured her that Dr. Mitchell was like an angel from heaven. Full of divine light, he would guide her out of the darkness of hysteria and back to health, but only if she followed his rules. Charlotte glanced sideways at the nurse and tried not to look ungrateful. She had read about Mitchell's practice and hoped for the best outcome. She, like most of the women who attended the clinic, was at the end of her rope.

Finally, the nurse dropped her off at Mitchell's office door and hurried back to work. Charlotte stared at the before-and-after pictures of the sick women. They seemed off and somewhat disquieting, like an exhibit at a circus freak show. But then, she felt like a freak, and she realized that here was where she belonged. She hoped that she could be healed, but it would be a difficult journey. She was not surprised. Her life had been full of strife and sadness up until this point.

Not long after Charlotte was born, her father abandoned his family. She was her mother's third child and one of two who survived. She had an older brother, Thomas. Apparently, the doctor told her mother that she would die if she tried to have another child, and upon hearing that news, Frederick Beecher Perkins left home. He did occasionally visit. Once, he brought Charlotte some black Hamburg grapes and her older brother a gun. His most lasting gift to Charlotte was a childhood spent in poverty living as an outcast sponging off other family members. There was a wide selection of relatives to choose from. Her great-grandfather was the Congregational pastor Lyman Beecher, and her great-aunts were Catherine Beecher and Harriet Beecher Stowe. Out of a sense of shame, her father's family marginalized her. She never got the education she yearned for, but she did inherit her father's tendency to run away from domestic life.

As a young girl, influenced by the popularity of her Beecher aunts, she decided to devote her life to social reform. She was an avid reader and studied anatomy, physiology, geology, and history. She also had a knack for drawing and earned money by selling her illustrations. To control her innate desire for nonconformity, at the age of fifteen, she started putting strict self-discipline into practice, including hard exercise. She took calisthenics and hygiene classes at the Providence Ladies Sanitary Gymnasium, often performing for her family and friends. Her workouts included running a mile, vaulting, jumping, climbing a knotted rope, walking on her hands, and gliding easily through the traveling rings. At age nineteen, while visiting the gym twice a week and running one mile each day, she began attending the newly opened Rhode Island School of Design. Her mother objected, but her father agreed to pay the fees. She even got her mother to make the following commitment:

I, Mary Perkins, do hereby agree . . . never to badger my beloved and obedient daughter on the subject of going to Art School, having given my full and free consent to her so doing.

At this time, Charlotte became more involved in the women's movement. She corresponded with Alice Stone Blackwell, assistant editor of the *Woman's Journal*, and they became friends. Her poetry and drawings were accepted for publication. Her first poem, "In Duty Bound," was published in December 1883.

Charlotte had not given much thought to getting married. But the charming and handsome bohemian artist Walter Stetson brazenly proposed marriage a mere three weeks after they met. He was drawn to her innocence, beauty, and straightforward way of speaking. He loved everything that was chaste in her. Even though he had a lusty reputation with impure women that he would never marry, he worshipped Charlotte as a goddess. Despite his youthful romanticism and artistic talent, it was obvious to everyone but Charlotte that he wanted a conventional marriage with a domestic wife who placed him at the center of her universe. Going against her mother's wishes, she resisted his proposal. Yet he was sweetly persistent and repeated his proposal for two years until she finally said yes.

For a few months, they lived a happy and busy married life. Stetson was an affectionate and attentive husband, helping with the cooking, cleaning, and shopping. Then Charlotte became pregnant and experienced severe morning sickness that continued throughout her pregnancy. Before giving birth, she wrote in her diary that she was "hysterical" on two occasions. Although she made every effort to enjoy being pregnant and appreciate her family and friends, she grew more and more ill. Nevertheless, a healthy daughter, Katharine Beecher Stetson, was born on March 23, 1885. After giving birth, Charlotte fell into a deep depression. She had everything that she was supposed to want: a loving husband, a healthy baby, a lovely home, and even a servant. Yet, Charlotte wrote, "I lay all day on the lounge and cried." A nurse tended the baby.

Charlotte remained depressed, needy, and vulnerable for two years. "Every morning the same hopeless waking," she wrote in her diary. "Retreat impossible, escape impossible." Moreover, she blamed herself. Her mother continually informed her daughter that she must stop being lazy and learn to bear it. The only time she felt normal was during travels away from home. Finally, the crying fits, frenzy, and physical exhaustion made it clear to her husband and mother that she needed help. A friend offered her one hundred dollars for travel expenses to seek help from the famous nerve doctor in Philadelphia. Before leaving, she wrote a lengthy letter to Mitchell describing her symptoms and expressing her respect for him as "the first authority on nervous disease."

"Dear Sir," she began:

I write this for you, fearing that I shall soon be unable to remember even this much. . . . My desire is to make you acquainted with all the facts of the case, that you may form a deeper judgement than from mere casual examination. To cure disease says Dr. [Oliver Wendell] Holmes, we must begin with the grandfathers. Here are mine.

After a brief description of her grandparents, she wrote the following about her parents:

Mother.

A sickly and delicate child, overdosed and petted. Abnormally affectionate and conscientious. Given up to die with consumption three times, but still lives. An intellect large in some directions but singularly limited in others. Highly talented in music but no perception of art or poetry. A deep thinker, but absolutely illogical. Is in every way an exaggerated type of the so called "feminine" qualities, love of husband home and children being almost manias. Highly religious.

My father.

Highly eccentric. Of a benevolent and reformatory disposition at first, but grew more solitary and morose with years. Brilliant intellect, an author, editor, librarian, etc. Also musical. Has not a superior in the county for general information. Had several love affairs but broke them off, one on the very eve of marriage. Finally married. Took separate rooms when the children came, could not be broken of his rest. Left his family after three years and has since lived alone. Boarded with a well loved sister awhile, but could not bear even such restraint, and returned to his room. Has neglected his wife who procured divorce. Neglected his children. Would take money his family needed to buy some precious book. Fine physique as a young man, but delicate lungs. Large brain, susceptible nerves, small moral sense. Very reserved and proud.

Charlotte's letter revealed her deepest fears about herself.

"Before marriage I had a very cheerful disposition, notably so," she wrote:

This agony of mind set in with the child's coming. I nursed her in slow tears. All that summer I did nothing but cry, save for times when the pain was unbearable and I grew wild, hysterical, almost imbecile at times. Late in 1885 I made a wild determination, weaned the child, borrowed money, and started to visit friends in California. Spent the winter there, getting perfectly well I thought. Came home in March. Had bronchitis six weeks and before that was over relapsed into the previous year's condition. . . . And there are mental symptoms, which alarm me seriously. . . . I beg of you not to laugh at me as every one else does. . . . I am an artist of sufficient merit to earn an easy living when well. I am a writer, a poet, a philosopher, in little. I am a teacher by instinct and profession. I am a reader and thinker. I can do some good work for the world if I live. I cannot bear to die or go insane or linger on [in] this wretched invalid existence, and be weight on this poor world which has so many now. I want to work, to help people, to do good. . . . There is something the matter with my head. No one here knows or believes or cares. . . . It is harder to write every day. I have given up my newspaper work little as it was. I can't think, I can't remember, I can't grasp an idea. But I could once. I shall have a fine night after writing this, but I fear every day to lose memory entirely. And maybe you can help me.

While she was gazing at the before-and-after pictures on the wall out-side of Mitchell's office, he appeared at his office door and escorted her inside. Without asking her how she felt, he promised her a "positive cure," provided that she gave up all control and life concerns to him. He wanted to make clear that, as her doctor, he was in complete control and that her feelings, questions, and worries did not matter. Charlotte nodded to indi-cate that she understood. Here was the great doctor, a formidable genius, and she would listen to him and get better.

Next, he said that he would assess her condition and then she could go settle into her room at the clinic. He quickly took her pulse, tempera-ture, height, weight. She was not as skeletal-looking as the women in the pictures, but she lacked much appetite. He told her that he wanted to encourage the disappearance of her angles and introduce more rounding curves. She may have wondered, like other women did, if Mitchell was going to take her picture. But he did not. After he finished his examina-tion, he sat at his desk and told her that she had neurasthenia, a very curable mental disease.

At his words, Charlotte felt great relief and relaxed into her chair. The torment she had suffered for years was made worse by well-meaning friends and family members who could not understand her pain and kept telling her to take care of the baby, attend to her household, and soothe her husband. In other words, they did not believe that she was sick. Mitchell told her that she had reached a state of "cerebral exhaustion." For many pa-tients, this statement alone, acknowledging the legitimacy of their ailments, restored their self-confidence and helped them recover.

Charlotte asked Mitchell if he had gotten her letter describing her symp-toms and the history of her condition and that, perhaps, her words would help him with his cure. His reaction shocked her. He said that he found the letter utterly useless. Moreover, the fact that she should imagine her obser-vations would be of any interest to him was an indication of her arrogance. Stunned, Charlotte left his office quietly with her nurse escort.

The next few weeks passed slowly. Once she was put to bed, fed the milk by comforting nurses, forced to eat endless amounts of raw beef soup and a diet full of fat and calories, rubbed, and electrified, she felt much fatter and a little better. After a while, even with the milk-drinking, she had trouble sleeping. Without any outside stimulation—reading, writing, or talking with friends—she became lost in daydreaming. She missed her daughter but still hated her mother. She wanted to sketch the amiable but dull-witted nurse who smiled with congratulations whenever Charlotte cleaned her plate. Apparently, they had to force-feed other patients.

As the days went by, the room seemed smaller. The white hospital walls inched closer to the bed, and the gray shadows in the corners of the room grew longer. During the hours of being immobile and alone, she might have wondered who else had rested in this bed. Hundreds of women had passed through these rooms, all in some state of need.

Mitchell, who visited with her at least once a day, started to become her adversary. Their conversations were boring, confusing, irritating, and provoking. He would be the kindly doctor one minute and a scolding brute the next. If she made a statement, he would interrupt and then contradict her. She began to lose confidence and perhaps started using the word *personally* to begin each sentence: "Personally, I think that" and so on.

Once she was fattened up, Mitchell began her "moral reeducation," which taught her how to keep her emotions under control. He told her that women should not share their feelings with others. It was a bad habit that only made matters worse and always bored their listeners—usually their husbands. To counteract women's emotional shortcomings, Mitchell encouraged order, control, and self-restraint. A woman should schedule every minute of every day, including sleep and leisure time. There was no place in the modern household for expressing feelings, spontaneity, or whimsy. Aspirations that threatened the tranquility of domestic life no longer constituted a threat; they were controlled and suppressed. Since her behavior was entirely dictated by rules established by her all-knowing doctor, she did not have to take any responsibility for her life. Mitchell's "reeducation" was a master class in sublimation.

But in Charlotte's case, the simplicity of her response stumped Mitchell. She seemed insincere. In reality, he could not see what she was thinking, and that frustrated him. However, she did not stay the normal six to eight weeks. After a month, Mitchell pronounced her cured and sent her home with these final instructions:

Live as domestic a life as possible. Have your child with you all the time. . . .
Lie down an hour after each meal. Have but two hours' intellectual life a day.
And never touch pen, brush or pencil as long as you live.

Mitchell gave this advice to a woman who was trained as a commercial artist and was beginning to forge a career as a writer. But because she had somewhat recovered, she returned home determined to follow his advice. For months afterward, she ignored her intellectual life, hid her papers and pens, and lived solely as wife and mother. She did this to feel better, but she continued to get worse.

During those months, the spectral image of Dr. Mitchell commanding her to behave haunted her subconscious. *Never touch pen, brush or pencil as long as you live.* His final words weighed her down like heavy chains and obliterated all hopes for a happy future. Inside, she was torn to pieces. She wanted to be well, to be good to her husband and daughter. But she yearned to pick up her brush or write a story. She had told everyone that the famous doctor had cured her. But in reality, trying to follow Mitchell's rules, Charlotte came perilously close to psychosis. She made a rag doll, hung it on a doorknob, and played with it like a child. She dreamed of traveling to Pasadena, California, to be with her best friend, Grace Channing. She tried to shop, cook, and clean. But her profound distress, fear, and paranoia grew, and she started crawling into closets and hunkering under beds, trying to get away from the overwhelming stress of obedience to Mitchell.

Finally, in the fall of 1887, Charlotte realized that she would not survive if she did not leave her self-created prison. She suddenly understood that the cultural demands placed on women by men like Mitchell were driving them mad. Making a profound effort toward self-preservation, she decided to "cast off" Dr. Mitchell and do exactly what she pleased. She and her husband separated—Walter very reluctantly. For the first time in her life, she openly defied the accepted rules of her world. A year later, with few marketable skills and little money, she took her toddler Katharine and went to California. Basking in the warmth of the sun on the West Coast, she began a new phase of her life.

∽

Throughout his career, Mitchell categorized his rest-cure patients as those who "recovered" and those who did not. There was no in between. In his black-and-white way of thinking, what took place at his clinics was more than healing. With each case, he was entering into a battle for the soul of a woman. Either the doctor reined in his patient's emotional desires and taught her how to exist in a masculine world or she was lost to the chaos of her feminine sentiment. For many women, he offered care and protection, a respite from the demands of an adult world, and a prescription for dealing with upsetting thoughts and desires. Rather than disappearing into hysteria, the Victorian woman could turn to her physician. If she followed his orders, she would be safe.

Mitchell's expertise arose from his knowledge of that shadowland called feminine will. He believed that he could see through the desires of almost every woman who entered his clinic and used that ability to manipulate her back into acceptance of her domestic role in life. He wrote that the woman who wanted to be helped would become the doctor's active ally, not a "passive fool." According to Mitchell, "the fools are to be dealt with by other moral drugs."

The Mitchell rest cure contained a complete pharmacopeia of "moral drugs" for stubborn women. For women who shirked their domestic duties, rest became imprisonment. A patient's continued obstinance called for retribution. Like the heroic knight in "The Hill of Stones," Mitchell retaliated with full force to destroy any inkling of her independence. If patients refused to eat, they were force-fed. The sponge baths, douches, and rectal enemas given by nurses became torment. In rare cases, Mitchell would spank her like a misbehaving child.

For Mitchell, there was no such thing as an independent woman. He literally could not imagine a woman being a successful doctor or lawyer. If women did succeed, it was only because they had stolen those powers from their fathers, brothers, or husbands. These beliefs left him with the constant dread of women gaining equality with men, ushering in eternal chaos. In this delusional state, he could not acknowledge that his rest cure had failed to help anyone. Difficult cases sometimes disappeared from his records, but not from history.

One of these cases was Jane Addams, who, in 1881, had started classes at the Woman's Medical College in Philadelphia. Shortly after her studies began, she realized that she was not suited for medicine and became very frustrated because she found little guidance or sympathy from her professors. For years, she had suffered from depression, and it grew worse while she was in medical school. In addition, she experienced pain from a curvature of the spine. A few weeks after the death of her beloved father, her depression and pain grew worse, and she entered Mitchell's hospital. He told her that her mental suffering, made worse by her spinal disease, was due to the stress of her education and diagnosed her with neurasthenia.

Jane was at the clinic for three months. The rest and constant massages temporarily alleviated her backache but did not improve her depression. She told Mitchell that she was not getting better and finally left the hospital of her own volition. Using her generous inheritance, she traveled to Europe to find her life's purpose. Along the way, she read Tolstoy's *My Religion* and learned how he had found meaning in living with the poor. In London, she visited the impoverished East End and Toynbee Hall, a settlement house where privileged college students lived and worked among the needy. These travels changed her life. She returned to America determined to make a difference.

In 1889, she cofounded Hull House in Chicago, which became famous for the settlement movement, social reform in low income, migrant neighborhoods that encouraged education and the alleviation of poverty. She became an important advocate for woman's suffrage and world peace and cofounder of the American Civil Liberties Union. Later in life, she became the first American women to be awarded the Nobel Peace Prize. It was fortunate for the world that she had not followed Mitchell's advice.

Mitchell never forgot Jane Addams and the failure of her case. In fact, not long after Jane established Hull House, he wrote a novel titled *Dr. North and His Friends,* about a beautiful hunchbacked girl who was always on the verge of depression and hysterical collapse. The other characters lamented that her intelligence would increase her disappointment because no man would marry a cripple. Dr. North claimed that she had been living in a world too stimulating for someone so "mentally eager and physically feeble." He then proceeded, over the next four hundred or so pages, to heroically restore her to health and happiness.

Charlotte and Jane had survived their encounter with Mitchell and gone on to better lives. Not all were so lucky. In 1888, Mitchell's good friend William Dean Howells, the renowned novelist and literary critic, sent his twenty-five-year-old daughter, Winifred, to Mitchell for care. Winifred had been a highly imaginative young woman and a good student and wrote delightful poetry. During her mid-teens, she experienced an illness that led to a mental breakdown. She started to lose weight. When orders to "eat, exercise, and be cheerful" failed, she was sent to a sanatorium. Over the next several years, she went through many different treatments, including several rounds of force-feeding and rest cures prescribed by other physicians, but she did not get better. Because she was openly emotional, very bright, and an avid reader who loved to write, her father concluded that she was highly susceptible to neurasthenia; she was overindulging her intellect and, as a result, weakening her feminine brain, which led to hypochondriacal delusions and extreme nervousness.

Howells's wife, Elinor, openly opposed his decision to put their daughter through yet another rest cure. But according to friends, Howells was exasperated by Winifred and decided she required some "bracing discipline with her therapy." Like Mitchell's most ardent fans, Howells believed without question in the doctor's methods. He told his father, "If you could once see Dr. Mitchell, you would see how he differed from all other specialists, and would not have a doubt but she was in the best and wisest and kindest hands in the world."

Because Winifred's case was extremely difficult, the cost to Howells was enormous, nearly two thousand dollars. When she arrived at the hospital in Philadelphia, she weighed fifty-seven pounds. As with his other patients, Mitchell gave her a thorough examination to rule out any organic illness. Once he declared the emaciated girl physically healthy, he began the same treatment that she had already received from other doctors—he would restore her physical strength through force-feeding and then treat the hysteria. He was determined to succeed where lesser men had failed.

But feeble Winifred proved to have a strong and sturdy will. From the outset of her treatment, she argued with Mitchell and told him that he was wrong, that something else was the cause of her illness. Over and over, she told him about her intense pain. He never listened. When she refused to eat, he began a brutal force-feeding regimen. He told her father about the regimen when they met for lunch in New York on November 30. Little Winny's condition was purely hysterical, he said, and would change when her body and brain were nourished. When Howells balked at the cruelty of the method, Mitchell assured him that as soon as Winny gave in to the treatment, which she surely would, she would begin to get better.

Because Winifred was not allowed any visitors, even family, Mitchell personally kept in touch with Howells about his daughter's condition. On

December 23, Mitchell lunched with Mr. and Mrs. Howells and told them enthusiastically that Winny had gained ten pounds. She was still very obstinate and complained often about her imaginary pain, but she did not "fight the feeding" anymore. On the whole, he was very hopeful.

On January 6, Mitchell reported that Winny was still very stubborn and had to, once again, be forced along the path to health with a very firm hand.

In late February, Mitchell moved Winifred to Merchantville, Pennsylvania, to one of his other treatment centers. He had established numerous clinics in and around Philadelphia, including "rest houses" managed by his employees trained in "nervous work."

Still being forced to eat, Winifred continued to weaken until, finally, her heart gave out. One week after she was transferred, she passed away. The death stunned Mitchell but did not surprise her father. Upon hearing the sad news from Mitchell, Howells wrote to his father, "I telegraphed you yesterday that our poor suffering girl had ceased to suffer. It was Saturday evening, at Merchantville, near Philadelphia, from a sudden failure of the heart."

Mitchell performed an autopsy on Winifred and discovered an "organic" ailment that caused her death. His diagnosis of her illness had been tragically wrong. After receiving the news from Mitchell, Howells replied that "the torment that remains is that perhaps the poor child's pain was all along as great as she fancied, if she was so diseased, as apparently she was." In other words, she had been telling the truth.

Even after this tragic event, Howells and Mitchell remained friends in public, but Howells must have suffered from his loss, since he had clearly loved his daughter. On June 7, he wrote Henry James, "You know perhaps the poor child was not with us when she died; she died homesick and wondering at her separation, in the care of the doctors who fancied they were curing her." And in a letter to Samuel Clemens, he wrote, "If she could have been allowed to read, I think the experiment might have succeeded."

There was never any investigation into Mitchell's treatment of Winifred. In fact, no record existed of her being admitted to his hospital, and all the case studies from that period mysteriously went missing. By sending her away to the facility in Merchantville, Mitchell hoped to finally break her will. She had become a small but relentless opponent. Instead of healing her, he gave her a terrible death.

～

Over the months, Charlotte's world had grown brighter. No matter what, she was now determined to live an unconventional life. After moving to California, she and her daughter, Katharine, lived with Charlotte's best friend, Grace Channing. Charlotte's husband, Walter, soon joined them. Slowly, over time, she encouraged a romantic relationship between her husband and her best friend. It worked! After she and Walter divorced, he married Grace, and Charlotte relinquished custody of Katharine to them. Charlotte reported in her memoir that she was happy for the couple, since Katharine's "second mother was fully as good as the first, [and perhaps] better in some ways."

Charlotte's career began to flourish. In 1890, she was able to give up her job as a saleswoman and make her living as a writer and public speaker, giving fiery lectures about the economic dilemma caused by women's dependence on men and stating that women should demand independence. She fought for social reform, and she continued to publish poems and essays in the *Woman's Journal*. But she still experienced a crushing depression at times, even while earning a living on her own. It was a darkness that had stalked her since giving birth to her daughter. She did not write in her journal for three years after undergoing the rest cure. Finally, one night, as the shadows grew closer, she began writing the autobiographical story that would cleanse the haunted remains of the treatment from her being and make her famous. She titled it "The Yellow Wall Paper."

The story was narrated by a young married woman suffering from a "nervous depression—a slight hysterical tendency" that her husband, John, a doctor, dismissed as "temporary." Like Mitchell, John was completely uninterested in his wife's assessment of her own condition. In order to "cure" her, John took his wife to the countryside for a "perfect rest." He rented a large, ramshackle, and isolated house. His wife asked if they could occupy the bedroom on the first floor that opened onto a piazza, but her husband chose the nursery on the second floor because there was room for two beds. Her bed was firmly nailed down, and though it sat near a window, there were bars on the window, and the walls were covered with hideous yellow wallpaper.

From the beginning, the young wife disagreed with her husband's

methods of confinement and constant rest. She believed that work and congenial company would be better for her. Yet she understood that there was
no escape from her situation, especially since her husband was a doctor:
"If a physician of high standing, and one's own husband, assures friends
and relatives that there is really nothing the matter but temporary nervous
depression—a slight hysterical tendency—what is one to do?"

Similar to Mitchell, her husband imposed a strictly regimented treatment: "I have a schedule prescription for each hour in the day," John told
her. Then he commanded her to not even think about her condition. His
sister, acting as Charlotte's nurse, watched over her constantly.

John "is very careful and loving, and hardly lets me stir without special
direction," the narrator commented. While he was gone all day to treat
other patients, she stayed in her bed, resting. "I'm really getting quite fond
of the big room, all but that horrid paper." But after days spent alone in the
room staring at the walls and through the bars of the window, she began to
feel worse. She pleaded with her husband to take her away, but he refused.
You're beginning to gain weight, he told her happily.

All day, every day, the young wife stared at the wallpaper, obsessing over
its ugly ornate patterns. She was starved of any other intellectual stimulation, so the wallpaper became a puzzle she had to solve. The narrator
positioned herself as an objective observer with a superior tone much like
Mitchell might use with a hysterical patient:

"It is dull enough to confuse the eye in following," she complained, "pronounced enough to constantly irritate and provoke study, and when you
follow the lame uncertain curves for a little distance they suddenly commit
suicide—plunge off at outrageous angles, destroy themselves in unheard-of
contradictions. . . . You think you have mastered it, but . . . it turns a back
somersault and . . . slaps you in the face, knocks you down and tramples on
you." She noted that the paper's "defiance of law . . . is a constant irritant to
a normal mind."

Frustrated by his wife's behavior, John threatened to send her to Mitchell
if she did not get well faster. This threat horrified her. John called her "his
darling and his comfort and all that he had," but he refused to listen to her
pleadings to leave the house and go back home. She was his "little girl." He
knew best.

As the treatment continued and her condition deteriorated, the obsessed
narrator grew increasingly threatened by the yellow wallpaper. There be-

gan to appear a "strange, provoking, formless sort of figure that seems to skulk about" within the paper itself. This figure looked like a woman. Then one day, the narrator noticed that many women were slithering like snakes behind the shapes in the wallpaper. The horror of the situation grew worse at night when John was there with her in the bed that was solidly nailed to the floor. In the dark, the pattern changed. It grew longer and straighter, resembling the bars on the room's windows, and the women in the wallpaper had become literally imprisoned.

She could not sleep. She never dreamed. All hope was lost. In a frantic attempt to escape her worsening situation, she began to scratch at the terrifying wallpaper, peeling it away to find "all those strangled heads and bulbous eyes and waddling fungus growths" that seemed like dead babies. She contemplated committing suicide but could not find anything to do it with and then decided that it would be wrong anyway. Her only remaining escape route was madness. Joining the creeping women, she began crawling in circles around the edges of the room, her shoulder always touching the wall so that she did not lose her way on her journey. As she crawled along the floor, she heard John at the locked door calling for her to open it. When she did not answer, he shouted for an ax to break it down.

"'John dear!' said I in the gentlest voice, 'the key is down by the front steps, under a plantain leaf!'"

After retrieving the key, he entered the room and, seeing the shattered condition of his wife, fainted to the floor. The story ended with her crawling over him and continuing on with the other creeping women around the room. They were freed from their wallpaper prison at last.

Charlotte felt elated but completely drained after writing her story. Never again would she attempt to write anything so personal. When the story was ready for publication, she mailed a copy to the famous author, editor, and literary critic who had recently become her mentor and champion: William Dean Howells, the father of Winifred and acquaintance of Mitchell. Charlotte never mentioned Winifred to her friends, and it is possible that she never knew about the young woman's tragic death.

Charlotte's first big break as an author had occurred a few months earlier when the *Nationalist* magazine published her poem "Similar Cases," a satirical review of people who resisted social change. Not long after its publication, Charlotte received a notable fan letter that changed her life:

DEAR MADAM,

I have been wishing ever since I first read it—and I've read it many times with unfailing joy—to thank you for your poem in the April *Nationalist*. We have had nothing since the Biglow Papers half so good for a good cause as "Similar Cases."

And just now I've read in *The Woman's Journal* your "Women of To-day." It is as good almost as the other, and dreadfully true.

Yours sincerely,

WM. DEAN HOWELLS

After Charlotte read the letter, waves of electric joy passed through her body. She had arrived. Having a mentor with the prestige and authority of Howells, a man who had been editor of *The Atlantic*, literary critic, and author of the Editor's Easy Chair column for *Harper's*, she finally felt like a real writer. Better yet, Howells was outspoken about the political rights of women and believed that they had the duties and therefore should also have the rights of citizens, including the right to vote. Even so, the genteel Howells mentoring the flamboyant Charlotte Perkins Stetson seemed like an improbable match.

When Howells received the "The Yellow Wall Paper," he forwarded it to his friend Horace Scudder, editor of *The Atlantic*, saying that it was a riveting piece of Gothic horror reminiscent of Poe. Scudder wrote in his rejection to Charlotte:

Dear Madam,

Mr. Howells has handed me this story.

I could not forgive myself if I make others as miserable as I have made myself.

Sincerely yours,

H. E. Scudder

After Scudder's sharp rebuff, Charlotte persevered, but to no avail. Everyone was drawn to her story, but no one wanted to publish such a controversial piece. No woman had ever written anything like it. Finally, Howells sent it to the *New England Magazine* and badgered the editor for days until he agreed to publish it. A few years later, Howells would include the story in his collection *Great Modern American Stories*; he introduced it as "terrible and too wholly dire" and said that at the time, the editor of *The Atlantic* was right: it was "too terribly good to be printed." Perhaps his interest was purely literary, but his continued support of Charlotte was meaningful. She would have been the same age as Winifred, and her straightforward and assertive personality along with her gift for writing might have reminded him of his daughter.

Upon publication, "The Yellow Wall Paper" was generally well received. Howells's support of Charlotte's writing enhanced its credibility and led to much publicity for the writer. In the spring of 1891, Lilian Whiting, journalist and editor of the *Boston Budget* and the *Boston Evening Traveller*, wrote a column about Charlotte that was reprinted in newspapers across the country: "There is no doubt that in Charlotte Perkins Stetson we have a new and brilliant creative genius whose work within the next decade will make a deep impression on imaginative art in American literature."

Charlotte received many notes from her readers, most of them favorable. A physician who at one time had been addicted to opium congratulated Charlotte and told her that, until the publication of her story, "There has been no detailed account of incipient insanity." She even sent a copy to Mitchell but never received a reply. Yet the story also stirred up controversy, especially within the medical profession; some kind of censorship was suggested but never implemented. Other readers were shocked by the vivid account of the mental breakdown of a middle-class wife and mother. One reviewer wrote that the story read "like the scrappy reminiscences of an opium debauch."

Charlotte's prominence as an author and feminist continued to grow. In 1893, she reconnected with her first cousin Houghton Gilman, a Wall Street attorney; the two would marry a few years later. But "The Yellow Wall Paper" was not recognized as a revolutionary feminist work until decades later. And as fate would have it, the story that Charlotte wrote and Howells helped to popularize would ultimately destroy the once-stellar reputation of Mitchell and his rest cure.

For decades, Mitchell continued to implement his rest cure as a way to reinforce the conventional role of women. His treatment was, indeed, an early form of brainwashing. But as time passed, modern women, like Charlotte, demanded more independence, better education, and professional work. These "New Women" of the late nineteenth century posed a grave threat to the social order, according to Mitchell and his peers. Preventing the higher education of women became his life's purpose.

Similar to the husband of the narrator in "The Yellow Wall Paper," Mitchell grew more and more obsessed by his cause. He stated that the only people with any authority to speak about women's schooling were male doctors. He railed against the numerous surveys conducted by university women that statistically refuted his belief that too much education made women sick. His private life grew more chaotic. Friends and family members simply avoided the topic; even his wife kept her opinions to herself while at home. One could say that he was becoming hysterical over the advancement of women.

Organizing to Win

TEN-YEAR-OLD MARJORIE JACOBI STOOD AMONG THE GIRLS' CLOTHES at B. Altman's department store watching for the menacing figure of the supervising floorwalker as her mother chatted nonchalantly with the shopgirls about their working conditions. While out buying clothes, Mary Putnam Jacobi and her daughter were covertly investigating the Ladies' Mile shopping district near Union Square for the New York City Consumers League.

Jacobi was a founding member of the Working Women's Society (later known as the Consumers League) and the organization's primary medical voice for labor reform. Led by Alice Woodbridge, a former retail clerk, and philanthropist Josephine Lowell, the league exposed the miserable working conditions for women in department stores, restaurants, textile mills, sweatshops, laundries, canneries, and candy factories.

Behind the glamorous decorations and beautiful inventory on display in the department stores, the shop clerks stood for hours on end without any breaks. They were never paid overtime. Owners diminished wages even more by imposing discretionary fines for any number of petty offenses. Rampant sexual harassment kept women employees constantly afraid. Foul-smelling lavatories with dirty, wet floors served both men and women and were often door-less, to prevent the girls from wasting time there. The cash girls had one of the worst jobs in the city. They toiled in hot, airless cellars under the strong glare of electric lights with hundreds of money carriers pouring waterfalls of coins on them, producing a deafening noise. Workers often fainted. At the end of the day, exhausted and hungry, they would ascend from the department-store cellars like reanimated corpses.

Following a systematic study of working conditions, the Consumers League created a "White List" of stores that paid a decent wage, required only daytime hours, provided sufficient breaks and clean conditions, and exhibited "humane and considerate behavior toward employees." The White List, published in the daily papers and mailed out to consumers, served to shame department stores and reform them by applying public pressure.

Jacobi had become a leading medical voice for labor reform, testifying in court about the negative impact of industrialism on the health of American women. Her research exposed the working conditions that led to disease and death and provided trade unions with the scientific information they needed to fight for workers' health and safety.

Jacobi's presence in the Consumers League gave the organization credibility. Famous for being the highest-paid woman in America—earning the astronomical sum of $50,000 per year (equivalent to over $1.5 million in 2023)—she was an established figure in the medical community. She held membership and leadership positions in a half a dozen or so different medical societies. Newspaper reporters referred to her expertise when writing about cures for anemia and promoting women's health issues. Her current research focused on neurology, including hysteria, and the continuing inquiry into sex differences. In her volume of research called *Essays on Hysteria* (1888)—a series of papers that she presented to neurologists at the New York Academy of Medicine—quoting the German neurologist Eulenberg, she confronted Mitchell's rest cure head-on:

> The predominance of hysteria among women depends, ultimately, far more upon the social conditions to which they are subjected, than upon uterine catarrhs and erosions. These conditions combine to arrest energy of will and independence of thought in women; to suppress impartial comparison of their own individuality with external objects; to restrain or suspiciously supervise all impulses to free action; and especially to obstruct and oppose any attempt at emancipation from the limits of a narrow and trivial existence.

Because Jacobi was curious about gender fluidity, she researched sexual identification as a way to prove that a woman's mental capacity was equal to a man's. Predating the discovery of sex hormones by more than a decade, she wrote case studies that explored gender equality and demonstrated that an individual's intelligence was unrelated to sex organs. In fact, she argued no one was ever completely feminine or masculine. Her research, of course, enraged men like Mitchell who would never consider themselves to be touched by a speck of "femininity." In response, male scientists continued to advertise the "fact" of male superiority.

In 1889, newspapers across the country carried Jacobi's reaction to a controversial article published in the *Forum* titled "Woman's Place in Nature" by scientific popularizer, biologist, and novelist Grant Allen. In the article, Allen claimed that "the males are the race." By "the race," Allen meant the wealthy and middle-class Caucasians, whose birth rates had fallen from just over seven children per woman in 1800 to about three and a half in 1900. To stem the threat of declining birth rates and preserve the "national health and vigor," Allen rejected the Victorian New Woman, who valued education, self-actualization, and career over marriage and family. He argued that motherhood was the only significant female function. The only true human beings were men; "all that is truly woman is merely reproductive."

An early advocate for eugenics and social Darwinism, Allen believed in "pure" reproduction in which the white female selected the strongest white male, weeding out the weak and deformed in order to reproduce a "divinely human" superman. He recommended that middle-class and wealthy women reduce or eliminate activities outside the home to make room for their most important duty: procreation.

Allen's proposal that women sacrifice their lives in order to procreate triggered a response almost as heated as the one to Edward Clarke's *Sex in Education*. "Must she keep right on reproducing a race of men which turns round and sets its heel upon her neck?" the editors of the *Woman's Standard* mused.

In her response, Jacobi, a proponent of both marriage and birth control, used her acerbic wit and knockout prose to reveal just how much she valued this man's opinion on women: "Mr. Allen's generalization curiously resembles the antique doctrine which, as physiologist, he would now repudiate, namely, that the female parent was simply and literally the soil upon which a seed was planted and developed independently into offspring." In England, "thinkers have . . . seen the necessity of limiting . . . reproductive activities, in order to secure greater comfort for those who are already born."

The scope of Mary's life had grown exponentially since she had won the Boylston Medical Prize more than a decade earlier. In 1880, she introduced a progressive course of study at the Woman's Medical College that was highly successful; two years later, she wanted to extend the progressive course of study from three to four years. That proposal proved to be too much for Emily Blackwell. She feared that students would drop out or, worse, not enroll at all. Out of frustration, Jacobi resigned from teaching at the Woman's Medical College in 1889, but she continued to work with Blackwell at the New York Infirmary. She also served as a visiting physician at St. Mark's Hospital and kept advising young women physicians through various medical associations.

And she refocused on her fight for coeducation at the best colleges. In early 1890, to her utter delight, an interesting opportunity arose that could give women medical students exactly what they needed to succeed.

It was an unusually warm day in mid-March when Jacobi traveled from New York to Philadelphia. As the train sped along, she enjoyed the view of the passing countryside. Already, the vibrant crocus blooms were piercing through the melting snow.

A few days earlier, Jacobi had received a surprising invitation from M. Carey Thomas, the bright, young dean of faculty and a professor of English at Bryn Mawr College. Thomas had unexpectedly invited her to discuss funding for a new medical school. Jacobi was glad to be traveling for a happy reason this time. A month earlier, she had gone to Boston to attend the funeral of her dear teacher Dr. Lucy Sewall, who had died from heart failure. Her lifelong companion, Dr. Zakrzewska, now seventy-one years old, had cared for Lucy until the bitter end. Zakrzewska, thank goodness, was still going strong.

At Philadelphia's Pennsylvania Station, she found her escort waiting among the electric trolley cars and horse-drawn hansom cabs. She enjoyed the fast horse that pulled the cab clacking down the brick streets, making it too loud to easily converse.

That afternoon, when they arrived at Bryn Mawr, located thirteen miles from downtown Philadelphia, a gym class was practicing archery outdoors. Believing that active girls were smarter students, Bryn Mawr had built the largest and best-equipped gymnasium of any woman's college in the country. Jacobi heartily approved, and she smiled and waved as she passed the students. Her niece attended the school, and Jacobi had previously toured the campus with her sister Amy.

Despite the endless discussions about the dangers of higher education for women, more and more parents were sending their daughters to college. While college education for all Americans was rare and costly, those families passionate about learning found ways to afford it for both their sons and daughters. Since the 1870s (after Jacobi had successfully refuted Clarke's *Sex in Education*), opponents of women's education had been waging a losing battle. In 1870, women accounted for 21 percent of all students enrolled in institutions of higher education. By 1890, that number had increased to 36 percent, and it was growing every year.

Sending a daughter away to college took courage. It defied every late-Victorian norm. Leaving home with trunks full of hatboxes, everyday clothes, ball gowns, and a tennis racket, the young woman traveled away from her parents to find adulthood and intellectual stimulation. In addition to a life free from household duties, she was learning to think on her own, and she wanted to establish a career before even considering marriage.

M. Carey Thomas had devoted her life to creating a women's college equal in all regards to the best men's colleges. Bryn Mawr's approximately 120 students and their professors formed intense bonds. In fact, college education among women was fast becoming a strong agency for social change. From the 1870s through the 1920s, between 40 and 60 percent of women college graduates did not marry, an astronomical number compared to only 10 percent of women overall who remained single. Women's colleges had created a basis for the generation of real female power. And the wielding of this power was the reason for Jacobi's visit today.

As the horse cab wove through the campus, Jacobi's escort explained that Dean Thomas lived at what had been christened "The Deanery," a cozy, eight-room Victorian cottage surrounded by tall trees and a mass of vines that nearly engulfed the front porch. When Jacobi arrived, several students were gathered on the porch steps talking with a woman who, except for her more elegant clothing, looked exactly like her students. It was Dean Thomas.

Martha Carey Thomas was the daughter of a Quaker family and had attended Quaker schools in her native Baltimore and in Ithaca, New York.

Her father, John Carey Thomas, a physician, accepted the unwavering feminism of her mother and her mother's sister Hannah Whitall Smith, a popular minister active in the Women's Christian Temperance Union. As a result of her mother's and aunt's influence, Carey grew up to be a fiercely independent upper-class white woman. While her mother and aunt went out on the streets to "preach to the unconverted," Carey studied. She read Herbert Spencer and, after entering his world of positivism and social Darwinism, found herself repulsed by the vulgar working class, whom she regarded as her natural "inferiors." She set out to create for herself a world of rare beauty populated by only the best women. In that quest, she would forcefully succeed.

Against her father's objections, M. Carey Thomas sought a college education and in 1877 was one of the first women to graduate from Cornell University. Intent on pursuing graduate work, she was allowed to enroll at Johns Hopkins University, where her father was a member of the board of trustees, but after her enrollment, she was refused admittance to classes. Frustrated, she traveled to Germany and studied at the University of Leipzig, but after three years, the school denied her a degree because she was a woman. She then applied to the University of Zurich, where she was admitted for the languages examination and was awarded a PhD summa cum laude in 1882. She wrote her successful dissertation on Swinburne with the help of her close friend and partner Mamie Gwinn. She spent another year working at the Sorbonne in Paris before returning to the United States. Two years later, at the newly opened Bryn Mawr College for women, she was appointed professor of English and became the first woman college faculty member in the country to hold the title of dean. At just thirty-three years old, Thomas had achieved fame and influence because of her restless, driving ambition. In this way, she was similar to Mary Putnam Jacobi.

Thomas was smiling down at her students when she saw the carriage pull up; she glided down the steps to meet Jacobi. It wasn't that Thomas was an ethereal-looking woman. She seemed more like a mythic, hardheaded creature whose entire life relied on wielding charm. Jacobi, at least, was instantly enchanted.

Once Jacobi was inside, a servant whisked away her small suitcase, and Thomas took her on a tour of the Deanery. Like the other buildings on campus, the home was Victorian Gothic, with steeply pitched roofs, pointed arches in the doors and windows, roof gables, delicate interlaced trim, and gargoyles. The rooms had an uncluttered simplicity with comfortable, sturdy furniture and a homey atmosphere. A brick fireplace on the first floor warmed the parlor and sitting room. Thomas had begun decorating the walls with the works of the best contemporary artists, and many of the light fixtures were from Tiffany. Over the years, she would expand the Deanery into a sprawling forty-six-room mansion that sometimes housed guests, students, and alumnae.

After Jacobi had changed out of her travel clothes, she joined Thomas in the parlor, eager to learn more about this idea for a new medical school. But first, Thomas wanted to know more about the current state of medical education for women. Jacobi revealed her frustrations: "America is the only country that has promptly granted women a legal right to practice medicine, and where the public has promptly secured them a clientele— yet where they have been compelled to stumble along without any hospital advantages worthy of the name, and upon educational curricula, uncontrolled, unsupervised by any competent authority, and which therefore has been usually quite incompetent. The situation is scandalously anomalous."

Jacobi explained that women's medical schools were still a cautious experiment that could fail at any time due to lack of students and funding. Because medicine was a constantly changing field where once innovative practices could be outdated in an instant, medical education had to grow and change too. That was why she saw women's medical schools as a temporary and makeshift way to measure competency in science and the medical arts. Feeling energized, Jacobi enjoyed telling her story to Thomas, a highly intelligent woman who listened intently and asked pertinent questions.

Thomas finally revealed the reason she had invited Jacobi to visit. Johns Hopkins University hoped to add a school of medicine to its hospital and create an institution at the forefront of medical research. However, the plans for the project had run into money problems.

Johns Hopkins had opened in 1876. Welcoming the school into the circle of elite universities, Harvard president Charles Eliot gave the opening address. The school's primary benefactor, philanthropist Johns Hopkins, a Quaker who wanted to advance public health and education in Baltimore, had bequeathed the school seven million dollars for a university, an affiliated hospital, a medical school, and an orphanage. At the time, it was the largest philanthropic donation in U.S. history.

Except for the fact that it did not include women, Hopkins's educational philosophy was extremely innovative for its day. He wanted a hospital subordinate to the needs of a university, but it took thirteen years to complete. Having recruited physicians of the highest stature for the hospital and medical school—chief physician William Osler, pathologist William Henry Welch, surgeon William Stewart Halstead, and gynecologist Howard Kelly—the hospital opened its doors in 1889. The completion of the medical school would finally fulfill the vision of its benefactor, but unfortunately, the funds intended for this purpose had been invested in the Baltimore and Ohio Railroad. When the railroad became financially unstable and stopped paying dividends to its stockholders, the medical school was put on hold, its faculty waiting in the wings. The school's president, Daniel Gilman, issued a desperate plea for a philanthropic partner, but the sole offer that arrived in his inbox was not the one he expected.

Although Thomas's father was an influential Hopkins trustee, like Harvard, Princeton, Columbia, and Yale, Hopkins did not accept women, and this policy had forced Thomas to travel to Europe for her graduate education. A proud and unyielding woman, Thomas never forgave the university for her humiliation. Now she had an opportunity to take sweet revenge. It seemed that the philanthropic offer that arrived in Gilman's inbox came from five Baltimore women who were good friends and heartfelt allies. Led by Carey Thomas, these young women saw the school's financial troubles as an opportunity to advance their cause of women's higher education.

Carey Thomas, Mary Elizabeth Garrett, Elizabeth (Bessie) King, Mary (Mamie) Gwinn, and Julia Rogers met on Fridays for stimulating and high-minded discussions about novels, plays, art, and essays. The fathers of all but Julia were on the board of trustees of the Johns Hopkins Hospital, the university, or both. The Friday Evening group read essays and recited romantic poetry by Shelley, Swinburne, and Gautier that left them full of "rapture and fire." While the opinionated Carey Thomas always dominated group discussions, the elegant Mary Elizabeth Garrett seemed to be more persuasive simply because she was the richest.

Mary Elizabeth was the only daughter and youngest child of John W. Garrett, who was president of the Baltimore and Ohio Railroad, the first major railroad built in America and the same organization that had stopped paying dividends and bankrupted the funding for Johns Hopkins's medical school. Due to her bright and inquiring nature, she was her father's favorite child, and he often said, "I wish Mary had been born a boy!" When he died in 1884, she inherited a fortune—more than two million dollars—and three lavish estates. She owned more property than any woman in America, and she vowed to use her money to help women. Now, her membership in the Friday Evening group had given her that opportunity.

As daughters of trustees, the group had direct access to the board's information and its reaction to the unfortunate delay in opening the medical school. Working with this confidential information from their fathers, they decided to establish the Women's Medical School Fund committee, charged with raising $100,000 for the endowment of the medical school on the condition that the trustees agreed to admit women. The choice of $100,000 was likely the result of back-and-forth negotiations between board members, who were supportive fathers, and their assiduous daughters.

The women's first order of business was to attract other activists to raise funds by installing a network of chapters across the country. This was the reason that Thomas had invited Jacobi to meet with her. The Friday Evening group needed leaders to run those chapters. The group had thought of Jacobi for New York, of course. Chapter leaders would be charged with convincing potential donors that the medical school was in fact going to open, that Johns Hopkins was willing to admit women, and that improving women's medical education in the United States was worth a contribution.

Jacobi expressed enthusiasm for the project. She felt that, with their wealth and insider connections, Thomas's group would have a much better chance for success than she, Emily Blackwell, and Zakrzewska had had nearly a decade ago when negotiating with Harvard. That loss was excruciating.

The next morning, Jacobi left Bryn Mawr fully expecting to be appointed to run the New York chapter. Unfortunately, Thomas had other ideas. While she held Jacobi's opinions on medicine in the highest regard, she found the older woman to be so personally unappealing that she wrote about it in a series of letters to Mary Elizabeth Garrett, who was also acquainted with the famous woman doctor.

"She is such a whimsical woman is she not?" she wrote in her first letter, referring to Jacobi. "And such a talker and so prejudiced against women and so little of a lady and altogether so disaffecting—Indeed I am going to give up hoping anything from clever women in [the] future . . . Dr. Jacobi gave me . . . her view on the subject of women's med[ical] education in no measured terms with an [amount] of plain speaking that will serve me instead of my annual dose of Zola."

Finding Jacobi ignorant of art and literature, Thomas expressed disappointment because Jacobi was otherwise "very clever in a very tedious way." This might be why Thomas preferred her friend "Miss Lyon" to head the New York chapter.

Yet there might have been another reason why Thomas found Jacobi so "unappealing." While outwardly claiming to be a positivist like Jacobi, in reality, over the years spent in Europe, Thomas had developed a clear sense of herself as one of the few true lovers of beauty, the most human of all human beings. Rough-minded working-class and poor people, Black people, Asian people, and native peoples were all relegated to just above the animals in her bigoted way of thinking. But perhaps the lowest of those in her opinion were the Jews. As a student in Germany, she wrote, "The Jews are the same now and were the same then, a most terrible set of people to my thinking." A few years later, she arbitrarily stopped accepting Jewish students at Bryn Mawr. This act along with her blatant loathing of "those people" so offended Mary Elizabeth Garrett that they did not speak for months. It was not until Thomas finally apologized and reopened Bryn Mawr to Jewish girls that the two women reconnected.

In 1890, around the same time that Thomas met with Jacobi, the *Jewish Exponent* charged her with continuing to limit the number of Jewish students, so the fact that Jacobi was married to a Jewish man and had given birth to half-Jewish children might have influenced Thomas's low opinion of the famous doctor.

Mary Elizabeth Garrett, however, supported Jacobi's role in their pursuit of opening the Johns Hopkins medical school to women. Garrett's genteel demeanor and soft smile hid an iron will that surprised even her closest friends. She was forbidden to enter the family business, but she nevertheless gained invaluable training as her father's personal secretary. She accompanied him on many of his business trips, recording his correspondence and watching him interact with some of the most influential businessmen of the time, including Andrew Carnegie, J. Pierpont Morgan, and Cornelius Vanderbilt. While Thomas was an ambitious schemer, Garrett could charm almost anyone into giving her what she wanted.

After Thomas's meeting to secure the backing of Jacobi, Thomas, Garrett, Mamie Gwinn, Julia Rogers, and Bessie King began the arduous task of creating a national Woman's Medical School Fund committee. Those who made donations would be called subscribers.

Because her father was president of the Johns Hopkins board of directors, Bessie King hosted the official launch for the Women's Medical School Fund committee, which took place on May 2, 1890. To publicize their mission and bolster their credibility, they would send press releases to newspapers and magazines, hold fundraising parties, and recruit the support of distinguished Americans. They subscribed to a newspaper-clipping service to keep track of the publicity they generated.

Under the auspices of the committee, the Friday Evening group authored and distributed a circular full of rhetoric meant to inspire immediate action. They went after society figures, writers, famous women, and female physicians by widely advertising the following stated mission: "In order to hasten the opening of the school, and to secure for women the most advanced medical education, it is proposed to raise the sum of $100,000 . . . All contributions will be regarded as conditional on a total contribution of $100,000, and on the acceptance of the condition by the Trustees."

After a few weeks of hard work publicizing the Woman's Medical School Fund, the self-assured women of the Friday Evening group began to worry. Even though publicity increased, donations remained stagnant. It seemed that those with money were not interested in women doctors. What would it take to convince them? The group launched its secret weapon. Mary Elizabeth Garrett put to use her stratospheric social standing to recruit subscribers from the nation's elite. She would go after the very highest of the high society, beginning with the First Lady herself, Caroline Harrison.

To keep her friends and other group leaders informed about her progress, Garrett wrote a series of letters, each beginning "Dear Girls."

April 29, 1890

Dear Girls,

Mrs. Bayard Smith declines to serve not because she is not interested, but because she is not willing to be on a committee unless she can work very hard and she is very feeble to undertake new work. She began by saying she did not think she believed in women physicians, doubted whether they had nerve enough . . . the experiment of letting them study medicine had never been tried & c. When some of these impressions were corrected, she changed her tune . . . and wound up volunteering to distribute circulars if I w'd send them to her.

On May 22, 1890, Garrett visited Washington, DC:

Dear Girls,

Not being far from Georgetown, I went to see Mrs. Billings (John Shaw); found her, and she agreed to ask about eight of the Washington list to join the committee; she is very much interested and ready I think to be very helpful . . . I then went . . . to Mrs. MacLean's . . . she also needed no conversion. . . . I asked her about Cincinnati and whether Mrs. Longworth and Mrs. Lars Anderson were as I thought the best people in Cinn to start the movement there if they would. Most emphatically she said they were. . . . As you may remember by arrangement, Dr. Brown came and gave me a great many points about California to take to Mrs. Hearst. I think it will be best for me to try again this week to see Mrs. Hearst.

However, not everyone was sympathetic to their mission:

I went to Mrs. Lincoln's . . . she refuses to serve on a committee, saying simply that she is not in sympathy with women studying medicine; that she could not argue or give any reasons that it was a feeling of prejudice and she thought there was no chance of her changing her mind. . . . Prejudice is certainly the most difficult thing to meet.

The Women's Medical School Fund committee established fifteen chapters, from New York to California. Each regional committee, led by a chairperson, secretary, and treasurer who were all prominent members of their communities, collected and recorded the funds. In Washington, First Lady Caroline Harrison served as chairperson; her address was listed as the White House. The committees sent their collected donations to a central bank account in Baltimore that would hold the money until all $100,000 was raised. Among those who joined the committee and made financial contributions were Jane Stanford, wife of Leland Stanford, founder of Stanford University and then a U.S. senator; Bertha Palmer, the queen of Chicago society, whose husband, Potter Palmer, had built the Palmer House Hotel; Louisa Adams, wife of former president John Quincy Adams; Julia Ward Howe; Alice Longfellow, daughter of poet Henry Wadsworth Longfellow; and novelist Sarah Orne Jewett.

In New York, despite Thomas's campaign against her, Jacobi, along with Emily Blackwell, led their chapter and recruited dozens of subscribers, including physicians' wives such as Mrs. Louis Agassiz, Mrs. William Osler, and, most surprisingly, Mrs. S. Weir Mitchell.

By October, with nearly seven hundred contributors, the chapters had raised over $50,000. To make up the rest, Garrett's gift was by far the largest: $47,787.50. Money continued to trickle in, and when the group sent their funds to the board, they had amassed $111,300.

The trustees of Johns Hopkins had watched their daughters' galactic fundraising efforts with wide-eyed amazement. On a public scale, it put to rest the idea that women were too fragile and muddled to organize a successful business venture. The trustees accepted the donation and signed a contract charging them with collecting the remainder of the $500,000 endowment needed to build the medical school. The contract also specified the condition that women must be accepted into Johns Hopkins's medical school and that the funds must be raised by February 1, 1892, or the group would withdraw their subscriptions.

To show off their victory, the founders of the Women's Medical School Fund and their proud fathers decided to hold a posh luncheon at Johns Hopkins Hospital and a reception at Mary Elizabeth Garrett's palatial home. Every notable committee member and chapter leader was invited.

∾

Traveling by train from New York, Mary Putnam Jacobi, Emily Blackwell, and Elizabeth Cushier arrived at Camden Station in Baltimore just before noon on November 11, 1890.

Known for her expertise in gynecology and surgery, Dr. Cushier had graduated from the Woman's Medical College in 1872, completed a year and a half of further studies at the University of Zurich, and was employed by the New York Infirmary as a surgeon and professor at the Woman's Medical College. She was the third woman invited to join the New York Academy of Medicine, after Dr. Mary Putnam Jacobi and Dr. Sarah McNutt. In her private practice, she treated, among many others, M. Carey Thomas. Cushier and Emily Blackwell were a couple and lived together in their home in Montclair, New Jersey. In a letter to Elizabeth Blackwell in 1888, Jacobi wrote about Cushier, "She is [. . .] a remarkable lovely woman, spirited, unselfish, generous and intelligent. I do not know what Dr. Emily would do without her. She absolutely basks in her presence; and seems as if she had been waiting for her for a lifetime."

When they stepped down from the train, the group of physicians were pleasantly surprised by the commotion taking place near the train tracks: Stately ladies dressed in serious business clothes—silk and wool muslin suits and afternoon frocks with fashionable hats from Paris—were roaming the platform, gathering their luggage and searching for their assigned carriages. Everyone seemed to be on the way to Johns Hopkins Hospital. To Jacobi, so many women traveling unescorted by husbands, sons, or brothers meant that times had indeed changed. She felt right at home.

She and the two other doctors found their carriage and joined the elegant procession of attendees moving up the wide avenue leading to the hospital. As the crowd of women poured into the hospital's entryway, they were greeted by receptionists who were surrounded by rows of vases and stands containing a forest of green palms, chrysanthemums, and other fragrant flowers. In the lobby, everyone passed by the receiving line of Mary Elizabeth Garrett, Carey Thomas, Bessie King, Mamie Gwinn, and others. The floors and wainscoting had been polished until they sparkled. Nurses were dressed in crisp white uniforms. Everything was in perfect order and ready to be scrutinized by important guests, among them First Lady Caroline Harrison and her niece Mary Dimmock.

Since Jacobi was one of five speakers featured at the luncheon, she, Emily Blackwell, and Cushier were seated near the podium. Others in attendance included Mrs. Robert P. Porter, wife of the superintendent of the census; Mrs. Billings, wife of the assistant surgeon general of the U.S. Army, and Clara Barton, president of the Red Cross Association, as well as the wives of governors, bankers, and newspaper editors. As introductions were made, eyes lit up with recognition and admiration, and soon everyone felt at home. It was as if they were building a wall of powerful women that could not be breached.

At a few minutes before two o'clock, after everyone had been presented to Mrs. Harrison and her entourage, Bessie's father, Francis T. King, escorted Mrs. Harrison down a long, covered corridor to the nurses' home at the south side of the hospital, where a great room had been prepared for the luncheon. It began with bouillon followed by Maryland-style terrapin, croquettes and peas, broiled oysters, celery salad, ice cream, cakes, and bonbons. The buzz of conversation and the clatter of dishes animated the room for over an hour, and when dessert was finished, Mr. King, president of the hospital trustees, stood to make an announcement.

"It gives me great pleasure to extend to you, on behalf of the trustees, a hearty welcome to the Johns Hopkins Hospital. Your presence here today on behalf of the committees which you have recently formed will be an epoch in the history of the Johns Hopkins University and Hospital and in the higher medical education of women in this country. Medical colleges for women have been successful, but a post-graduate course, the same that men have, is greatly needed, and I hope through your efforts and ours that we will soon be able to give it here."

Then he introduced Dr. Mary Putnam Jacobi. Her dark eyes sparkled as she stood to speak.

"I do not think I shall be accused of exaggeration by any of the ladies on whose behalf I speak when I say that this is really a great occasion. . . . We are here today under the inspiration of two ideas. . . . There is, in the first place, the idea that medical education properly belongs to a university; that it is an intellectual matter, and not a mere trade, to be practiced for pecuniary profit; and then there is the further idea, and which more especially concerns us, that women are to participate to the full in this intellectual aspect of medicine, and to follow it to the highest plane of intellectual development to which it can be carried. . . . But here it is the women themselves who have been aroused to feel the necessity of these higher intellectual opportunities for women and to exert themselves personally and energetically to secure them. For the munificence of the noble woman who has initiated this enterprise, for the generous energy of the others who have so nobly sustained her, we medical women do feel especially and profoundly grateful."

To enthusiastic applause, Jacobi took her seat. Two more board members spoke, and when they had finished, Mr. King invited everyone to inspect the hospital. The male doctors acted as guides and escorted small parties around the teaching hospital. After the tours, guests boarded carriages that drove them to Mary Elizabeth Garrett's house at the corner of Monument and Cathedral Streets for a reception with Mrs. Harrison. These events sparked enormous attention in the newspapers.

During the following weeks, flush with the success of this first great fundraising event, chapter members waited breathlessly for the board members to collect the remaining $500,000, due in February. However, time passed without any movement on the part of the board members, and distress began to seep into conversations; soon overt frustration arose.

The board members' failure to act, like a rumbling earthquake, triggered a crack in the foundation built by the Women's Medical School Fund. Opposition to women attending the Johns Hopkins medical school gained strength. A queasy feeling that the same beguilement, gaslighting, and ensuing disillusionment that Jacobi, Blackwell, and Zakrzewska had experienced when Harvard University reneged on its promise haunted those subscribers to the Women's Medical School Fund. So many colleges had been opened to women and then closed, so many promises remained unfulfilled, that women like Zakrzewska had chosen not to join the celebration at the Johns Hopkins Hospital, calloused toward the whims of men.

Corresponding with a friend in Baltimore who had contributed to the present cause, Zakrzewska cautioned her against being too hopeful. Don't expect too much, she advised. She did not receive a reply from her friend until after the reception at Johns Hopkins. Full of hope, her friend acknowledged Zakrzewska's wise words of caution but also included a vow to remain ever vigilant.

"However, I agree with you," she told Zakrzewska, "that we must watch carefully, and if there should ever be a sign of trying to evade you may depend on us to fight it out."

Combat Zones

BALTIMORE, 1890

A S THE FUNDRAISING DRAGGED ON, SOME OF THE JOHNS HOPKINS trustees started to question their decision to admit women. According to Martha Carey Thomas, university president Daniel Coit Gilman preferred not to have a medical school at all if it meant admitting women. He was secretly hoping that a wealthy male donor would step forward and supply the entire $500,000. "Only a man of large means and of large views will be likely to appreciate the situation," Gilman stated. And if no benefactor appeared, then Gilman was willing to have no school at all.

His clandestine search for a male patron sparked action from others who did not want women admitted to Hopkins. It began with an editorial in New York's *Medical Record*.

On November 15, 1890, the anonymous author of the "The Temptation of Johns Hopkins" argued that the trustees' acceptance of the gift of $100,000 had been a disastrous move. This careless act would "seriously impair the prestige and limit the usefulness of the university's medical school." Potential male students would go elsewhere simply because of "the disillusioning propinquity of lady medicals." Persuaded by sentiment—a father's love for his child—Dr. James Carey Thomas, attorney Charles Gwinn, and board president Francis King had simply not been able to resist the enticement of their daughters Carey, Mamie, and Bessie. According to the author, "the persistent nagging" of the Baltimore ladies succeeded in bribing the poor, henpecked trustees into the unfortunate decision of admitting women.

Weeks later, *The Nation* criticized the board of trustees' foolish decision. After all, Johns Hopkins University refused to admit women (and would continue do so until 1970). Other newspapers ran editorials in agreement with *The Nation*, suggesting that the gullible Women's Medical School Fund members had been tricked, and they would suffer defeat when the school failed to open. Word spread quickly that the women had made an enormous mistake.

As an avid reader of both the *Medical Record* and *The Nation*, S. Weir Mitchell watched the drama unfold with great interest. The most celebrated doctor in America saw his chance to intervene. His plan, if successful, could intensify the disruption and dampen any hopes that a medical school accepting women would be opened at Hopkins in the near future, if ever.

∽

In the late nineteenth century, the popularity of scientific cures had given rise to widespread medical celebrity. The lives of prominent physicians like Mitchell were exciting, and newspapers covered them regularly. A few months before the Johns Hopkins medical school agreement, the American Press Association distributed an article nationwide titled "Famed as Physicians: New York's Leading Practitioners of the Healing Arts." Spanning three columns and featuring illustrated portraits, the article included "Dr. Barker's Power of Diagnosis," "Dr. Sayre's Plaster Jacket," and "A Capable Female Doctor."

"Ranking easily among the great physicians of New York, Dr. Mary A. Putnam-Jacobi is an example of what a woman may do if she has the brains and the perseverance," the article reported. It described her long journey to prominence, from her schooling in Paris to being elected the first female member of the Academy of Medicine. It ended with the assurance that, while brilliant, Jacobi was still the perfect lady: "She is the wife of Dr. Abraham Jacobi, and it will interest women to know that she is one of the best housekeepers in New York."

Whether or not Jacobi excelled at housekeeping did not matter. Citizens going about their daily lives in places such as Lima, Ohio, Atchison, Kansas, and St. Helens, Oregon, were reading about the gifted woman doctor who was as competent as any man. It normalized the idea of women as physicians and acted as necessary ammunition in the battle for coeducation. If the Women's Medical School Fund was to claim success, it needed every bit of help.

The same APA article about famous New York physicians also included a paragraph on Dr. George F. Shrady, assistant surgeon in the U.S. Army during the Civil War and consulting physician to hospitals throughout New

York. He had become famous by attending General Grant on his deathbed and President Garfield after he had been shot. Most important, Shrady was the founding editor of the *Medical Journal*.

Jacobi had published articles in Shrady's *Medical Journal* since she was a student in Paris. As a member of the Women's Medical School Fund committee and a famous doctor, she was the obvious choice to confront these voices of opposition that were emerging in print. She replied to "The Temptation of Johns Hopkins" in the *Medical Journal* with mockery: "It will no longer be possible to absolutely deprive the best intellect in the one sex of the necessary opportunities which are freely accessible to the most mediocre capacities in the other. . . . The universities of France, Switzerland, Italy, Denmark, Norway, Sweden, and Belgium have not found their 'prestige impaired and their usefulness limited' by the admission of women to their just share in educational privileges. Why should the Johns Hopkins University be more impeded than they?"

Jacobi then scolded the author for belittling the great public spirit exhibited by Mary Elizabeth Garrett and the other women who contributed funds meant for the "intellectual benefit of their own sex" as "persistent nagging." Few people ever questioned the endowments made by wealthy men to Harvard and Cornell, she jabbed.

In response to *The Nation*'s editorial, however, even stronger action was necessary. In February 1891, *Century* magazine published a set of open letters, later distributed as a pamphlet titled "The Opening of the Johns Hopkins Medical School to Women." The *Century*, an illustrated monthly that also printed fiction from such notable authors as Mark Twain and Henry James, had the highest circulation of any periodical in the country.

Readers opening the pamphlet turned past the title page to find an illustration of a serene Florence Nightingale staring up at them. The distinguished list of authors writing in public support of women in medicine surprised and amazed everyone: James Cardinal Gibbons, the popular Catholic priest and advocate for labor rights who had recently been appointed archbishop of Baltimore; Mary Putnam Jacobi, M.D.; Josephine Lowell, founder of the New York Consumers League; Charles F. Folsom, M.D., secretary of the Massachusetts state board of health; M. Carey Thomas; and William Osler, M.D., chief physician at Johns Hopkins Hospital.

When James Cardinal Gibbons proclaimed that, because women had long served as midwives, he saw nothing wrong with women doctors, it made a solid impact. In fact, it was "important to the well-being of society that the study of medicine by Christian women should be continued and extended. . . . The prejudice that allows women to enter the profession of nursing and excludes them from the profession of medicine cannot be too strongly censured, and its existence can be explained only by the force of habit." Cardinal Gibbons believed that the influence of numerous well-trained female physicians would lead to nothing less than "the moral regeneration of society."

In her essay, Jacobi breezed through the recent history of American women in medicine, claiming that they were excluded from American medical schools for the "same ingenuous reason which led them to keep the standard of medical education as low as possible": profit. "The more students, the more pay; but the more severe the conditions of matriculation and graduation, the fewer the students. Similarly, it was feared that the admission of women would be unpopular among students, known to be as tenacious of their 'dignity' as they were careless of their instruction," Jacobi said bitingly. Since then, the modern European view of medicine, driven by science and laboratory research, had arrived in America, and the study of medicine had grown into a profession so complex that it required "an intellectual and material resource greater than . . . for any other branch of education." Since women were denied entrance to the top medical schools in America, they were forced to travel to Europe to obtain the quality education necessary to practice medicine.

Josephine Lowell, known as the "grand dame of the social reformers," wrote a gripping tribute to the most sympathetic and womanly of physicians, Susan Dimock, who had graduated with a medical degree from the University of Zurich in Switzerland in 1871, the same year that Jacobi had graduated from the École de Médecine. In 1872, Dimock became a resident physician under Zakrzewska at the New England Hospital for Women and Children, specializing in obstetrics and gynecology. She was renowned for her precise surgical skills and for developing the first graded school of nursing in the United States. At age twenty-eight, while traveling in Europe, she tragically drowned when the SS *Schiller* ran aground and sank off the coast of the Scilly Isles. At her funeral in Boston, eight renowned male physicians, including Henry Bowditch and Samuel Cabot, served as pallbearers. To many women stricken with illness, physicians like Susan Dimock "may come as a savior," Josephine concluded.

Charles Folsom, the venerated physician and defender of public health care, wrote that the first great university to give women medical students the same advantages as men was "likely to find it profitable to do so."

Carey Thomas argued that medical science and technology had become so costly, women's schools could not sustain the expense involved. And since most American hospitals barred women from clinical training, Johns Hopkins Hospital would provide just that. Furthermore, Thomas pointed out that Hopkins would open the first *graduate* school of medicine. "In graduate study, where the students are necessarily mature in age, richer in knowledge, fewer in numbers, tried and sifted by the tests of examinations, of perseverance, of life with its embarrassments, hindrances, and vicissitudes, the disadvantages of coeducations are at a minimum, and its advantages are at a maximum."

Perhaps the most persuasive essay was written by the chief physician at Hopkins, William Osler. His public support was critical. Osler observed that the École de Médecine in Paris now offered the utmost freedom to women in all departments. "At lectures and demonstrations it was evident every day that the hearers and seers were considered as students only, quite irrespective of sex," he wrote. "Their success is shown by the increasing number of those who obtain positions as interns. . . . The question at issue is really one of principle. . . . If any woman feels that the medical profession is her vocation, no obstacles should be placed in the way of her obtaining the best possible education."

The *Century* essays, especially Dr. Osler's, impressed readers and strengthened the fight for coeducation. Moreover, the Women's Medical School Fund, with its cross-country network of famous women, was once again recruiting supporters and scouting for funds. If the Johns Hopkins board members were not up to meeting the terms of their agreement, the Women's Medical School Fund would do it for them.

It was at this moment that Mitchell made his move. The target: his close friend Dr. William Osler.

⤙

Osler's parents, the Reverend Featherstone Lake Osler and Ellen Free Pickton Osler, were Anglican missionaries who emigrated from England to Bond Head, Canada, near Toronto, in 1837. The second youngest in a family of nine children, Willie Osler loved sports and reading, and from an early age, he exhibited a talent for well-planned practical jokes. In college, at age sixteen, he got himself arrested and charged with assault by tormenting the school's unpopular matron. Feeling repentant, he declared to his parents that he would become a minister. Instead, he ended up enrolling in medical school at McGill University in Montreal.

After receiving his M.D. in 1872 at the age of twenty-one, he traveled to Europe for postgraduate training and worked with the eminent pathologist Rudolf Virchow in Berlin. Returning to Montreal in 1874, Osler became a professor at McGill, teaching histology and pathology. A popular instructor with limitless enthusiasm and a youthful, innovative teaching style, he, assisted by his students, volunteered to do all the autopsies at Montreal General Hospital. Eventually, Montreal General hired him as an attending physician as well. Over time, Osler developed expertise in a wide range of diseases.

In 1884, Osler surprised his colleagues by applying for the recently vacated chair of clinical medicine at the University of Pennsylvania's medical school. He was gaining international recognition as a premier physician and wanted to advance in his profession. In addition to publishing his research in journals and presenting at association meetings, he had just been elected a fellow of the Royal College of Physicians of London. At the time of his application, Osler was in Leipzig, and Mitchell was traveling in Europe with his wife.

As a University of Pennsylvania trustee, Mitchell was tasked with interviewing Osler. When they met in London, fifty-five-year-old Mitchell was skeptical that the thirty-five-year-old Osler would meet the older man's high standards for genteel refinement. When Osler ate a piece of cherry pie and disposed of the cherrystone with his spoon rather than his fingers, he passed the test. Mitchell recognized him as "a kindred spirit," someone who was a passionate bibliophile, loved laboratory research, and had a rare expertise in pathology.

Like Mitchell, Osler had a penchant for social climbing. He married Grace Revere, the great-granddaughter of Paul Revere, in 1892. And both men believed the white man to be supreme among all races. Mitchell saw himself reflected in the younger man, and he immediately began campaigning for Osler to be awarded the position. It worked. Despite the fact that Osler was a foreigner, he won the chair.

Throughout Osler's years in Philadelphia, Mitchell served as his mentor and friend. When the new 110-bed Infirmary for Nervous Diseases was completed in 1887, Mitchell helped secure Osler's appointment to the facility. While there, Osler read Mitchell's writings, held long discussions with him about the rest cure, and pondered the secrets of its success—namely, the proper godlike demeanor of the physician over his patients. As medical professionals, they formed an intimate brotherhood. Then, in 1889, Osler accepted the position as the first physician in chief of the new Johns Hopkins Hospital, and he left Philadelphia for Baltimore.

That same year, Mitchell wrote that coeducation was "abominable for many reasons, but for physiological reasons, I think it foolish and absurd; as for others, I think it needless. You put a woman—a girl—in a class with men—or lads. Her wants and her menstrual disabilities she is forced by modesty to hide, or control, or defy." It became all about her needs, not his, and eventually, the young men would receive no education at all, according to Mitchell. Even those readers enraptured by Mitchell's writing may have wondered how a woman could "defy" her monthly period.

Mitchell simply refused to accept that his good friend Osler would allow the "abomination" of coeducation at Johns Hopkins. He feared that this lapse in judgment would ruin Osler's career. To save his friend, he decided to write a novel—serialized every month in the *Century* magazine, right in the middle of the controversy—as an opportunity to disparage women doctors, put a halt to the Hopkins fiasco, and get Osler back to Philadelphia. He believed that this work of fiction, that he supposed would be read by millions, would do the most damage. It was called *Characteristics*. Episodes ran from December 1891 through July 1892.

"This book is a broken record of portions of the lives of certain friends of mine, and of what I, Owen North, physician, have seen and heard," Mitchell's novel began.

Mitchell hoped to attract Osler's attention by the theme of his book: character development. An advocate of self-control, or balance, akin to Seneca's philosophy of Stoicism, Osler believed that if physicians were to practice with a clear head and kind heart, they should always maintain a cool, unflustered demeanor.

Characteristics employed as a framing device a group of four men telling entertaining and enlightening tales. In the first two chapters, the narrator, Owen North, recalled how he was paralyzed from a bullet that had pierced his spine during the Civil War. He spent an agonizing year recovering from paralysis. Even though he could walk again, he had become addicted to morphine. Resisting the help of friends, he recovered on his own purely through a stoic strength of character.

In the second half, Dr. North, who was now thirty-seven and an assistant surgeon in the army, met Alice Leigh, a twenty-four-year-old with an "unusual force of character" who strongly believed that a woman "of fortune and intellect" should have a career. Rather than the feminine choices of music, sketching, or helping the poor, she wanted to become a doctor, so she sought advice from Dr. North. A back-and-forth conversation between North and Alice began and continued for pages about her desire to help people, to learn science, and achieve something. Not wanting to "wound this gentle girl, with her honest longings," he resisted disappointing her. But at the same time, he could not imagine this "handsome, high-minded girl with her exquisite neatness and delicacies of sentiment and manner amidst the scenes and work which belong to the life of the student of medicine."

When she persisted in her longing, North finally quieted her by saying, bluntly, that women were not as good as men at doctoring even if they had exactly the same education. In fact, women who became doctors damaged themselves and the country. "I never saw a woman who did not lose something womanly in acquiring the education of a physician. I hardly put it delicately enough: a charm is lost." Alice responded that charm did not matter, and North said, "You cannot think that. You would lose the power to know that you had lost something. That is the real evil."

Mitchell's prose was stylized and overly dramatic. In fact, the entire exchange between Alice and Dr. North resembled those fanciful conversations enacted by Mitchell's favorite professor from medical school, Dr. Charles Meigs, where the moral physician subdued the bewildered little lady and cured her of any worldly desires besides raising children. To rescue young Alice from the awful fate of becoming a doctor, North gallantly pursued her hand in marriage.

꩜

After reading the final installment of Mitchell's book in the *Century*, Jacobi was, once again, furious at the doctor whose ego was stretched so wide that he thought his amateurish writing was as expert as his practice of medicine. Mitchell had once compared his poetry to Walt Whitman's. As his patient, Whitman appreciated Mitchell's medical care but described his writing as "a little bitter," "non-vital," and so "stiff at the knees" that his words "don't quite float along freely with the fundamental currents of life, passion."

Jacobi would agree. But what angered her the most about Mitchell was not his tedious prose. It was his intentional cruelty. It was clear that Mitchell absolutely understood the heartbreak and frustration women felt in their unfulfilled desire for change. He saw it in his practice and had documented it as a cause of neuroses and hysteria. But like most men of his time, Mitchell placed the health of women well below the needs of men. A woman's pain did not matter.

In her response to *Characteristics*, Jacobi excoriated Mitchell's "habit" of assuming that all women were like his sickest patients. She derided his narcissistic assumption that the "most delightful" aspect of "womanly charm" was her ability to attract the attention of men, not her intelligence. With biting sarcasm, Jacobi highlighted his frivolous pursuit of fiction by dismantling the lack of scientific evidence, logic, and detail in his writing:

> You do not state in "characteristics" why medicine, above all other pursuits, should have this deteriorating effect upon feminine attractiveness. Nor suggest why occupations that are so necessarily stimulating to the personal sympathies which I believe to be the real basis of what is most legitimately feminine, should be capable of warping feminine character. These occupations, like any others which are serious and responsible, must tend to diminish coquetry; but how can they lessen the power of sympathy, the maternal instinct, which is at least as powerful and valuable an instinct as coquetry? Far be it from me to suggest that coquetry be banished from, or eradicated out of the world. But surely there will be women enough left for its development and exercise, even if the present handful of female physicians were multiplied ten or twentyfold.

Jacobi next revealed that she had known for years that Mitchell had stolen her research. She cited her essay on cold pack and massage in anemia that was published a "year before the appearance of your little book on Fat and Blood." Her book contained a good many precise studies and suggestions that "proved to be quite identical with many of yours." And she did not stop with Mitchell. She provided a list of other male doctors who had "appropriated" her work, noted simply as a way to dispute Mitchell's idea of female incapacity:

Again, in 1876 I developed a theory of rhythmic nutritive processes in connection with menstruation, which has been subsequently confirmed by such men as Hegar in Germany, and also by some English observers. But in America this is scarcely heard of, although certain phrases I formulated, as the "supplementary wave of nutrition," have been adopted without acknowledgment.

And once more: several years ago, and while gynecologists were still generally dominated by the teaching of Thomas and Emmet that the endometrium either did not exist, or was insignificant, or could not be treated, I published a rather elaborate paper asserting that all pelvic disorders necessarily started from the endometrium, that it and the cortex of the ovary formed a continuous germinal membrane, and that the lymph spaces originating on the endometrium were the channels of infection exciting all peri-uterine disease. . . . Today these very same ideas have suddenly rushed to the front: but because of the more powerful theoretical turn which Dr. Polk [dean and professor of gynecology at Cornell University Medical School] gave to the matter, he is credited with the entire priority and originality, and my earlier demonstration and argument is never mentioned.

In her final paragraph, she taunted him:

Let me ask you once more: have you ever had an opportunity of watching a woman originally "charming" deteriorate under the influence of medicine? If not, how do you know that those whom you have met, medical and charmless, were not always so, even before they had taken the fatal plunge? . . . I would not venture to write so long a letter, were it not that I believe you will soon be at Newport and at leisure for idleness.

Mitchell never wrote back or acknowledged Jacobi's letter. In later years, he did pursue friendship with her husband. However, as Jacobi was a celebrity doctor who was part of New York's high society, her words would have stung him. He would have found her free use of sarcasm and irony supremely irritating and her use of the word *idleness* exceptionally insulting. Mitchell was being called out on his ineptitude and bad manners. By a woman.

Even worse, his scheme to persuade Osler to return to Philadelphia was failing.

～

During the serialization of *Characteristics*, the deadline of February 1, 1892, for the board of trustees to contribute the remaining funds for the medical school passed without being met. It looked like the school might never become a reality.

Then, on December 22, 1892, Mary Elizabeth Garrett decided to put a halt to the drama. Employing an imperial style that she had learned from her father, she wrote a letter to the Johns Hopkins trustees:

> In the resolutions of your board of trustees, adopted on October 28, 1890, it was provided that the medical school of your university should be opened when a general fund had been accumulated for its establishment and maintenance amounting to not less than $500,000.
>
> In the minutes of your board of trustees, adopted on April 30, 1891, it was stated that the university would have in money and property applicable to its medical school fund when it received the Woman's Medical School fund the sum of $178,780.42. This sum, because of subsequent payments, outstanding collectable amounts, and the interest accrued thereon, may now be safely assumed to be $193,023.
>
> It is necessary, therefore, that the general fund referred to should be increased by the sum of $306,977 to insure the opening of your medical school. I now place this amount of $306,977, payable as hereinafter provided, at the disposal of your board of trustees for the use of its medical school.

She added several conditions to her gift. First, all funds would revert back to her if the university ever discontinued a medical school devoted to the education of both men and women. Second, a Women's Fund Memorial Building should be constructed, and the terms of their gift must be printed each year in the course announcements. Third, a six-woman committee would oversee and provide counseling to the women studying in the medical school. And finally, expressing concern about the poor state of current medical education, Garrett stipulated that the medical school should be exclusively a four-year graduate-school course leading to the degree of doctor of medicine and "that there shall be admitted to the school those students only who by examination or by other tests equally satisfactory to the faculty of the medical school . . . have proved that they have completed the studies included in the preliminary medical course."

During the next week, the Women's Medical School Fund committee in charge of publicity made sure that dozens of newspapers across the country announced the agreement with the headline "A Chance for the Girls." The *Baltimore Sun* ran an article on December 30, 1892, that extended across two full columns with the headline "Miss Garrett's Gift" and several subheads: "She Presents $306,977 to Johns Hopkins Medical School; It Will Open in October, 1893. Women to Be Received and Educated upon the Same Terms as Men."

No matter what the headlines proclaimed, December 1892 was just the beginning of final negotiations. On Christmas Eve, Mary Elizabeth Garrett and the trustees gathered at the home of C.J.M. Gwinn and voted to accept Garrett's offer but with an exception. The requirement for a four-year graduate-level medical school, rather than the three-year undergraduate standard, was too stringent. Daniel Gilman expressed grave concern that the specifications would limit the number of incoming students and bankrupt the school. Osler joked that they were lucky to be professors, since they surely could not be admitted as students. This threatened to do what Mitchell could not: change Osler's mind.

Next, trustees expressed concern that they would lose control over the administration of the school. Garrett asserted that her contract allowed for complete control by the school administration over curriculum as long as it met the basic standards of a four-year graduate institution outlined in her agreement. The trustees, unaccustomed to making business deals with a woman, accused her of asserting too much control. She refused to make any changes and left the room in a huff.

These tumultuous back-and-forth negotiations continued for more than six weeks. Secret meetings among faculty members and malicious lies and misunderstandings among the trustees, Johns Hopkins, and the Friday Evening group members led to widespread animosity. Garrett became so upset by the process that Thomas had to take over the conversations with board members. "I often sat up all night preparing campaign broadsides," she wrote to a friend. The whole event seemed more like a Gothic melodrama than business negotiations.

Then, on February 15, 1893, Garrett composed a final letter that modified the terms of her endowment. In plain language, she reassured the trustees that in no way would her terms interfere with the operation of the university. She granted the right to the university "to make such changes in the requirements for admission . . . or to accept such equivalents . . . as shall not lower the standard of admission." In another paragraph, she stated that "it will be observed that by the tenor of these terms no university course will be in any way modified by any conditions attached to my gift."

By this time, most of the faculty members had come to support the strict admission requirements stipulated in the contract. Professor William Welch had changed his colleagues' minds by declaring that Hopkins could take the lead in a great reform of medical education by requiring thorough undergraduate preliminary training in the courses that lay at the foundation of medical science: biology, chemistry, and physiology. Welch believed that the policy would increase not only the reputation but the prosperity of the medical school. Welch won the day.

On February 20, Garrett and the trustees signed the requirements-for-admission contract, agreeing that "the aforegoing statement and terms are fully approved by me, Mary E. Garrett. Feb. 20, 1893. 9:30 am."

The Johns Hopkins medical school owed its existence to Mary Elizabeth Garrett and her generous endowment. When the school opened several months later, three of the eighteen students in the first class were women, and their number continued to increase each year. In addition to being the first prominent medical school to admit women and men on equal terms, Johns Hopkins was the first graduate-level medical institution with a four-year program. The high standards set by Garrett in her endowment were gradually adopted by other American medical schools and soon became the modern standard. She and the Friday Evening group and those women who rallied to support their cause had changed the face of American medicine.

∽

For months afterward, Mitchell fretted over Osler's irrational devotion to women doctors. What had gotten into his young protégé? Mitchell would never know, but if he had learned the real reason for Osler's "weakness toward women," it would have left him dumfounded.

More than a decade earlier, in June 1880, twenty-nine-year-old Osler traveled from McGill University in Montreal, where he was a professor of medicine, to New York to attend the thirty-first annual convention of the American Medical Association, held in the meeting hall of the YMCA building. Nearly a thousand delegates from every state in the nation presented dozens of papers on subjects ranging from recommendations about the adoption of the metric system to the approval of the formation of a national board of health.

In obstetrics, Dr. Marion Sims reported on four cases of epileptic attacks in women that he believed were due to a menstrual-cycle malfunction. Sims described how he surgically removed their ovaries and noted that he had cured two, killed one, and the fourth was still experiencing attacks. Osler watched Sims's presentation with suspicion. In his notebook, he wrote: "Many of the leading gynecologists were conspicuous by their absence during [Sims's] discussion. Why does not some bold surgeon introduce the operation of gelding for many of the troubles to which the sterner sex are victims?"

In the next section, Osler watched D. L. Thompson, pharmacist and homeopathic doctor, read his paper titled "Classification of Remedies." Although extremely popular at the time, homeopathy was considered to be quackery by the AMA. A spirited discussion followed the presentation. One of Thompson's chief critics was Dr. Mary Putnam Jacobi.

Osler listened to Jacobi logically dissect Thompson's paper and then dismantle his arguments and was stunned by the intellectual force of her attack. Like hearing recorded sounds on a phonograph or viewing electric lighting for the first time, watching Jacobi argue succinctly about medicine was an experience completely foreign, somewhat terrifying, but also delightful. She sounded like a man, yet, being a petite, attractive woman in her late thirties, a wife, and a mother, she had a most feminine presence. She maintained evenhanded composure and a sincere yet thoughtful facial expression. She was exhibiting the best part of Stoicism.

In this moment, his belief about women's capabilities began to change. In the article he authored for a Canadian medical journal about the convention, he wrote briefly that "the clear, logical manner in which [Jacobi] explained her ideas on the subject was a most agreeable treat." In fact, watching Jacobi argue for science altered young Osler forever.

A Partnership of Women

MARJORIE JACOBI WAS TURNING SIXTEEN NEXT MONTH, ON December 28, and her family had already begun decorating for the upcoming birthday-holiday parties. Soon, the great walnut staircase that was her home's centerpiece would have thick holly branches and brightly colored red and gold tinsel woven throughout. A majestic fir, suitably decorated, would greet visitors in the entryway.

Abraham, who rarely gave his daughter gifts because she received dozens every year from Mary and her other Putnam relatives, was planning a surprise for Marjorie this year: two volumes of his collected works that he had intended to give to his son, Ernst. Of course, giving medical books to a girl on her sixteenth birthday, especially a girl who enjoyed parties and fashionable clothes, was not a well-thought-out plan. In many ways, Abraham remained disconnected from his home life, devoting his time to his medical practice and visiting with his best friend and next-door neighbor, Carl Schurz.

There were few differences between the two Jacobi doctors regarding medical or sociological matters, but one of them would occasionally fail to share the other's enthusiasm for a cause. This happened in the case of suffrage. Mary had fully embraced the vote for women, but Abraham remained quietly neutral, unlike Schurz, who was stridently opposed to women voting. Mary and Schurz had heated debates, but Abraham would not discuss the subject. That's why, on the afternoon of November 19, 1893, he was surprised and a bit flustered when Susan B. Anthony arrived at their home for Sunday dinner.

At the time, Anthony was staying in New York City with friends after her long journey west, visiting Kansas, Ohio, and the Chicago World's Fair. In Chicago, women had taken part in building the exhibits, spoken at events, and served in leadership roles. The expansive Woman's Building was designed by a woman architect and exclusively featured women's accomplishments. Anthony had commented that the World's Fair exhibition did more for the suffrage movement than twenty-five years of agitating.

Mary Putnam Jacobi had never met the suffrage leader and had expressed open frustration at not being invited to participate in official events. But when she received a note from Susan asking if they could meet, she responded immediately with a dinner invitation. That evening, they both enjoyed a warm and friendly conversation; Abraham excused himself early and disappeared into his study. The two women discussed medicine and women's rights and praised the life of their mutual friend Lucy Stone, who had passed away the previous month at the age of seventy-five. Anthony was two years younger than Stone. With her silver hair, commanding chin, and sparkling eyes, she seemed vibrant and strong.

After dessert, Jacobi proposed that they talk business in the parlor and escorted Anthony across the imposing entryway with its marble floor and twenty-foot ceiling and up the walnut staircase to the large and comfortably furnished parlor. Jacobi was filled with curiosity. In the past, she and the suffrage leadership had not seen eye to eye. She rejected the sentimentality of the old guard of suffragists, including Anthony. For example, suffragists campaigned against medical vivisection, a practice that Jacobi implemented herself and publicly supported, labeling women as "the sex most sensitive to moral and humane considerations."

Jacobi also opposed them on a key issue: alcohol prohibition and temperance reform. In a heated debate with Lucy Stone's daughter, Alice Stone Blackwell, in the pages of the *Woman's Journal*, Jacobi wrote that temperance "imperil[ed] the logic of woman suffrage" by making it seem that women were interested only in emotional issues. It would be more "rational" to address abuse in general rather than attacking the bad behavior of individuals. Suffragists should be guided by logic, not emotion, pragmatism, not moralism. Jacobi knew this difference of opinion had prevented her from being asked to officially join the cause. She was thus intensely curious about the reason for Anthony's presence in her parlor this evening.

It turned out that the suffrage icon wanted to talk about Colorado. Twelve days earlier, on November 7, men went to the polls there and enthusiastically gave women the right to vote. Colorado became the first state in America to enact women's suffrage by popular referendum. *This shall be the land for women*, its citizens shouted in celebration. Part of the secret behind the vote's success was the quiet force of Denver's wealthy women, including Margaret "Molly" Brown and Elizabeth "Baby Doe" Tabor, who provided vital financing and strong public support for the cause. This win had given Anthony an idea for New York.

She wanted to launch a massive house-to-house petition-signing campaign throughout the state to expand support for suffrage. Starting the following month, her committee planned to send out thousands of letters, circulars, and pamphlets and simultaneously hold meetings in all of the state's sixty counties. Women would canvass their neighborhoods with petitions and gather signatures. These petitions would be presented at the New York Constitutional Convention being held in the spring. Suffragists wanted to make a very simple change to the state's constitution that would legalize the vote for women: elimination of the word *male* as qualification for voting. In order to achieve these goals, Anthony asked Jacobi to take the lead in raising $50,000 to pay for an army of statewide canvassers.

Surprised by the request, Jacobi sat for a minute gathering her thoughts. It was not her expertise in science and medicine that Susan was seeking but the influence of her social standing and wide network of wealthy friends. Even though Anthony was known as a brilliant strategist, the Napoléon of the women's rights movement, Jacobi was not so sure about the feasibility of this idea. While Anthony, a plain-spoken Quaker, was the first great woman politician, she was in a foreign land when it came to New York City's gilded class.

"I think such a canvass would be impossible," Jacobi told Anthony matter-of-factly. "Few persons would sign a petition so presented, and their names would have little influence."

When Anthony did not comment, Jacobi offered up her own idea. Instead of canvassing the rich door to door, Jacobi volunteered to recruit a few upstanding women who would then attract other supporters. The key was to arouse sufficient interest among society women with large circles of friends; they would, in turn, invite their friends over for "parlor meetings" where they could discuss the cause and sign petitions. The main ingredient to her plan was personal influence. This strategy would be in addition to the regular volunteer canvassing efforts throughout the rest of the state. Of course, the importance of New York City was obvious. The city's 1.7 million residents was almost one-third of the state's total population.

By the time Jacobi finished speaking, Anthony was smiling. She liked the idea and agreed to take it to Jean Greenleaf, president of the New York State Woman Suffrage Association. A few days later, Jacobi received word that her plan had been adopted and that she should proceed immediately. She would report her progress at intervals to Greenleaf.

Thus commenced the 1894 battle for New York.

Difficulties arose immediately. The first woman Jacobi approached seemed ideal. She was deeply interested in political and social matters and had participated effectively in public affairs, and she would have been interested in suffrage except for one thing: the 35,000 prostitutes working the streets in New York City. Between 5 and 10 percent of women in nineteenth-century New York City were sex workers. She had no desire to let these ignorant and irresponsible women vote. The next woman Jacobi asked was convinced that suffragists were coarse, ill-dressed "hyenas in petticoats" and she was terrified to be seen with them. Now Jacobi understood the fight ahead of her. It was imperative that elite women overcome these prejudices along with the fear that their endorsement of the cause might end up being sensationalized in the newspapers.

Jacobi decided to take the first step herself. She invited thirty women into her home to meet Josephine Shaw Lowell, founder of the Consumers League, and hear her talk about the proposed amendment to New York's constitution for women's suffrage. As an added incentive, she invited Elizabeth Cady Stanton, whose father, Daniel Cady, had been one of the largest landowners in New York. Stanton was from the same class of women as the others at the meeting and would put attendees at ease.

Lowell opened by giving a succinct overview of suffrage in New York. After she finished, Jacobi asked each attendee to express her own view of the situation, and several of the delicate ladies turned pale with fright. Apparently, these high-society women had not ventured into the public sphere since they were debutantes. They quivered and their voices shook as they dared, for the first time, to make a speech before an audience. But the longer they spoke, the easier it became, and soon the gathering turned very animated. The remarks of the few who opposed suffrage received sharp comebacks from those in favor. Finally, Jacobi asked Stanton to close the meeting. The elderly activist, though fragile in health, was a master orator. Her warm words of encouragement along with the strength of her presence elevated the attendees' determination to act. They were given copies of the petition and asked to hold parlor meetings with their own circle of friends.

For her next meeting, Jacobi invited Lillie Devereux Blake, novelist, Civil War correspondent, and president of the New York City Woman Suffrage League. Blake was famous for her protest in 1886 at the unveiling of the Statue of Liberty. Blake and her army of women displayed banners and flags from railings, sang, and shouted into megaphones to draw attention to the greatest hypocrisy of the day: A woman's image had been chosen to represent the ideal of Liberty, yet women possessed few legal rights in America.

Blake and Susan B. Anthony were contentious friends. They disagreed on the essential purpose of the women's movement. Blake preferred a wider scope of reform, including full social, political, and economic equality as well as access to higher education, while Susan wanted to concentrate only on suffrage. Like Jacobi, Blake argued that gender roles, acquired through learned behavior and cultural reinforcement, were unnatural and that women and men from any race shared a common, fluid nature. Women were equal to men and should be allowed to vote. Anthony believed that it was only white women who possessed the superior moral authority and unique, separate nature that demanded empowerment through suffrage. But for the sake of New York, the two joined forces. Blake was a vivacious presence at Jacobi's meeting that day, inspiring several of Jacobi's friends who had been indifferent to the cause to sign the petition and become active.

The next meeting was held in the home of Catherine Abbe, a society matron and historian who was married to a prominent surgeon. That day, Jacobi, Abbe, and four other notable women—Eleanor Butler Sanders, Lucia Gilbert Runkle, Lee Haggin, and Adele M. Fielde—decided to form the Volunteer Committee, an organization similar to the New York City Woman Suffrage League but meant to oversee the upper-class parlor meetings. Representing a mixture of inherited wealth and new money, all of these women traveled comfortably in high society.

Eleanor Butler Sanders, a philanthropist and socialite, was married to Reverend Henry M. Sanders, leader of the popular Madison Avenue Baptist Church. Her great-niece was Eleanor Butler Roosevelt. Lucia Gilbert Runkle, a celebrated journalist for the *Tribune*, was the widow of an esteemed lawyer and an editor of the *Library of the World's Best Literature*

Selections. Lee Haggin, an influential supporter of the arts, was married to the son of a millionaire mine owner and horse breeder. And Adele M. Fielde, a famed biologist who had made significant contributions to the study of ants, had gained her social status through missionary work in China. She was the only unmarried woman on the Volunteer Committee. All of these society ladies fully expected to use their influence to persuade numerous wealthy men and women to sign a suffrage petition.

While the original aim of the parlor meetings was to allow everyone present to speak her mind on suffrage, soon it became customary for the entire meeting to be carried by half a dozen speakers. Members of the Volunteer Committee, especially Runkle, Fields, and Jacobi, often made presentations. These women managed to secure the signatures of two of the most prominent women representing new money in New York City: Laura Spelman Rockefeller, married to John D. Rockefeller, and Olivia Sage, wife of financier and businessman Russell Sage. In turn, both Laura and Olivia opened their homes to the cause.

Other supporters came from old wealth. At one meeting, a reporter from the *Herald* counted almost ninety representatives of the Four Hundred— the most aristocratic New Yorkers—an unprecedented occurrence. Twenty-four-year-old Margaret Chanler, William B. Astor's great-granddaughter and Caroline Astor's great-niece, showed up at meetings and held a few of her own. She was most concerned that the government taxed her property without a care for her political voice. Her concern proved valid after Mary and other volunteers collected information about the taxable real estate in New York owned by women—more than six hundred million dollars' worth of property, not including New York City. Once those records were added, the amount more than doubled.

Chanler's presence attracted other young society women, who brought an emotional energy that approached melodrama when they spoke about their own future as women in America. For Jacobi, the spirited preaching at these gatherings reminded her of the days of the great religious revival in New York that followed the Panic of 1857. But these young women were "carried off their feet" by a wave of social feeling that made them fight over who would hold the next parlor meeting.

When these younger, more fashionable women began to appear, so did the press, and the goal of the newspapers was to increase sales by fomenting spectacle. Reporters labeled the middle-class activists in the New York

City Woman Suffrage League as the "regulars" and the elite wealthy activists as the "volunteers." The regulars were referred to as "females" and the elites "ladies." Wealthy advocates complained that their work had nothing to do with those regular suffragists. "You see, we are not like the Woman Suffrage League," one woman explained to the press. "We do not want advertising. We shun it. . . . We want enfranchisement, not notoriety."

The New York City Woman Suffrage League set up its base of operations at 10 East Fourteenth Street, right in the middle of the bustling high-end shopping district. Meant to attract wealthy shoppers, the office sometimes intimidated those who wandered inside. The walls covered with maps of the city and an organizer's desk "piled up with stationery, printed blanks and official-looking documents" gave the premises a no-nonsense "business-like air."

Twenty blocks away, on the corner of Fifth Avenue and Thirty-seventh Street, the Volunteer Committee transformed Sherry's, a gilt-edged restaurant where the wealthy gathered for elaborate dinners, dances, and charity events, into its headquarters. During suffrage meetings, the committee placed one elegant table in the middle of the room for campaign materials. Ornate chairs and divans surrounded the table so that interested people could leisurely view the materials. A sign outside the restaurant invited passersby to come in and "Please Sign the Petition." Best of all, they served five p.m. tea. It was a perfect command center for rich people. As one journalist reported, it took sublime "political skill" for these women to place "their citadel on the crest of Murray Hill" instead of "trailing their skirts in the byways of the city."

Eager to capture information about the celebrities attending the meetings at Sherry's, reporters lined up along the street and waited until someone from the gilded class arrived. Then they galloped toward the restaurant like hounds after a fox. Journalists even showed up at the parlor meetings around town. According to one correspondent, "Dr. Mary Putnam Jacobi [was] on the warpath for woman suffrage."

The reporting on suffrage was unprecedented. In the first months of 1894, *The New York Times* increased its coverage by 82 percent. The intensity of this reporting evoked strong reactions, especially from those who opposed the vote for women. But not even the savvy members of the Volunteer Committee could have predicted the next turn of events.

In mid-April 1894, *The New York Times* reported on the formation of a new anti-suffrage organization in Brooklyn; a group of women had met to protest the "obligation of suffrage." A week later, some affluent Manhattan women followed suit. Powerful socialites from the oldest New York families emerged like matriarch spiders ready to defend their clan; J. P. Morgan's wife, Frances; Sarah Hewitt, the wife of New York City's former mayor Abram Hewitt; Helena Gilder, wife of the editor of *Century Illustrated Monthly Magazine*; Edith Wharton's sister-in-law Mary Cadwalader Jones; and Catharine C. Hunt, married to architect Richard M. Hunt, joined the resistance. These women had decided to defend the existing order.

As Jacobi stated in her final report to Jean Greenleaf, "Thus when every one was talking about the suffrage, and little else, people who disdained or dreaded the suffrage began to bethink themselves, then to bestir themselves," insisting that political equality would challenge the "divinely ordered differences" between the sexes and deprive women of the special privilege of not voting. Ironically, many of those opposed to suffrage participated in the same charities as their ballot-supporting peers and in some cases were related to each other.

Eager to revel in the growing conflict, newspapers enthusiastically reported on the "civil war" among the elite women of New York City. Jeering headlines read "The Merry War Goes On," "Traitors in the Woman's Camp," and "Woman Against Woman." According to Jacobi, the whole thing had become comical. The elite women who opposed suffrage proceeded to copy the Volunteer Committee by opening their headquarters at the luxurious Waldorf Hotel, where they circulated a petition. Their rules, however, prohibited any male signatures, an action that would limit the number of total signatures but emphasized that it was the women themselves who did not want the vote.

One reporter suggested that these opposing groups were living in a version of the fairy-tale Cinderella with Jacobi acting as the "Fairy Godmother," granting wishes by bringing to life the "fashionable campaign" of Cinderella. For years, those fighting for woman's suffrage "had been sneered at, hustled aside, and made the laughing stock of the general public." Then along came Dr. Mary Putnam Jacobi, "a woman of wealth, social position and culture." Like the Fairy Godmother, she has turned suffrage into "the belle of the political ball."

The wealthy suffragists with their crystal slippers were already at the ball making eyes at the princely goal of enfranchisement when the ugly "anti-suffragist" stepsisters arrived from Brooklyn to break the spell. At the same time, the middle-class New York City Woman Suffrage League members, described as "old-timers," "downcast but dogged," were "working like beavers" toward suffrage. Subsequently, the Volunteer Committee was at odds with its sister "anti-suffrage" elites and depicted as poor collaborators with the middle- and working-class "old-timers."

Denying that the "signature of a society woman" was more important than "that of a business woman or a stenographer or a seamstress or any other woman," Jacobi opened their exclusive Sherry's headquarters to all New Yorkers twenty-one years of age or older. To calm any fears about the hoi polloi, Jacobi assured her fellow committee members and wealthy suffragists that "educated" women would assert leverage over "poorer and more ignorant women" when it came to voting. For example, the Volunteer Committee often referred to census data showing that the African American population in New York was so small that enfranchising Black women would not threaten the status quo. These elite suffragists found comfort in imagining that their class would provide political leadership for all women when they won the vote. But they would not win at all if they did not find a way to dig down and cooperate with each other.

The New York Constitutional Convention was quickly approaching. Veteran suffragists like Elizabeth Cady Stanton and Lillie Devereux Blake reminded their constituents that their common goal was enfranchising *all* women and that collaboration among groups was essential for winning. To encourage solidarity, Jacobi invited members of the New York City Woman Suffrage League to the Volunteer Committee's parlor meetings. Gathering more and more signatures for the convention being held in Albany was their only goal. The two groups combined ranks, engineered immense enthusiasm, and scheduled two massive gatherings to showcase their cooperative spirit right before the convention. The first was a by-invitation-only meeting held at Sherry's in early May. The city's chamber of commerce president served as the master of ceremonies. Proprietor Louis Sherry welcomed each attendee until two thousand people were crammed into several rooms. An additional thirteen hundred were turned away. During the event, volunteers gathered signatures and notable members gave speeches. Conflicting lectures echoed throughout the venue, and one person commented that she could stand between two rooms and hear a different speech with each ear.

A few days later, suffragist leaders held a larger gathering at the Cooper Union's Great Hall. An eager audience packed the auditorium. In a show of strength, leaders for both the New York City Woman Suffrage League and the Volunteer Committee sat together on the stage, with Elizabeth Cady Stanton in the spotlight. Reporters from every New York newspaper stood scribbling notes. Reverend Henry M. Sanders, Eleanor Sanders's husband, opened the meeting with the affirmation, "We believe in woman suffrage very much as a matter of mathematical truth warranted by a sense of justice and fair play." The audience responded with loud applause. Other speakers followed, but when seventy-seven-year-old Elizabeth Cady Stanton was introduced, the rafters shook as the people cheered. The older suffragists madly waved their white handkerchiefs. Stanton's voice rang clear as she spoke. "The State has no right to abolish the suffrage for any class of people. . . . It is said that the brain of man is already overweighted, and a new element must be brought in to help him meet the questions of the day. This new power is woman." Every woman present felt her heart bursting with pride and hope.

After the meeting, attendees poured into corridors, examined the suffrage literature, and signed the petition books displayed on tables. A large sign announced that petitions would be available at Sherry's for signatures until May 15, when the campaign's war room would shift to Albany, the location of the constitutional convention.

~

On May 8, 1894, delegates from across New York assembled for the first day of the state's fourth constitutional convention. The 175 delegates had been elected during the November 7, 1893, New York state election, with five from each senatorial district and fifteen at-large delegates. The convention would last the entire summer and adjourn on September 29.

Joseph H. Choate, the convention president, appointed a committee in charge of suffrage amendments, but none of the men on this committee supported the idea of women voting. After the May 15 deadline, volunteers submitted petitions, each tied with a yellow ribbon, to the committee. Convention members stacked the volumes on the secretary's table, where they made an imposing appearance. The numbers were impressive. The New York State Woman Suffrage Association turned in petitions with over

332,000 names. In addition, the New York Federation of Labor submitted a "memorial" representing 140,000; the Labor Reform Conference had 70,000; several trade unions had collected 1,396; and Granges delivered 50,000—a grand total of 593,544 for suffrage. In comparison, the anti-suffragists, or "Remonstrants," as they called themselves, submitted the signatures of 15,000 women.

Susan B. Anthony and Jean Greenleaf made the opening suffrage addresses at the convention on May 24. One week later, on May 31, Mary Putnam Jacobi was the first to address the assembly of convention delegates, followed by Lillie Devereaux Blake, Harriette Keyser, and Margaret Chanler.

In her speech, Jacobi presented key arguments as to why the delegates at the constitutional convention should strike the word *male* from the state constitution and vote for suffrage. Every seat in the assembly chamber was claimed by the champions and opponents of woman suffrage in New York. The men appointed to the suffrage committee sat in the well of the assembly chamber. Susan B. Anthony had joined the New York suffrage contingent in the front row, and they all wore orange delegate ribbons, the color of "feminine ballot seekers." Jean Greenleaf introduced Jacobi, and the crowd cheered!

Jacobi approached the podium, where she was engulfed by sunlight streaming through windows. "A small, dark, unobtrusive woman of 52 years, always robed in funeral black and with manners more brusque than suave," was how one reporter described Jacobi. Since most of the journalists present had not attended medical association meetings, none of them had ever heard Jacobi speak. She looked so petite and feminine, they hoped that she would not collapse into embarrassing hysterics. But when she concluded her hour-long discourse, these same journalists reported her presentation as "erudite, logical and dignified" and "a masterful plea for woman suffrage that was without doubt one of the most remarkable speeches ever made by a woman." The next edition of the *Woman's Journal* printed her entire address, claiming that "all the way through she was heartily applauded." It was a call to action:

Gentlemen, it is with a deep sense of the momentous importance of our errand that we present ourselves before you on this occasion. Never in the history of the world has a greater question been submitted to a deliberative body for discussion than that which we now pray you to consider. Other conventions, in this and other lands, have framed constitutions for a State—have laid down laws for a people, have enfranchised social classes—have even called entire nations into being. But we ask you to consider that part of the State about which constitutions have been silent—to enfranchise a class so immense that it constitutes the full half of all social classes; to call into political existence a vital half of the nation, which hitherto, though personally, socially, and legally recognized, has been politically non-existent.

Jacobi continued by telling listeners that the enfranchisement of women in New York would be "momentous," but she also assured them that the votes of women would imply "no sudden shock or overturning of established order." She redirected the suffrage question from one based on sex to one based on evolution and class. The convention allowed for the "orderly evolution of complex modern societies" to make necessary and fundamental changes.

Borrowing the provocative language of race and class common to the suffrage campaign and among the white men present, she cited women's "evolution . . . in contrast to the regression of the nation's male masses."

No matter how well-born, how intelligent, how highly educated, how virtuous, how rich, how refined, the women of to-day constitute a political class below that of every man, no matter how base-born, how stupid, how ignorant, how vicious, how poverty-stricken, how brutal. The pauper in the almshouse may vote; the lady who devotes her philanthropic thought to making that almshouse habitable, may not. The tramp who begs cold victuals in the kitchen may vote; the heiress who feeds him and endows universities may not. . . . The white woman of purest blood, and who, in her own person, or that of mother or grandmother, has helped to sustain the courage of the Revolutionary war, to fight the heroic battle of abolition, and to dress the wounds of the Rebellion,—this woman must keep silence.

Jacobi also spoke on behalf of working women in industry, the "poor and weak women" who were unvoiced and defenseless when it came to political representation, especially the three thousand women teachers in New York City who deserved proper representation on school-related issues. Legally, women were now "distinct individuals" who controlled their own earnings, owned property, paid taxes, inherited and bequeathed money, and represented themselves in court. Even with these rights, women had no individual voice in politics, which Jacobi called a "monstrous anomaly."

She received a standing ovation. Suffragists felt energized. Victory was here at last.

Days passed, and the night before the delegates would vote on suffrage, Jacobi called together her colleagues from the Volunteer Committee. Expecting a last-minute pep talk, Catherine Abbe, Eleanor Butler Sanders, Lucia Gilbert Runkle, Lee Haggin, and Adele M. Fielde huddled around Jacobi. But she was not smiling. In fact, her message was bleak. After witnessing some of the debate over enfranchisement and listening to delegates' more private discussions, she was convinced that the suffrage amendment would fail.

The committee members shook their heads in disbelief. But Jacobi had gone through the siege of Paris. For her, failure meant opportunity. From the ashes of bitter loss would arise something new and better.

Jacobi declared that the amendment would fail out of ignorance. Most women were ignorant of how government worked. Thus, it was imperative to raise women's understanding of politics and how it affected their lives. In her logical way, she proposed that the existing committee should reorganize and focus on creating education that would prepare women for intelligent participation in public and civic affairs. That night, Jacobi and the other members present agreed to dissolve the Volunteer Committee and replace it with the League for Political Education.

The next day, the suffrage amendment failed in a vote of ninety-seven to fifty-eight. The women had hoped for support from Republicans in particular, but party politics worked against them. Most who voted against the amendment agreed with Francis M. Scott of New York City, who proclaimed to the chamber: "I vote, not because I am intelligent, not because I am moral, but solely and simply because I am a man."

⟳

After returning home, Jacobi got to work expanding the arguments from her convention speech into a treatise, *"Common Sense" Applied to Woman Suffrage*, which was published by G. P. Putnam's Sons in 1894. Intended for a middle-class audience, the book took its title from Thomas Paine's revolutionary pamphlet "Common Sense," equating the cause of suffrage with the American Revolution.

Members of the League for Political Education, the forerunner of the League of Women Voters, paid a fee of two dollars per year. Its first education course was a study of John Fiske's *Civil Government of the United States* with an extensive outline prepared by Jacobi. Some students described it as a "catechism" because it was a thorough introduction and took so long to complete. The league networked with other women's organizations and urged them to integrate suffrage as part of their regular activities so that it became a normal part of any woman's club or charitable organization.

The campaign for suffrage had altered the trajectory of Jacobi's life. Over the next few years, she fought for humanitarian causes and against the corruption and influence of political machines. She continued to advocate for women's health, drawing a line from women's freedom to the fate of American civilization. In her dual role as physician and activist, she recommended an active girlhood that included education and exercise.

⌒

In 1901, Jacobi joined an expedition west to Yellowstone National Park. She stayed for a week, and on the final day, she decided to "indulge in a hot bath in the geyser water." Squinting at the sunlight reflecting off the scalding-hot springs, Jacobi gathered up her bathing skirt and dipped herself carefully into the water. The shocking 140 degrees Fahrenheit along with the pungent sulfur smell made her wince, but soon she was in up to her neck luxuriating in the warmth that relaxed her bones.

Not far from where she was bathing, a succession of terraces that resembled a rock-strewn, alien world rose some ten stories high, formed by the outflow of geothermal springs. The flinty white material that looked like melting snow covering the terraces was calcium carbonate, better known as limestone. Bacteria that fed on sulfides in the water were the source of its foul odor. The hotter the water, the stronger the smell, so when Dr. Mary Putnam Jacobi looked at the caking limestone terrace or inhaled the hot spring's rancid scent, she must have imagined a symphony of cells performing effortlessly at a microscopic level.

In the morning, she would begin her journey back home, which included a thirty-six-hour train ride. She was looking forward to seeing her newborn granddaughter, Ruth. Marjorie, who had graduated from Barnard College in 1899, had gotten married the next year to a delightful young friend of the family, George McAneny, and given birth to a healthy baby nine months later. Jacobi had instilled in her daughter a sense of justice, advising her to be "absolutely truthful" and "gentle while strong." Above all, she told Marjorie, "Never . . . allow your liberty to be taken away from you by anyone." Marjorie had selected a husband who reflected all of those qualities her mother valued, including truthfulness, freedom, and quiet strength. A reformer and budding politician, McAneny often joined Jacobi in advocating for the New York City Consumers League.

That night, after a light supper, Jacobi climbed into bed feeling pleasantly exhausted.

In the middle of the night, her eyes flew open.

She stared at the wood-beamed ceiling where, during the week, wasps had tried to build a nest that she kept knocking down with a broom. The back of her head was splitting with pain. Someone was moaning. Tears filled her eyes when she realized that she was the one making those whimpering sounds. She tried to cover her mouth but could not move her arm.

It took all the strength she had to push herself up to a sitting position. When her torso was finally upright, her stomach began to churn. The stillness in the pitch-black room gave way to violent spinning, and nausea engulfed her entire being. Using all her remaining strength, she managed to swing her legs to the floor and find the chamber pot just in time. She vomited up everything in her stomach. When the nausea finally subsided, she collapsed back into bed. Never in her life had she felt so afraid and helpless.

The next day, she remained in bed, took phenalgine for the pain, and gradually recovered. But weeks later, when she was back in New York and seeing patients in her medical practice, her throbbing headaches returned along with some nausea. She began recording her symptoms, how long they lasted, and how often they occurred. Now she was the patient—and the doctor.

～

A few months after returning from Yellowstone, she was in her office getting acquainted with a new patient, Charlotte Perkins Gilman. Recently married to Houghton Gilman, a Wall Street attorney, Gilman had a new home on the Upper West Side of Manhattan that was within walking distance of Jacobi's office. When Jacobi discovered that she and the famous author were neighbors, she wrote to Gilman offering to treat her "brain trouble." Despite her happy marriage, Gilman still suffered from dark periods of depression. She could not think, speak, or even rise from her bed on some days. Since she made her living by writing and speaking publicly, a career that kept her traveling most of the year, her "brain trouble" was debilitating. In fact, she had accumulated debt because she was unable to work. More than anything, she wanted to pay what she owed without relying on her husband.

Gilman was now at the height of her powers. Her book *Women and Economics: A Study of the Economic Relation Between Men and Women as a Factor in Social Evolution*, published in 1898, had made her internationally famous. Jacobi agreed with its central thesis wholeheartedly: since human women, unlike any other female creature on earth, were forced to depend on men for their food, this dependence turned marital sex into an economic exchange between husband and wife. Nowhere in nature was the female supported by the male throughout her life except among humans.

Jacobi welcomed Gilman to her office with a warm handshake, expressing great admiration for her work. She listened carefully while Gilman described her symptoms, then explained to her that she wanted to try an experimental treatment that might help lessen her brain fog and sadness. Jacobi asked Gilman if she minded being part of an experiment because, so far, none of her current patients with similar symptoms had agreed to it.

Gilman said that Jacobi could do anything she wanted, with one condition. She had never forgotten how Mitchell had openly scoffed at her written account of her own symptoms when she underwent his "rest cure." In fact, his authoritative demands had made her depression worse. This time, she wanted to be included as an active participant. And Gilman had come prepared. She pulled out a long "fever-chart." She had drawn parallel lines to show the progression from normal days to melancholia, "the years marked off with brief notes as to condition; and a wavering red line along the stretch of it, with a few peaks and many deep valleys, the average generally below normal."

Jacobi looked over the chart. Unlike the Blackwell sisters or other women doctors who thrived on emotional connections with patients, Jacobi rejected sentiment and advised her students to study each case "as coolly, impartially, abstractly, as if it were a problem in algebra." Jacobi believed that emotional connections to patients could lead to incorrect diagnoses and treatment. Similar to Mitchell's, her approach was the opposite of collaboration. This time, though, Jacobi charted a new course for herself. Gilman was one of Mitchell's so-called failures. Considering Jacobi's own very public disagreement with Mitchell and her criticism of his rest cure, her treatment of Gilman's mental condition would have symbolic repercussions. Thanking Gilman for the helpful fever chart, she agreed to a cooperative relationship. Gilman later wrote that Jacobi was the "most patient physician I had ever known." She "seemed to enter into the mind of the sufferer and know what was going on there."

Perhaps Jacobi's ideas about patient care had softened because her own baffling illness was getting worse. She had cared for bodies other than her own for most of her adult life. Now, the pain she suffered made her acutely aware of her own frailty. She understood the fear and frustration that Gilman was facing.

Today, though, Jacobi was full of enthusiasm. Pulling out her stethoscope, she told Gilman that they should get started right away with a thorough physical examination. Jacobi took her vital signs, drew blood for analysis, and obtained a urine sample. She let Gilman tell her all about herself, about her misery and pain, asking occasional questions and making notes in a chart. After Jacobi completed the examination, Gilman agreed to visit her office several times a week.

Two days later, Jacobi had Gilman relax on the exam table while she applied electrotherapy to her solar plexus in order to stimulate digestion. Then she had her drink a mixture of phosphoglycerates in wine to promote digestion, assimilation, and nutrition. She gave Gilman a notebook for recording any changes to her digestion.

At the next appointment, Jacobi explained that they would start the project of regenerating her cerebral activity. Like the child first learning to think and read, "forms and colors are the elements of all visual impressions. . . . It is upon forms and colors, therefore, that both perceptions and memory must first be exercised." She explained that her method would wake up Gilman's inert brain and get it working again through incremental, supervised, irrelevant tasks. Gilman spent the session on the floor in Jacobi's office constructing simple shapes with a set of Froebel Blocks for children.

After several days of block building, Jacobi asked Gilman to construct a particular shape. Then she knocked it down and told Gilman to rebuild the exact same shape from memory. They repeated this exercise for the next few sessions. Then, increasing the difficulty, Jacobi asked Gilman to draw maps of any familiar place, rooms, street corners, anything.

After map drawing, Gilman moved on to reading, first simple and then more complex books, finally ending up with E. B. Wilson's *The Cell in Development and Inheritance*, a textbook introduction to cell biology. Following Jacobi's advice, Gilman returned to writing her current manuscript, *Human Work*, a complex discussion of her organic vision of society. At the same time, Jacobi assigned Gilman a regimen of physical exercise that included learning the popular new sport of basketball and joining a team playing at Barnard College. As Gilman wrote, she felt the joy of physical exertion during which her misery and pain and shame seemed to fade into a remote past.

Jacobi and Gilman worked together for several weeks as their friendship grew. When Gilman felt that she had absorbed the knowledge and skills she needed, she left, feeling refreshed and better able to cope with her life.

She was not content to let her unique healing experience under Jacobi's care fade away. In a short story titled "Dr. Clair's Place," she brought to life the benevolent treatment of women provided by Dr. Clair at her sanatorium in Southern California. For the weakest patients, Dr. Clair offered simple rest in comfortable chairs. Those wanting more could read books, magazines, and newspapers in the library. "There were all manner of easy things to learn to do: basket-work, spinning, weaving, knitting, embroidery; it cost very little to the patients and kept them occupied. For those who were able there was gardening and building—always some new little place going up, or a walk or something to make." There was music, dancing, swimming, and even mountain climbing. None of this was compulsory, and her visitors "enjoyed life" every day.

But the most important benefit of Dr. Clair's place was not her benevolent medical treatment, according to Gilman. It was the wonderful people "who lived up there with work and interests of their own, some teachers, some writers, some makers of various things, but all Associates in her wonderful cures" where women learned how to earn their own living through meaningful work. "And out of the waste and wreck of my life—which is of small consequence to me," Gilman's narrator wrote, "I can myself serve to help new-comers. I am an Associate. . . . And I am Happy!"

Not long after Jacobi finished treating Gilman, she received word that her friend and mentor Dr. Marie Zakrzewska had died after a long illness. At the funeral, Zakrzewska's farewell letter was read to the mourners: "I do not think that my name . . . will be remembered. Yet the idea for which I have worked . . . must live and spread. . . . I desire no hereafter. I was born; I lived; I used my life to the best of my ability for the uplifting of my fellow creatures; and I enjoyed it daily in a thousand ways."

Jacobi understood exactly what Zakrzewska meant. While pursuing the study and practice of medicine, Jacobi and her mentors Drs. Elizabeth and Emily Blackwell, Dr. Ann Preston, and Zakrzewska confronted head-on society's need to keep women bound to the idea that they were inherently sick. Along the way, they found self-actualization in doing good work. As these pioneering women discovered, the antidote for any affliction, physical or mental, was the freedom to participate fully in a life well lived.

Epilogue

The Last Victory

*Vague longings beset me. I imagine great things and
glorious deeds; but Ah! The vision passes like a fleeting
dream and the muddy reality is left behind. I would be
great. I would do deeds, so that after I had passed into
that world, that region beyond the grave, I should be
spoken of with affection so that I should live again in
the hearts of those I have left behind me.*

—MARY PUTNAM, AGE TEN

IN THE SPRING OF 1902, JACOBI'S HAND TREMORS AND HEADACHES
grew worse. Just as Charlotte Perkins Gilman had kept a daily record
of symptoms, Jacobi wrote down her own. But she needed help. That winter, she welcomed the assistance of Emily Dunning, her new intern and
a recent medical school graduate. Emily was among the last students to
attend the Women's Medical School of the New York Infirmary. With a
heavy heart, Emily Blackwell had decided to close the women's college and
merge with Cornell's medical school after that university began accepting
women in 1898.

Emily Dunning had decided at fourteen that she wanted to be a nurse.
Her family had fallen on hard times, and when a friend of the family
suggested that Emily might earn a living as a milliner's apprentice, her
mother, who could not imagine her exceptionally bright daughter reduced
to making hats, said, "That settles the question. You are going to go to college." Emily's sister was a classmate of Marjorie Jacobi and suggested contacting Marjorie's mother, the famous doctor.

Jacobi saw potential in young Emily Dunning and advised her to go to college and study science. She suggested that if Dunning studied hard and made the effort, she might become a doctor rather than a nurse. It was the right advice for Dunning. She earned her medical degree in 1901 and began applying for clinical internships. Even though she received the highest grade on the entrance assessment for an internship at Gouverneur Hospital in New York City, the hospital rejected her application because she was a woman. The large city hospitals still refused to accept women for clinical work.

Two years earlier, in an address before the Women's Medical Association of New York, Jacobi had called for her colleagues to organize strong coalitions to fight prejudices against women doctors at city hospitals. She acknowledged that it would be a bitter struggle, but she urged women to keep applying at the hospitals and be willing "to go up again and again to be knocked down" until they finally claimed victory. Now, determined to help her gutsy protégée win a hospital appointment, Jacobi decided to lead that fight. She campaigned for every prominent physician who had supported her career to write letters of recommendation for Dunning. In addition, Jacobi used her personal connections to gather support from local politicians and religious leaders.

While continuing to apply for a position at hospitals, Dunning gained valuable clinical experience as Jacobi's assistant. The celebrated physician spent hours sharing the breadth of her knowledge, the careful steps she took for diagnosis, and the varied means of treatment available. She covered every topic, even the controversial practice of birth control. Finally, in the spring of 1902, Dunning won a competitive appointment as an intern at Gouverneur Hospital. She would be the first woman to work as an emergency doctor in New York.

Newspaper headlines announced: "Woman on an Ambulance: Exciting Experiences in Store for Surgeon Emily Dunning." She would be working in the rough neighborhood east of the Bowery, an area where even some male interns refused to go. After receiving the news, Dunning expressed her gratitude to Jacobi, whose delight was unbounded. Dunning would begin her internship in January. Until then, she continued to work with Jacobi, who needed the young doctor's help more than ever. Because of the progression of her illness, she had decided to close her practice at the end of the year.

Her pain was worsening. She was having more attacks that forced her to remain in bed. "Most frequently upon rising after sitting a long time," she wrote, "perhaps especially in the evening, I would fall to the floor, and experience considerable difficulty in getting up again." But what most disturbed her, to the point of heartbreak, were the psychological changes. "I began to lose the initiative which had formerly been so active with me. . . . It seemed as if a gauze veil were thrown over all the objects in which I had formerly been so intensely interested." Jacobi had diagnosed herself with a brain tumor.

In the 1880s, she had joined other physicians in an effort to distinguish signs of brain tumors from symptoms of nervous disease. She had published her conclusions in her book *Essays on Hysteria* (1888) in a section titled "Tumors of the Brain." Except for experimental surgeries, treatment options were minimal. For the past year or more, Jacobi had suspected that she was suffering from a fatal disease. She had come to terms with the inevitability of her own death, but coming to the end of her career was different. She was sixty years old and if she had been healthy, she would have continued to work for another decade. When the time came to close her office, Jacobi had Emily Dunning at her side. She finalized patient records and ended her lease. For the sake of her mentor, Dunning remained stoic, but each moment seemed incredibly sad. Jacobi grew exhausted, and at the end of the day, Dunning escorted her home. Marjorie had insisted on taking care of her mother as her illness progressed, and Jacobi had moved in with her daughter and son-in-law at 19 East Forty-seventh Street, where she would live for the rest of her life.

After Dunning started her hospital internship, Jacobi kept track of her progress and periodically sent notes of encouragement. In 1904, the day after she finished her residency, Dunning married another physician, Benjamin Barringer. Jacobi surprised Dunning on the eve of her marriage by delivering her wedding present in person, arriving with her attendant in a spiffy new automobile. Even though she ordinarily used a wheelchair, she gripped her attendant's arm and climbed slowly up the high front stoop. She handed Dunning a small suede leather box. Upon opening it, Dunning found Jacobi's social card, MRS. A. JACOBI, and beneath it, one hundred dollars in gold.

⤙

Jacobi spent the last years of her life analyzing her own illness. Abraham took little part in her health care. In 1903, Helen Baldwin, a New York

Infirmary physician, became her doctor, and to familiarize Baldwin with the case, Jacobi began writing a clinical account of her disease. She included her years of documentation, starting with the dates of her first symptoms. She noted even the smallest physical changes, her various drug regimens, and the development of other signs of the tumor. At first, the narrative had a simple title: *Case*. But as her condition got worse, it became part memoir and part clinical report. She retitled it *Description of the Early Symptoms of the Meningeal Tumor Compressing the Cerebellum, from Which the Author Died. Written by Herself*; it was published in 1906, the year that she died.

In true form, Jacobi would have the final word.

Abraham, whose life had been filled with such profound loss, found joy spending time with his two grandsons, Herbert and Arnold. In the spring of 1906, his best friend, Carl Schurz, died from pneumonia. Upon hearing of Schurz's death, Jacobi said, "The heaviest blow has fallen," referring to the shock to Abraham. Three weeks later, Jacobi passed away at the age of sixty-three in her daughter's Manhattan home on June 10, the anniversary of her son's death more than twenty years earlier.

On January 4, 1907, members of the Women's Medical Association of New York City, led by committee chairman Dr. Annie Sturgis and secretary Dr. Emily Dunning Barringer, held a memorial to honor Jacobi's life in the big hall of the Academy of Medicine. Young girls in white dresses acted as ushers while a string quartet played uplifting music. Jacobi herself had not liked listening to music, but she appreciated its function. Eminent men and women celebrated her career. Felix Adler, founder of the Ethical Culture Society, spoke of her contributions to education and as an individual whose "humane interest remained supreme." Florence Kelley, director of the Consumers League, described Jacobi's efforts on behalf of working women. Dr. Elizabeth Cushier spoke of Jacobi's insightful teaching and mentoring of women medical students and her many contributions to women in medicine. And Richard Watson Gilder, editor of the *Century*, praised her writing talents.

The eminent Dr. William Osler, recently appointed Regius Professor of Medicine at the University of Oxford in England, extolled Jacobi's legacy and her influence on the "emancipation of women" in the medical profession. "The value . . . of a human life may be gauged by the influence, the heliotropic potency which it exercises on its fellows. Position, wealth, reputation are as nothing in comparison with this truly solar gift of calling out the best that is in those about us. To many in this country she, whose memory we do honor to-night, stood as a bright particular star in the firmament of the profession." Osler proclaimed that he was waiting for "a woman in the profession with an intellect so commanding that she [would] take rank with the Harveys, the Hunters, the Pasteurs, the Virchows, and the Listers." This woman "will be of the type of mind and training of Mary Putnam Jacobi."

The Alumnae Association of the Woman's Medical College of Pennsylvania celebrated Jacobi's life with a memorial tablet that was placed in the main hall. At the unveiling ceremony where school alumnae remembered her pioneering spirit, Charlotte Perkins Gilman spoke about her own connection to Jacobi's life and thanked the great physician for helping to restore her intellectual and physical vitality.

In 1925, the Women's Medical Association of New York City continued Jacobi's legacy by publishing her selected writings in *Mary Putnam Jacobi, M.D.: A Pathfinder in Medicine* (New York: G. P. Putnam's Sons). That same year, Jacobi's sister Ruth Putnam published *Life and Letters of Mary Putnam Jacobi* with an introduction by their brother Haven. In 1950, Jacobi's life was dramatized on a Philadelphia radio program, *Within Our Gates,* as part of a campaign in support of the Woman's Medical College of Pennsylvania.

Hollywood depicted the life of Jacobi's protégée Emily Dunning Barringer in a film called *The Girl in White* (1952), starring June Allyson, based on Barringer's memoir, *Bowery to Bellevue: The Story of New York's First Woman Ambulance Surgeon.* The actress Mildred Dunnock portrayed a character named Marie Yeomans, a teacher based on Mary Putnam Jacobi.

Abraham lived for thirteen more years, until the age of eighty-nine. During that time, he rarely publicly recognized Mary's work in medicine, even in lengthy statements made to his biographer. In Bolton Landing, New York, the Abraham Jacobi and Carl Schurz Memorial Park recognized their public friendship, but Mary Putman Jacobi and her extraordinary life at Lake George remained unacknowledged.

While Jacobi did not survive to see the passage of woman's suffrage, her activist legacy lived on. Nine years after her death, on the eve of another New York Constitutional Convention in 1915, state suffragists published a new edition of *"Common Sense" Applied to Woman Suffrage* so Jacobi's words could inspire a new generation of feminists. Two years later, after a massive protest by suffragists during which women were arrested and imprisoned, New York voters passed an amendment to New York's constitution granting women the right to vote.

Jacobi did live long enough to see her hopes for women in medicine become reality. At the time of her death, seven thousand women were serving as physicians. More women were graduating from medical schools and being accepted into hospital clerkships, especially in New York City, Philadelphia, and Chicago. The American Medical Association formally began accepting women in 1915. Women's medical societies gained strength.

Yet, when the Woman's Medical College of the New York Infirmary closed its doors in 1900 to merge with Cornell, a group of women medical professors lost their jobs permanently. Like Hopkins, Cornell refused to hire women. By 1904, 61 percent, or 97 out of 160, of medical schools admitted women. By 1920, 75 percent were coeducational. By 1944, the only medical schools that did not admit women were St. Louis University, Georgetown, Dartmouth, Harvard, and Jefferson. Harvard Medical School admitted its first twelve women in September 1945 and hired a female professor in 1947. St. Louis University and Georgetown University followed in 1948. S. Weir Mitchell's alma mater, Jefferson Medical College in Philadelphia, was the last to admit women, in June 1960.

The Woman's Medical College of Pennsylvania, where Ann Preston graduated and later served as dean, remained open, employing women professors and surviving periods of instability and crisis until 1970, when it became a coeducational institution known as the Medical College of Pennsylvania.

The New England Hospital for Women and Children was renamed New England Hospital in 1951 when, due in part to financial difficulties, it welcomed men as well as women and children. In 1969, the hospital became the Dimock Community Health Center, named after Susan Dimock, the beloved resident doctor who drowned in the shipwreck of the SS *Schiller*. The clinic's restored complex is listed as a National Historic Landmark, and all the buildings are named after women.

The New York Infirmary for Indigent Women and Children remained in operation at its location in Stuyvesant Square until it merged with Beekman Downtown Hospital in 1981 and moved to Lower Manhattan, where it became known as the New York Downtown Hospital. Following a merger with New York–Presbyterian Hospital in 2013, it was renamed New York–Presbyterian Lower Manhattan Hospital. An affiliate of Weill Cornell

Medical College, the hospital serves as Lower Manhattan's only emergency department south of Fourteenth Street and treats tens of thousands of patients annually.

The percentage of women in medicine rose to 6 percent in 1910 and declined after that until 1950, when women physicians again reached 6 percent. At the same time, women's interest in medicine kept growing stronger, and their applications to medical schools rose steadily. Studies performed in 1966 noted that the number of women applicants had increased over 300 percent between 1930 and 1966 while the number of male applicants increased 29 percent. Yet the proportion of women accepted decreased and that of men increased. Open discrimination against women flourished. It was common practice for medical schools to immediately reject half of the female applicants solely on the basis of sex. During that time, men formed "old-boy" hiring networks that prevented top women graduates from securing positions in choice residency programs. Until the 1970s, the percentage of women in medicine remained steady at only 7 percent. For Black women, it was nearly impossible to gain entrance into medical schools. In 1970, only about 2 percent of physicians were Black women.

Things began to change with the rise of the feminist movement in the late 1960s. After the passage of Title IX in 1972, which prohibited discrimination in education based on sex, women's enrollment in medical schools more than tripled. By 1990, the number of women physicians had grown by 310 percent. According to the American Medical Association, by 2019, more than 50 percent of all applicants accepted into medical schools were women. Yet racial discrimination remained appalling. Only 4.6 percent of the women accepted were Black.

Today, 60 percent of practicing physicians under age thirty-five are women. Women make up over 85 percent of all ob-gyns. Not surprisingly, 82 percent of physicians over age sixty-five are men. Because of the growing need for primary-care practitioners, the roles of physician assistants (66.4 percent women) and nurse practitioners and midwives (89.2 percent women) are growing even more significant.

Jacobi's research into women's health, especially her Boylston Medical Prize study, compelled other women to follow in her footsteps. In the first decade of the twentieth century, physician Clelia Duel Mosher and psychologist Leta Stetter Hollingworth continued Jacobi's research and her efforts to depathologize menstruation, providing empirical data that proved women's intellectual capacity. But Jacobi's most notable work in neurology, her radical rejection of gender dichotomies and promotion of ideas about gender fluidity, was truly visionary. A new generation of women physicians and scientists began integrating the sciences with new genetic information on sex chromosomes and gender studies to challenge prevailing notions of sex differences.

If Jacobi were alive today, she would likely be a member of the Neuro-Genderings Network, an international group of scholars formed to critically evaluate how research on sex differences in the brain is produced. Representing a broad range of disciplines such as neuroscience, the humanities, gender and queer studies, feminist science studies, and science and technology studies, the network argues that, in the area of sex differences, science cannot be separated from politics, echoing Jacobi's own conclusions. These feminist scholars analyze and confront popular research on biological determinism and gender essentialism that basically agrees with Edward H. Clarke in asserting that a woman is simply a product of her biology. Prominent members include Daphna Joel, a neuroscientist and neurofeminist best known for her research showing that there is no such thing as a male or female brain, and Rebecca Jordan-Young, author of *Brain Storm: The Flaws in the Science of Sex Differences*, a critical analysis of research supporting the theory that psychological sex differences in humans are "hardwired" into the brain.

Jacobi would also be at the forefront of those who oppose the catastrophic *Dobbs v. Jackson* ruling outlawing abortion, a decision embedded deeply in the nineteenth century and the white man's malevolent sense of racial superiority. Writing for the majority, Justice Alito stated, "Procuring an abortion is not a fundamental constitutional right because such a right has no basis in the Constitution's text or in our Nation's history." In so doing, he and four other conservative justices resurrected Dr. Horatio Storer, referring almost exclusively to the legal decisions made in the mid-1800s during his antiabortion crusade. Before that time, abortion was legal and ordinary. According to men like Storer, "A woman's ovaries belong to the commonwealth; she is simply their custodian." Her sole occupation, much like a guardian overseeing a trust fund, is to protect the womb and its output at all costs.

The battles that Mary Putnam Jacobi and the first women physicians fought are being fought again today. Not only would Jacobi be on the front lines, she would be advocating for a consolidation of power in order to win, creating networks and supporting political candidates and organizations that fight for abortion rights. As Jacobi often advised: Risk everything, work hard, and reach for the stars. But most of all, organize.

Acknowledgments

M Y GRANDFATHER LEO THOMAS WAS A SUPREME TELLER OF TRUE tales. At holiday dinners and family gatherings, he held us all spellbound during meals, chatting about his life adventures and finishing his plate of food at the same time. Listening to Grandad's stories, I learned about fly-fishing at night, native stone architecture, and Tiger, the dauntless female cat who kept the movie theater my grandparents owned mice-free. I am grateful to Grandad, and to my mother, who inherited his ability for sharing that creative spark with me.

I want to thank my husband, Andy Newberg, for crafting my fabulous author website and reading story drafts. I'd like to thank my brother, David, and his wife, Gayla, and my vivacious nieces, Katie and Grace, for their encouragement and support. My sister, Rosalind, shared her marketing expertise. And Holly Heston, my friend and confidante, read early drafts and provided valuable comments.

This book would not have existed without the nurturing support of my superb agent, Mackenzie Brady Watson, and the brilliant team at Stuart Krichevsky Literary Agency. I am deeply indebted to Elisabeth Dyssegaard, my amazing editor, who shepherded the manuscript through to completion. I am grateful for her dedication and enthusiasm in bringing this story to life. Many thanks to my intrepid copy editor, Tracy Roe, whose medical expertise and meticulous edits heightened the quality of this book. To those at St. Martin's Press, whose passion and hard work made this manuscript into a stunning book, your efforts are much appreciated. I also want to thank Katie Adams for her expertise and assistance in developing the initial book proposal.

I am indebted to the scholars and biographers whose research helped pave the way for this book. In addition, I am grateful for the help from the archivists I contacted at the Alan Mason Chesney Medical Archives and the Schlesinger Library at Harvard Library. I could not have written this book without access to online sources at the National Archives, *The New York Times*, Drexel University's Legacy Center College of Medicine Archives, and many others.

Last, for helping me to maintain focus and stay conditioned and sane while writing this book, I want to thank my exercise therapist, Lindsey Long, and massage therapist, Jessica Caine. And to my cat family—Neo, Déjà vu, Penelope, Jingle, and Opie—you all are purring angels who keep me grounded every day.

Notes

Epigraph

ix **"Since 1848":** Mary Putnam Jacobi, *"Common Sense" Applied to Woman Suffrage: A Statement of the Reasons Which Justify the Demand to Extend the Suffrage to Women, with Consideration of the Arguments Against Such Enfranchisement, and with Special Reference to the Issues Presented to the New York State Convention of 1894* (New York: G. P. Putnam's Sons, 1894).

ix **"I said I":** Silas Weir Mitchell, *Characteristics* (New York: Century, 1915), 264.

Prologue: A Desire to Heal

3 **Lawrence Summers:** Sam Dillon, "Harvard Chief Defends His Talk on Women," *New York Times*, January 18, 2005, https://www.nytimes.com/2005/01/18/us/harvard-chief -defends-his-talk-on-women.html#:~:text=The%20president%20of%20Harvard%20Uni- versity,regretted%20if%20they%20were%20misunderstood.

3 **Jordan Peterson:** See Jordan Peterson's *Maps of Meaning: The Architecture of Belief* (New York: Routledge, 1999); *Twelve Rules for Life: An Antidote to Chaos* (Toronto: Random House Canada, 2018); *Beyond Order: Twelve More Rules for Life* (Toronto: Random House Canada, 2021).

3 **believed that her hormones:** Mel Robbins, "Hillary Clinton and the Clueless Hor- mone Argument," CNN.com, April 21, 2015, https://www.cnn.com/2015/04/20/opinions /robbins-hillary-clinton/index.html.

3 **got her period:** Lara Rutherford-Morrison, "Why This Letter About Hillary Clinton Is Wrong," *Bustle*, October 17, 2016, https://www.bustle.com/articles/189974-hillary-clinton -cant-be-president-because-of-menstruation-claims-this-letter-to-the-editor-but-thats.

4 **"Two treatises":** Ken Armstrong, "Draft Overturning *Roe v. Wade* Quotes Infamous Witch Trial Judge with Long-Discredited Ideas on Rape," ProPublica, May 6, 2022, https: //www.propublica.org/article/abortion-roe-wade-alito-scotus-hale.

Part One: Beginning

5 **"Unknown things":** Mary C. Putnam, "Theorae ad Lienis Officium" ("Theories with Regard to the Function of the Spleen") (medical-school thesis, Female Medical College of Pennsylvania, 1864), https://drexel.primo.exlibrisgroup.com/view/UniversalViewer /01DRXU_INST/12344620660004721?xywh=-3204,-226,10037,5003&r=0.

Chapter 1: A Moral Imperative

7 **On a typical day:** Blackwell advertisement, *New-York Tribune*, October 13, 1851, https: //www.newspapers.com/article/new-york-tribune-blackwell-advertisement/90830230/.

7 **rejected by twenty-nine:** "Dr. Elizabeth Blackwell Biography," Hobart and William Smith Colleges, www.hws.edu/about/history/elizabeth-blackwell/biography.aspx.

7 **With few exceptions:** Elizabeth Blackwell, *Pioneer Work in Opening the Medical Profession to Women: Autobiographical Sketches* (London: Longmans, Green, 1895), chapter 3.

8 **attended medical school:** Blackwell, *Pioneer Work*, chapter 3.

8 **While attending the medical college:** Blackwell, *Pioneer Work*, 178–179.

8 **Influenced by the charismatic:** Janice P. Nimura, *The Doctors Blackwell: How Two Pioneering Sisters Brought Medicine to Women—and Women to Medicine* (New York: W. W. Norton, 2021), 21–28.

9 **called himself D.K.:** D.K., "The Late Medical Degree to a Female," *Boston Medical and Surgical Journal* 40, no. 3 (February 21, 1849): 58–59.

9 **"As to females":** Justus, "The Late Medical Degree at Geneva," *Boston Medical and Surgical Journal* 40, no. 4 (February 28, 1849): 87.

9 **"unprincipled men":** Blackwell, *Pioneer Work*, chapter 5.

10 **Blackwell opened:** Ruth Abram, *Send Us a Lady Physician: Women Doctors in America, 1835–1920* (New York: W. W. Norton, 1985), 81.

11 **"Many sensitive women":** Edwin Fussell, "Valedictory Address to the Graduating Class of the Female Medical College of Pennsylvania, At the Tenth Annual Commencement, March 13, 1861," Philadelphia: J.B. Chandler, Printer, 1861, 7.

11 **These Quaker men:** Steven J. Peitzman, *A New and Untried Course: Woman's Medical College and Medical College of Pennsylvania, 1850–1998* (New Brunswick, NJ: Rutgers University Press, 2000), 1.

11 **fifty policemen:** Peitzman, *A New and Untried Course*, 6.

11 **the courageous escape:** "Temple Professor Uncovers Lost Literary Gold with 'Cousin Ann's Stories for Children,'" *Daily Local News*, February 8, 2011, https://www.dailylocal.com/2011/02/08/temple-professor-uncovers-lost-literary-gold-with-cousin-anns-stories-for-children/.

11 **"To My Little Readers":** Ann Preston, *Cousin Ann's Stories for Children* (Philadelphia: J. M. McKim, 1849).

11 **women's destiny:** Susan Wells, *Out of the Dead House: Nineteenth-Century Women Physicians and the Writing of Medicine* (Madison: University of Wisconsin Press, 2001), 61–68.

12 **"cult of true womanhood":** Barbara Welter, "The Cult of True Womanhood: 1820–1860," *American Quarterly* 18, no. 2 (1966): 151–74, https://doi.org/10.2307/2711179.

12 **Preston maintained:** Wells, *Out of the Dead House*, 61–68.

13 **"All these evils":** Charles D. Meigs, *Females and Their Diseases: A Series of Letters to His Class* (Philadelphia: Lea and Blanchard, 1848), 19, https://archive.org/details/femalestheomeig/page/18/mode/2up?q=evils.

13 **"The question is":** Walter Channing, *Remarks on the Employment of Females as Practitioners in Midwifery* (Boston: Cummings and Hillard, 1820), 4.

14 **"For this Misfortune":** John Tennent, with contributions from Benjamin Franklin, *Every man his own doctor, or, The poor planter's physician*, fourth edition (Philadelphia: Re-printed and sold by B. Franklin, near the market, 1736), 40. See Medicine in the Americas, 1610–1920, National Library of Medicine Digital Collections, http://resource.nlm.nih.gov/8111161.

14 **a good midwife:** Regina Morantz-Sanchez, *Sympathy and Science: Women Physicians in American Medicine* (Chapel Hill: University of North Carolina Press, 1985), 12.

14 **bar men from:** Morantz-Sanchez, *Sympathy and Science*, 17.

14 **Technological developments:** Morantz-Sanchez, *Sympathy and Science*, 17.

15 **the few hundred:** Morantz-Sanchez, *Sympathy and Science*, 19.

15 **Benjamin Franklin helped:** Morantz-Sanchez, *Sympathy and Science*, 16.

15 **practicing midwifery provided:** Morantz-Sanchez, *Sympathy and Science*, 18.

15 **"It is obvious":** Channing, *Remarks on the Employment of Females as Practitioners in Midwifery*, 7.

16 **"first and happiest fruits":** Channing, *Remarks on the Employment of Females as Practitioners in Midwifery*, 21.

17 **"Will you please inform":** Meigs, *Females and Their Diseases*, 199–200.

18 **woman "has a head":** Meigs, *Females and Their Diseases*, 47.

18 **Dean Holmes said:** Myra C. Glenn, *Dr. Harriot Kezia Hunt: Nineteenth-Century Physician and Woman's Rights Advocate* (Amherst: University of Massachusetts Press, 2018), 55.

19 **applied to Harvard:** Glenn, *Dr. Harriot Kezia Hunt*, 82–85.

19 **"When civilization":** Harriot Kezia Hunt, *Glances and Glimpses, or Fifty Years Social, Including Twenty Years Professional Life* (1856; repr., Chicago: Sourcebooks, 1970), 218.

20 **"by nature, better qualified":** "Editor's Table," *Godey's Lady's Book* (August 1851): 122–23.

20 **Harriot Hunt joined:** Glenn, *Dr. Harriot Kezia Hunt*, 127–28.

21 **Her brother Henry:** Nimura, *The Doctors Blackwell*, 119.

21 **"This medical solitude":** Nimura, *The Doctors Blackwell*, 175.

Chapter 2: A Tale of Two Hospitals

22 **"revolutionary tendencies":** Marie Zakrzewska, *A Woman's Quest: The Life of Marie E. Zakrzewska, M.D.* (1924; repr., New York City: Arno Press, 1972), 16.

22 **Marie's eyes:** Zakrzewska, *A Woman's Quest*, 17.

24 **Ernst Horn:** Arleen Marcia Tuchman, *Science Has No Sex: The Life of Marie Zakrzewska, M.D.* (Chapel Hill: University of North Caroline Press, 2006), 50.

24 **"women will now":** Zakrzewska, *A Woman's Quest*, 67.

24 **they sailed from:** Zakrzewska, *A Woman's Quest*, 72.

24 **"I have at last":** Zakrzewska, *A Woman's Quest*, 109.

25 **Hunt met the young:** Hunt, *Glances and Glimpses*, 347.

26 **"all sorts of":** J. Marion Sims, *The Story of My Life* (New York: D. Appleton, 1884), 209.

26 **"She fell with":** Sims, *The Story of My Life*, 231.

26 **on her knees and elbows:** Sims, *The Story of My Life*, 234.

26 **"ransacked the country":** Sims, *The Story of My Life*, 236.

27 **eighteen-year-old Lucy:** Brynn Holland, "The 'Father of Modern Gynecology' Performed Shocking Experiments on Enslaved Women," History.com, August 29, 2017, https://qa.history.com/news/the-father-of-modern-gynecology-performed-shocking-experiments-on-slaves.

27 **"Lucy's agony":** Sims, *The Story of My Life*, 238.

27 **"I thought she was":** Sims, *The Story of My Life*, 238.

27 **"He is thoroughly":** Nimura, *The Doctors Blackwell*, 180.

27 **saying that his success:** Charles Meigs, "Cure of a Vesico-Vaginal Fistual," *The Medical Examiner, and Record of Medical Science*, Volume 7, edited by Francis Gurney Smith and J. B. Biddle (Philadelphia: Lindsay & Blakistion, 1851). 655.

28 **She was not fooled:** Nimura, *The Doctors Blackwell*, 196.

28 **underwent thirty operations:** G. J. Barker-Benfield, *The Horrors of the Half-Known Life: Male Attitudes Toward Women and Sexuality in Nineteenth-Century America* (New York: Routledge, 2000), 102.

28 **"The blood affected me":** Nimura, *The Doctors Blackwell*, 154.

28 **"As this movement":** Nimura, *The Doctors Blackwell*, 175–76.

29 **"architect of the vagina":** Barker-Benfield, *The Horrors of the Half-Known Life*, 91.

29 **compared him to:** Barker-Benfield, *The Horrors of the Half-Known Life*, 101.

30 **appointed Mrs. Brown:** Zakrzewska, *A Woman's Quest*, 226.

30 **called the wedding:** *Newport [RI] Daily News*, September 2, 1873, 2.

30 **"Suffering womanhood":** Mary Putnam Jacobi, "Woman in Medicine," in *Woman's Work in America*, ed. Annie Nathan Meyer (New York: Henry Holt, 1891), 155–56.

31 **Zakrzewska, while applauding:** Zakrzewska, *A Woman's Quest*, 183.

31 **drawing-room talk:** Elizabeth Blackwell, "An Appeal in Behalf of the Medical Education of Women," 1856, Elizabeth Blackwell Papers, Library of Congress, https://crowd .loc.gov/campaigns/blackwells-extraordinary-family/elizabeth-blackwell-subject-file /mss1288001281/mss1288001281–2/.

31 **well-connected Harriot Hunt:** Zakrzewska, *A Woman's Quest*, 197–98.

32 **At the opening ceremonies:** Zakrzewska, *A Woman's Quest*, 212.

32 **the south and east:** Robert McNamara, "New York's Most Notorious Neighborhood," ThoughtCo.,March7,2021,https://www.thoughtco.com/five-points-ny-notorious-neighborhood -1774064.

32 **"homelike" establishment:** "What the Lady Doctors Are Doing," *New York Times*, July 24, 1857.

32 **Zakrzewska depended on:** Zakrzewska, *A Woman's Quest*, 196.

33 **a thousand maternal deaths:** Max Roser and Hannah Ritchie, "Maternal Mortality," Our World in Data, 2013, https://ourworldindata.org/maternal-mortality.

33 **late stages of pregnancy:** Laura Helmuth, "The Disturbing, Shameful History of Childbirth Deaths," *Slate*, September 10, 2013, https://slate.com/technology/2013/09/death-in -childbirth-doctors-increased-maternal-mortality-in-the-20th-century-are-midwives-better .html.

33 **Less than an hour:** Zakrzewska, *A Woman's Quest*, 219.

33 **doctors in that hospital:** Zakrzewska, *A Woman's Quest*, 219.

Chapter 3: Awakening

35 **Putnam ancestors:** Carla Bittel, *Mary Putnam Jacobi and the Politics of Medicine in Nineteenth-Century America* (Chapel Hill: University of North Carolina Press, 2009), 3–4.

35 **published single women:** Ruth Putnam, ed., *Life and Letters of Mary Putnam Jacobi* (New York: G. P. Putnam's Sons, 1925), 359.

36 **annual report:** "Annual Meeting of the New-York Infirmary for Indigent Women and Children," *New York Times*, January 28, 1862.

37 **Elizabeth Blackwell herself:** Bittel, *Mary Putnam Jacobi*, 33.

37 **nicknamed "Minnie":** Putnam, *Life and Letters*, 13.

37 **"see Thackeray":** Anna B. Warner, *Susan Warner ("Elizabeth Wetherell")* (New York: G. P. Putnam's Sons, 1909), 373.

37 **sign on the front door:** Putnam, *Life and Letters*, 32.

38 **"Tomorrow I shall":** Putnam, *Life and Letters*, 25.

38 **At age fifteen:** Putnam, *Life and Letters*, 51.

38 **moderately religious:** Bittel, *Mary Putnam Jacobi*, 19.

39 **"masculine millennium":** Bittel, *Mary Putnam Jacobi*, 19.

39 **the young pastor:** Bittel, *Mary Putnam Jacobi*, 19–20.

39 **questioning her faith:** Bittel, *Mary Putnam Jacobi*, 28.

40 **the word *laboratory*:** "New Biological Methods in the 19th Century: The Rise of Laboratory Biology; the Cell Theory; Experimental Physiology," School of International Liberal Studies, Waseda University, Tokyo, Japan, updated September 2023, http://www.f.waseda.jp /sidoli/HMELS_05_New_Biology.pdf.

41 **panicked response:** Putnam, *Life and Letters*, 60.

42 **"Women of New York":** "To the Women of New York," *New York Daily Herald*, April 27, 1861.

42 **three thousand:** "The Women and the War," *New York Daily Herald*, April 30, 1861.

42 **"God bless you":** "The Women and the War," *New York Daily Herald.*

42 **Wartime physicians:** Paige Gibbons Backus, "Female Nurses During the Civil War: Angels of the Battlefield," American Battlefield Trust, October 20, 2020, updated June 1, 2021, https://www.battlefields.org/learn/articles/female-nurses-during-civil-war#:~:text =Not%20only%20did%20they%20provide,them%2C%20and%20reading%20to%20them.

43 **qualified female recruits:** "From Battlefield to Bedside: Great Nurses of the Civil War," Roswell Park Comprehensive Cancer Center, May 6, 2020, https://www.roswellpark .org/cancertalk/202005/battlefield-bedside-great-nurses-civil-war.

43 **president (Dr. Valentine Mott):** Julia Boyd, *The Excellent Doctor Blackwell: The Life of the First Woman Physician* (London: Thistle, 2013), 226.

43 **appointed Dorothea Dix:** Boyd, *The Excellent Doctor Blackwell,* 227.

43 **understandably bitter:** Boyd, *The Excellent Doctor Blackwell,* 227.

43 **regular hospitals refused:** Nimura, *The Doctors Blackwell,* 229.

44 **fifteen thousand women:** "Nursing," Women and the American Story, New-York Historical Society Museum and Library, accessed August 9, 2023, https://wams.nyhistory.org/a -nation-divided/civil-war/nursing/.

44 **constant dangers of serving during wartime:** "Nursing," New-York Historical Society Museum and Library.

44 **represented 91 percent:** Patricia D'Antonio and Jean C. Whelan, "Counting Nurses: The Power of Historical Census Data," *Journal of Clinical Nursing* 18. no. 19 (October 2009): 2017–24.

44 **Boston's most affluent:** Glenn, *Dr. Harriot Kezia Hunt,* 181.

44 **protest having to pay taxes:** Glenn, *Dr. Harriot Kezia Hunt,* 92–93.

45 **Female Medical College:** Pamela Curtin, Taylor Geer, and Alona Sleith, "Ann Preston, M.D., Historical Marker," Clio: Your Guide to History, May 17, 2021, https://theclio.com /tour/2001/26.

45 **formal nurse-training:** "From Battlefield to Bedside," Roswell Park Comprehensive Cancer Center.

45 **three hundred dollars:** "This Day in History: July 13, 1863: New York City Draft Riots and Massacre," Zinn Education Project, accessed July 20, 2023, https://www.zinnedproject .org/news/tdih/draft-riots/.

46 **capture of New Orleans:** Patrick Kelly-Fischer, "'New Orleans Gone and with It the Confederacy'—The Fall of New Orleans," Emerging Civil War, May 31, 2022, https: //emergingcivilwar.com/2022/05/31/new-orleans-gone-and-with-it-the-confederacy-the -fall-of-new-orleans/.

46 **1.3 million:** Gary L. Miller, "Historical Natural History: Insects and the Civil War," Montana State University, https://www.montana.edu/historybug/civilwar2/gallnippers .html#:~:text=There%20were%20over%201.3%20million,the%20disease%20were%20com- paratively%20lower.

46 **Haven's worried family:** Putnam, *Life and Letters,* 63–64.

46 **slavery in Louisiana:** Kelly-Fischer, "'New Orleans Gone.'"

47 **"true and loyal citizen":** Putnam, *Life and Letters,* 65.

47 **childhood ponies:** Putnam, *Life and Letters,* 65.

48 **"Sarah Contraband":** Putnam, *Life and Letters,* 85.

48 **spoke to a group:** Putnam, *Life and Letters,* 65.

48 **Freedmen's Commission:** Bittel, *Mary Putnam Jacobi,* 35.

48 **he wrote back:** Putnam, *Life and Letters,* 67.

Chapter 4: Setbacks

50 **"hen medics":** Peitzman, *A New and Untried Course,* 2.

51 **"When dealing with":** Bittel, *Mary Putnam Jacobi,* 41.

51 **presented an overview:** Bittel, *Mary Putnam Jacobi*, 42.

52 **an unambitious man:** Carol B. Gartner, "Fussell's Folly: Academic Standards and the Case of Mary Putnam Jacobi," *Academic Medicine* 71, no. 5 (May 1996).

53 **"Miss Putnam's tickets":** Gartner, "Fussell's Folly," 472.

54 **Ann Preston thanked:** Gartner, "Fussell's Folly," 472.

54 **allowing Putnam to graduate:** Gartner, "Fussell's Folly," 473.

54 **Fussell resigned:** Gartner, "Fussell's Folly," 473.

55 **changed the college's name:** Peitzman, *A New and Untried Course*, 28.

55 **Rebecca Cole:** "Dr. Rebecca J. Cole," Changing the Face of Medicine, last updated June 3, 2015, https://cfmedicine.nlm.nih.gov/physicians/biography_66.html.

55 **that Dr. Cole was:** Leila McNeill, "Race in America: The Woman Who Challenged the Idea That Black Communities Were Destined for Disease," *Smithsonian Magazine*, June 5, 2018, https://www.smithsonianmag.com/science-nature/woman-challenged-idea-black -communities-destined-disease-180969218/.

56 **was Lucy Sewall:** Rhoda Truax, *The Doctors Jacobi* (Boston: Little, Brown, 1932), 35–36.

56 **hospital was full:** "The Attractions of Boston for Sick Women: Letter to the Editor," *Vermont Phoenix*, October 6, 1865; Truax, *The Doctors Jacobi*, 36.

56 **emergency visits:** Truax, *The Doctors Jacobi*, 36.

57 **lived at the hospital:** Virginia G. Drachman, *Hospital with a Heart: Women Doctors and the Paradox of Separatism at the New England Hospital, 1862–1969* (Ithaca, NY: Cornell University Press, 1984), 76.

57 **Interns entered:** Drachman, *Hospital with a Heart*, 77–78.

57 **first in Boston:** Tuchman, *Science Has No Sex*, 211.

57 **quiet laboratory:** Truax, *The Doctors Jacobi*, 37.

58 **government's collector:** "Putnam, George Palmer," *The National Cyclopaedia of American Biography*, Volume II (New York: James T. White, 1892), 388–389.

58 **fifteen-year-old Bishop:** Truax, *The Doctors Jacobi*, 38.

58 **"See how the water":** Truax, *The Doctors Jacobi*, 40.

58 **And she answered:** Truax, *The Doctors Jacobi*, 40.

58 **October of 1864:** Truax, *The Doctors Jacobi*, 38.

59 **"It's only the excitement":** Truax, *The Doctors Jacobi*, 41.

60 **quietly dread:** Truax, *The Doctors Jacobi*, 44.

60 **Shylock image:** John Higham, "Social Discrimination Against Jews in America, 1830–1930," *Publications of the American Jewish Historical Society* 47, no. 1 (September 1957): 9.

60 **"The whole thing must end":** Truax, *The Doctors Jacobi*, 52.

Chapter 5: Revolutionary

62 **Help of Elizabeth:** Putnam, *Life and Letters*, 95.

63 **the old nurse Hester:** Putnam, *Life and Letters*, 129.

63 **a key ally:** Putnam, *Life and Letters*, 104.

63 **wrote her parents:** Putnam, *Life and Letters*, 107.

63 **She bragged:** Putnam, *Life and Letters*, 128.

64 **complained to her mother:** Putnam, *Life and Letters*, 111.

64 **fourth clinic:** Putnam, *Life and Letters*, 121.

64 **Paris correspondent:** Bittel, *Mary Putnam Jacobi*, 61–62.

64 **reading Rousseau's:** Putnam, *Life and Letters*, 105.

64 **revered philosopher:** Karen Offen, *The Woman Question in France, 1400–1870* (New York: Cambridge University Press, 2017).

65 **"French prejudices rest":** Putnam, *Life and Letters*, 121.

65 **"I knew well enough":** Putnam, *Life and Letters*, 121.

65 **short, thick-set:** Putnam, *Life and Letters*, 187.

65 **"Why, Monsieur":** Wells, *Out of the Dead House*, 169.

66 **Tragedy was:** Putnam, *Life and Letters*, 132.

67 **In 1865, Bernard:** Bittel, *Mary Putnam Jacobi*, 53.

67 **chemical palace:** Peter J. T. Morris, *The Matter Factory: A History of the Chemistry Laboratory* (London: Reaktion Books, 2015), 149–50.

67 **"encountered frequently":** Putnam, *Life and Letters*, 140.

68 **Based on several:** Bittel, *Mary Putnam Jacobi*, 60.

68 **duchess of Orleans:** Putnam, *Life and Letters*, 95.

68 **packed with students:** Putnam, *Life and Letters*, 130.

69 **Emily introduced her:** Putnam, *Life and Letters*, 150.

70 **"If you wish yourself":** Putnam, *Life and Letters*, 152.

70 **masked his political:** Bittel, *Mary Putnam Jacobi*, 67–68.

71 **On November 23:** Bittel, *Mary Putnam Jacobi*, 63.

71 **Putnam was referred to:** Putnam, *Life and Letters*, 158.

71 **"Duruy law":** "The Duruy Law for Primary Education, 1867," Foundation Napoléon, March 2017, https://www.napoleon.org/wp-content/uploads/2016/04/duruyloi_1867–2017 _bibliographie_gallica_en.pdf.

72 **At dinner:** Putnam, *Life and Letters*, 158–59.

72 **"Write me a letter":** Putnam, *Life and Letters*, 159.

72 **received an invitation:** Putnam, *Life and Letters*, 166.

73 **three days later:** Putnam, *Life and Letters*, 168.

73 **letter to her parents:** Putnam, *Life and Letters*, 167.

74 **wrote to Monsieur Danton:** Bittel, *Mary Putnam Jacobi*, 65.

74 **hurried across the street:** Putnam, *Life and Letters*, 180.

75 **more than science:** Truax, *The Doctors Jacobi*, 76.

75 **patriarch Dumesnil:** Truax, *The Doctors Jacobi*, 91.

76 **fascinated by volcanoes:** Rebecca West, *Survivors in Mexico* (New Haven, CT: Yale University Press, 2003), 175.

76 **"red-hot":** Truax, *The Doctors Jacobi*, 80.

76 **"salt of the earth":** Truax, *The Doctors Jacobi*, 80.

76 **earning the two hundred:** Putnam, *Life and Letters*, 149; see also Bittel, *Mary Putnam Jacobi*, 75

77 **"Monsieur M.":** Putnam, *Life and Letters*, 282.

77 **"to my marrying":** Putnam, *Life and Letters*, 162.

78 **"Thank you very much":** Putnam, *Life and Letters*, 199.

78 **"My only trouble":** Putnam, *Life and Letters*, 132.

78 **the American woman:** "Women and Medical Colleges," *Health Reformer* 4, no. 9 (March 1870): 163.

79 **"Et bien":** Putnam, *Life and Letters*, 227.

79 **"Sir, I studied":** Putnam, *Life and Letters*, 227.

79 **"Well, I couldn't":** Putnam, *Life and Letters*, 227.

79 **sailed past:** Putnam, *Life and Letters*, 231.

80 **"first had failed":** Putnam, *Life and Letters*, 231.

80 **rushed to the courtyard:** Putnam, *Life and Letters*, 232.

80 **letter to her mother:** Putnam, *Life and Letters*, 222.

81 **anger toward:** Bittel, *Mary Putnam Jacobi*, 77.

81 **her friend Monsieur:** Truax, *The Doctors Jacobi*, 105.

81 **taken prisoner:** Putnam, *Life and Letters*, 256.

82 **Dr. Emily Blackwell:** Truax, *The Doctors Jacobi*, 106.

82 **shutting out:** Ellen Hampton, "'Circle of Iron and Fire': Americans in Paris During the 1870–71 Franco-Prussian War," Historynet, July 15, 2021, https://www.historynet.com /americans-in-paris/.

82 **"so much suffering":** Hampton, "'Circle of Iron.'"

82 **horses had been:** Hampton, "'Circle of Iron.'"

82 **bombs exploded:** Putnam, *Life and Letters*, 277.

82 **population starving:** Hampton, "'Circle of Iron.'"

83 **On March 18:** Hampton, "'Circle of Iron.'"

83 **"the crowning defeat":** Putnam, *Life and Letters*, 256.

84 **"You have reached":** Truax, *The Doctors Jacobi*, 117.

84 **"now *docteur*":** Putnam, *Life and Letters*, 286.

84 **fatty acids:** Putnam, *Life and Letters*, 291.

84 **the French newspaper:** Putnam, *Life and Letters*, 289–91.

85 **advance of science:** Bittel, *Mary Putnam Jacobi*, 85.

Part Two: Backlash

87 **"It is inevitable":** Mary Putnam Jacobi, "Mental Action and Physical Health," in *The Education of American Girls*, ed. Anna C. Brackett (New York: G. P. Putnam's Sons, 1874), 259.

Chapter 6: A Mistaken Ally

89 **uncovered statistics:** Frederick N. Dyer, *The Physicians' Crusade Against Abortion* (New York: Watson Publishing, 2005), 3.

90 **"body of jealous":** "Reviews and Notices," *Cincinnati Medical Observer* (Cincinnati: E. B. Stevens, 1857), 129.

90 **AMA appointed Storer:** See Nina Renata Aron, "The Father of American Gynecology Fought to Criminalize Abortion in the 1850s," Timeline, March 27, 2017, https://timeline.com /horatio-storer-criminal-abortion-c433606491da; Richa Venkatramen, "Horatio Robinson Storer (1830–1922)," Embryo Project Encyclopedia, September 21, 2020, https://embryo.asu .edu/pages/horatio-robinson-storer-1830–1922. For a thorough discussion of how Storer and the AMA criminalized abortion, see Carroll Smith-Rosenberg, *Disorderly Conduct: Visions of Gender in Victorian America* (New York: Oxford University Press, 1985), 217–44.

90 **drawn from racial fears:** Ramtin Arablouei and Rund Abdelfatah, "Abortion Was Once Common Practice in America. A Small Group of Doctors Changed That," NPR, June 6, 2022, https://www.npr.org/2022/06/06/1103372543/abortion-was-once-common-practice -in-america-a-small-group-of-doctors-changed-th?f=&ft=nprml; Michele Goodwin, "The Racist History of Abortion and Midwifery Bans," July 1, 2020, ACLU, https://www.aclu.org /news/racial-justice/the-racist-history-of-abortion-and-midwifery-bans.

90 **"be filled by":** Horatio Robinson Storer, *Why Not? A Book for Every Woman* (Boston: Lee and Shepard, 1866), 85.

91 **letter to Zakrzewska:** Zakrzewska, *A Woman's Quest*, 337.

91 **139 Cedar Street:** Tuchman, *Science Has No Sex*, 118.

92 **"Rock Garden":** Zakrzewska, *A Woman's Quest*, 458.

92 **"My love for her":** Zakrzewska, *A Woman's Quest*, 9.

93 **"grossest indelicacy":** Zakrzewska, *A Woman's Quest*, 272.

94 **"sunny, airy house":** Zakrzewska, *A Woman's Quest*, 293.

94 **exhibit empathy toward:** Zakrzewska, *A Woman's Quest*, 315–16.

95 **"Let he who":** Tuchman, *Science Has No Sex*, 163.

95 **"milk metastasis":** Druin Burch, "When Childbirth Was Natural, and Deadly," Live Science, January 10, 2009, https://www.livescience.com/3210-childbirth-natural-deadly.html.

95 **the first half:** Burch, "When Childbirth Was Natural."

95 **"Doctors are gentlemen":** Burch, "When Childbirth Was Natural."

96 **seemed to exist:** Tuchman, *Science Has No Sex*, 206–7.

96 **conservative physician:** Mary Roth Walsh, *Doctors Wanted: No Women Need Apply* (New Haven, CT: Yale University Press, 1977), 113.

96 **"nervous strain":** Horatio Robinson Storer, "To the Directors of the New England Hospital for Women," *Boston Medical and Surgical Journal* 75 (1867): 191.

96 **"During July":** Zakrzewska, *A Woman's Quest*, 338.

97 **competitor J. Marion Sims:** Walsh, *Doctors Wanted*, 115.

97 **inventing an operative:** Barker-Benfield, *The Horrors of the Half-Known Life*, 98.

97 **"hazardous operations":** Zakrzewska, *A Woman's Quest*, 339.

97 **"results of Storer's":** Walsh, *Doctors Wanted*, 112.

98 **following resolution:** Walsh, *Doctors Wanted*, 112.

98 **"Having received":** Storer, "To the Directors of the New England Hospital for Women," 191.

99 **"testing the ability:** Storer, "To the Directors," 192.

99 **According to the AMA:** Barker-Benfield, *The Horrors of the Half-Known Life*, 80.

100 **he footnoted:** Walsh, *Doctors Wanted*, 111.

100 **"habitually thievish":** Aron, "The Father of American Gynecology."

100 **institutionalized his wife:** Aron, "The Father of American Gynecology."

100 **married her sister:** "Biographical Sketch," Horatio Robinson Storer Papers, 1829–1943, Massachusetts Historical Society, last updated March 2005, https://www.masshist.org/collection-guides/view/fa0001.

100 **he persuaded:** Aron, "The Father of American Gynecology."

Chapter 7: Closed Energy System

101 **won her battle:** Peitzman, *A New and Untried Course*, 34.

101 **the amphitheater was:** Wells, *Out of the Dead House*, 194.

101 **Male students from:** Wells, *Out of the Dead House*, 195.

102 **"Go tomorrow":** "Current Topics of the Town: A Pioneer in the Medical Education of Women Describes Student Battles Once Waged About Them," in Ann Preston and Eliza J. Wood Armitage, Scrapbook of Newspaper Clippings, Ledger, and Math Exercises, image 34, accessed May 26, 2023, https://drexel.primo.exlibrisgroup.com/discovery/fulldisplay?context=L&vid=01DRXU_INST:01DRXU&search_scope=MyInst_andCI_ResearchOnlyInventory&tab=Everything&docid=alma991015166037504721. See also, "'Go tomorrow to the hospital to see the She Doctors!'" The Legacy Center, Drexel University College of Medicine Archives and Special Collections. Philadelphia, PA. https://drexel.edu/legacy-center/blog/overview/2012/february/go-tomorrow-to-the-hospital-to-see-the-she-doctors/.

102 **disguised an:** Peitzman, *A New and Untried Course*, 47.

102 **"Hat! Hat!":** "Our Philadelphia Correspondence," in Preston and Armitage, Scrapbook, image 6.

102 **"Boys, we will":** "Pioneers in the Face of Adversity," May 26, 2023. http://lcdc.library.drexel.edu/islandora/object/islandora:1347.

103 **"Gentlemen":** "Our Philadelphia Correspondence," in Preston and Armitage, Scrapbook, image 6.

103 **"What can you see":** "The Late Scene at the Pennsylvania Hospital," *Philadelphia Evening Bulletin*, 1869, Drexel University College of Medicine Archives and Special Collections, https://doctordoctress.org/islandora/object/islandora:1347/record/islandora:1658.

103 **"Was there a":** "The Late Scene at the Pennsylvania Hospital," *Philadelphia Evening Bulletin*.

104 **"gauntlet of":** "The Press: Moral Carditis," in Preston and Armitage, Scrapbook, image 8.

105 **"jeering incident":** Wells, *Out of the Dead House*, 208.

105 **petition against:** Wells, *Out of the Dead House*, 197.

105 **Medical College said:** Wells, *Out of the Dead House*, 198.

106 **"all the qualities":** "Clarke, Edward Hammond," *A Cyclopedia of American Medical Biography, Comprising the Lives of Eminent Deceased Physicians and Surgeons from 1610 to 1910* (Philadelphia: W. B. Saunders, 1912), 184.

106 **Vice President Wilson:** "Vice-President Wilson," *Chicago Tribune*, August 8, 1873.

106 **lungs hemorrhaged:** "Clarke, Edward Hammond," *A Cyclopedia*.

106 **joined the crowd:** "Obituary, Dr. Edward Hammond Clarke," *Boston Globe*, December 2, 1877.

107 **approached him about:** "Obituary, Dr. Edward Hammond Clarke," *Boston Globe*.

107 **touring the Charité:** Tuchman, *Science Has No Sex*, 174.

108 **"read with sorrow":** "The Medical Students: To the Editor of the Press," in Preston and Armitage, Scrapbook, image 14.

108 **"dullest village":** "A New Yorker at the Pennsylvania College," *New York World*, November 13, 1869, in Preston and Armitage, Scrapbook, image 13.

108 **a bath was:** Edward H. Clarke, "Medical Education of Women," *Boston Medical and Surgical Journal* (1869): 346.

109 **"shameless herd":** "The Other Side," Drexel University College of Medicine Archives and Special Collections, 2023, https://doctordoctress.org/islandora/object/islandora%3 A1347/record/islandora%3A1718.

110 **"recent occurrences":** Clarke, "Medical Education of Women," 345.

110 **"same right to":** Clarke, "Medical Education of Women," 345.

110 **two paintings:** Kimberly A. Hamlin, *From Eve to Evolution: Darwin, Science, and Woman's Rights in Gilded Age America* (Chicago: University of Chicago Press, 2014), 26.

111 **"these wretched":** Storer, *Why Not?*, 69–70.

111 **cheered Darwin:** Hamlin, *From Eve to Evolution*, 39.

111 **"number of scientific":** Hamlin, *From Eve to Evolution*, 38–39.

111 **"the scientists of today":** Hamlin, *From Eve to Evolution*, 39.

112 **"law of the conservation":** Cynthia Eagle Russett, *Sexual Science: The Victorian Construction of Womanhood* (Cambridge, MA: Harvard University Press, 1989), 11.

112 **"the physiological cost":** Herbert Spencer, *The Study of Sociology* (New York: D. Appleton, 1896), 341.

112 **"somewhat less of":** Spencer, *The Study of Sociology*, 341.

112 **"lagged behind men":** Russett, *Sexual Science*, 11.

113 **improper digestion:** Edward H. Clarke, *Sex in Education* (Boston: James R. Osgood, 1875), 40.

113 **"upon whom Nature":** Clarke, *Sex in Education*, 54.

113 **"not to educate girls":** Silas Weir Mitchell, *Wear and Tear, Or: Hints for the Overworked* (Philadelphia: J. B. Lippincott, 1871).

113 **"observation confirms":** Clarke, *Sex in Education*, 61.

114 **"'till menstruation'":** Charles West, *Lectures on the Diseases of Women* (Philadelphia: Henry C. Lea, 1867), 48.

114 **"There have been instances":** Clarke, *Sex in Education*, 39.

114 **Clarke endorsed:** Clarke, *Sex in Education*, 157.

114 **called "agene":** Clarke, *Sex in Education*, 93–94.

115 **Darwin had taken:** Russett, *Sexual Science*, 2.

Chapter 8: The Science of Love

116 **"a scientific spirit":** Putnam, *Life and Letters*, 235.

116 **"until now, women":** Mary Putnam Jacobi, *A Pathfinder in Medicine,* ed. Women's Medical Association of New York City (New York: G. P. Putnam's Sons, 1925), 482.

117 **"microscopic shred":** Jacobi, *Pathfinder,* 462.

117 **science had no:** Zakrzewska, *A Woman's Quest,* 67.

117 **used vivisection:** Jacobi, *Pathfinder,* 222, 291–94.

118 **forty students:** Bittel, *Mary Putnam Jacobi,* 103.

118 **health-care institutions:** Bittel, *Mary Putnam Jacobi,* 104.

118 **Students complained:** Bittel, *Mary Putnam Jacobi,* 100–101.

118 **make the study:** Bittel, *Mary Putnam Jacobi,* 104.

119 **"there was no limit":** Putnam, *Life and Letters,* 323.

120 **honorary secretary:** Truax, *The Doctors Jacobi,* 125.

120 **Grand Central Depot:** Christopher Gray, "Streetscapes/Grand Central Terminal: How a Rail Complex Chugged Into the 20th Century," *New York Times,* June 21, 1998, section 11, page 5.

120 **Tenement House Act:** "Tenements," History.com, April 22, 2010, updated October 10, 2019, https://www.history.com/topics/immigration/tenements.

120 **living in New York:** Truax, *The Doctors Jacobi,* 125.

120 **Her mother, Victorine:** Truax, *The Doctors Jacobi,* 127.

121 **many supporters:** Truax, *The Doctors Jacobi,* 127.

121 **hung a plaque:** Putnam, *Life and Letters,* 310.

122 **clinical professor:** Truax, *The Doctors Jacobi,* 137.

122 **Born in Prussia:** Bittel, *Mary Putnam Jacobi,* 155–56.

123 **almost two years:** Bittel, *Mary Putnam Jacobi,* 158.

123 **"helpless sort":** Bittel, *Mary Putnam Jacobi,* 158.

123 **transformed himself:** Bittel, *Mary Putnam Jacobi,* 160.

123 **child mortality:** "Child Mortality Rate (Under Five Years Old) in the United States, from 1800 to 2020," Statista (2023), https://www.statista.com/statistics/1041693/united -states-all-time-child-mortality-rate/#:~:text=Child%20mortality%20in%20the%20 United%20States%201800%2D2020&text=The%20child%20mortality%20rate%20in,it%20 to%20their%20fifth%20birthday.

124 **"small satisfaction":** Truax, *The Doctors Jacobi,* 138.

124 **"Let it not be":** Truax, *The Doctors Jacobi,* 139.

125 **"The crane":** Truax, *The Doctors Jacobi,* 146.

125 **not a Jew:** "Ostracism of Hebrews: The Wife of Dr. Abraham Jacobi Excluded from a Staten Island Hotel," *New-York Tribune,* May 31, 1880.

126 **"My 'Herr Doctor'":** Putnam, *Life and Letters,* 311.

127 **"My Dear Mary":** Putnam, *Life and Letters,* 306.

128 **moved forward:** Bittel, *Mary Putnam Jacobi,* 105.

Chapter 9: Battle Lines Are Drawn

129 **Established in 1868:** Julia A. Sprague, *History of the New England Women's Club from 1868 to 1893* (Boston: Lee and Shepard, 1894), 3–17.

130 **decided to break away:** Allison Lange, "Suffragists Organize: American Woman Suffrage Association," National Women's History Museum, Fall 2015, https://www.crusade forthevote.org/awsa-organize.

130 **wholehearted approval:** Sally G. McMillen, *Lucy Stone: An Unapologetic Life* (New York: Oxford University Press, 2015), 34.

131 **Public high schools:** "Edward Hammond Clarke and the Chance for Girls," New England Historical Society, 2023, https://newenglandhistoricalsociety.com/edward-hammond -clarke-chance-girls/.

131 **582 colleges:** Barbara Miller Solomon, *In the Company of Educated Women* (New Haven, CT: Yale University Press, 1985), 44. For a discussion of the push for higher education of women in the latter half of the nineteenth century, see pages 43–61.

131 **informed the ladies:** My description of this scene was developed from Henry B. Blackwell, "Sex in Education," *Woman's Journal* 3, no. 51 (1872): 404, and Clarke, *Sex in Education*.

131 **"woman can do":** Clarke, *Sex in Education*, 13.

132 **"Our present system":** Blackwell, "Sex in Education."

132 **"are indirectly affected":** Clarke, *Sex in Education*, 24.

132 **Within her body:** Clarke, *Sex in Education*, 38.

132 **"house within a":** Clarke, *Sex in Education*, 37.

132 **Scientific evidence:** Clarke, *Sex in Education*, 157.

133 **"course of education":** Blackwell, "Sex in Education."

133 **"race suicide":** Clarke, *Sex in Education*, 139.

133 **give examples:** Clarke, *Sex in Education*, 61.

134 **Holmes expressed:** Blackwell, "Sex in Education."

134 **towering academics:** For information about Holmes's, Eliot's, and Agassiz's eugenics research, see "Scientific Racism," Harvard University, 2023, https://library.harvard.edu/confronting-anti-black-racism/scientific-racism; Adam S. Cohen, "Harvard's Eugenics Era," *Harvard Magazine* (April 14, 2016), https://www.harvardmagazine.com/2016/03/harvards-eugenics-era; and Michael Cook, "Harvard's Dark Past as the 'Brain Trust' of American Eugenics," BioEdge, 2022, https://bioedge.org/enhancement/harvards-dark-past-as-the-brain-trust-of-american-eugenics/.

134 **at Oberlin:** Blackwell, "Sex in Education."

134 **Spanish proverb:** Blackwell, "Sex in Education."

135 **wisely against:** "Clarke, Holmes Against the Co-Education of Women," *Boston Globe*, December 23, 1872.

136 **thick rubber gloves:** Walsh, *Doctors Wanted*, 119.

136 **Reviews across the country:** "Sex in Education," review of *Sex in Education* by Edward H. Clarke, *Boston Globe*, October 31, 1873; "Literary," *Chicago Evening Post*, November 15, 1873; "What We Think of Dr. Clarke's Book in California," *Woman's Journal* (November 29, 1873): 378.

136 **Clarke joined:** Tuchman, *Science Has No Sex*, 174.

137 **In St. Giles:** "Higher Education of Woman: A Paper Read by T. W. Higginson Before the Social Science Convention, May 14, 1873," *Woman's Journal* 4, no. 21 (May 24, 1873): 161.

138 **thrown open:** "Collegiate Education for Women," *Jeffersonian*, June 12, 1873.

138 **"mother University":** "The Education of Girls: What a Professor of Vassar College Has to Say on the Subject," *Selinsgrove Times-Tribune*, May 30, 1873.

138 **adamantly opposed:** "Co-Education of the Sexes," *Decatur Local Review*, June 12, 1873.

139 **"requires special":** "Higher Education of Women," *Chicago Tribune*, May 25, 1873. Also, "John and Jane at Harvard," *New York Daily Herald*, May 24, 1873.

140 **"are the enemy":** "Co-Education of the Sexes," *Decatur Local Review*.

140 **"scared away":** "John and Jane at Harvard," *New York Daily Herald*.

140 **on this account:** "Higher Education of Women," *Chicago Tribune*.

Chapter 10: Counterattack

142 **local newspapers:** "Putnam," *Brooklyn Daily Eagle*, July 28, 1873.

142 **diatribes against:** Truax, *The Doctors Jacobi*, 166.

142 **imposing entryway:** Truax, *The Doctors Jacobi*, 164.

143 **nicknamed him:** Truax, *The Doctors Jacobi*, 164.

143 **Haven noticed:** Truax, *The Doctors Jacobi*, 164.

143 **George Palmer Putnam:** Truax, *The Doctors Jacobi*, 165.

144 **"It's only sightseeing":** Truax, *The Doctors Jacobi*, 167.

144 **journey, they took:** Truax, *The Doctors Jacobi*, 167.

144 **beyond Caldwell:** Truax, *The Doctors Jacobi*, 168.

145 **big "knob of":** Truax, *The Doctors Jacobi*, 168.

145 **for fifty dollars:** Bittel, *Mary Putnam Jacobi*, 165.

146 **childhood mortality:** Bittel, *Mary Putnam Jacobi*, 179.

146 **"the intelligent passenger":** A. Jacobi, *Infant Diet*, Revised, Adapted, and Enlarged to Popular Use by Mary Putnam Jacobi, M.D. (New York: G. P. Putnam's Sons, 1875), v.

146 **edition was advertised:** Bittel, *Mary Putnam Jacobi*, 179.

146 **"the humane":** Eugene P. Link, "Abraham and Mary P. Jacobi, Humanitarian Physicians," *Journal of the History of Medicine and Allied Sciences* 4, no. 4 (1949): 383, http://www.jstor.org/stable/24619157.

146 **"a revolutionist":** Link, "Abraham and Mary P. Jacobi," 388.

146 **nutritional process:** Mary Putnam Jacobi, *The Question of Rest for Women During Menstruation* (New York: G. P. Putnam's Sons, 1877), 161, 173, 211, 224.

147 **Jacobi organized:** Bittel, *Mary Putnam Jacobi*, 221.

147 **Brackett had grown:** Norma Kidd Green, "Brackett, Anna Callender," in *Notable American Women: A Biographical Dictionary*, ed. Edward T. James (Cambridge, MA: Belknap Press of Harvard University Press, 1971), 217–18.

148 **male physicians:** S. Weir Mitchell, *Doctor and Patient* (Philadelphia: J. B. Lippincott, 1909), 153.

148 **Clarke "relates":** Jacobi, "Mental Action and Physical Health," 266.

149 **"this argument":** Jacobi, "Mental Action and Physical Health," 266.

149 **contention that studying:** Jacobi, "Mental Action and Physical Health," 267.

149 **"possess neither":** Jacobi, "Mental Action and Physical Health," 270.

149 **process of ovulation:** Jacobi, "Mental Action and Physical Health," 272.

150 **she compared Clarke:** Jacobi, "Mental Action and Physical Health," 261–62.

150 **she died from:** Truax, *The Doctors Jacobi*, 178.

150 **"I always felt":** Putnam, *Life and Letters*, 318.

151 **deeply impressed:** "American Women: Their Health and Education," *Westminster and Foreign Quarterly Review* (1874): 220.

151 **books, titled:** Brackett, *The Education of American Girls*, ed. Anna C. Brackett; Julia Ward Howe, ed., *Sex and Education: A Reply to Dr. E. H. Clarke's "Sex in Education"* (Boston: Roberts Brothers, 1874); Eliza Bisbee Duffey, *No Sex in Education, or An Equal Chance for Both Girls and Boys* (Philadelphia: J. M. Stoddart, 1874); George Fisk and Anna Manning Comfort, *Woman's Education and Woman's Health: Chiefly in Reply to "Sex in Education"* (Syracuse, NY: T. W. Durston, 1874).

151 **covert plan:** Duffey, *No Sex in Education*, 117.

151 **accused Clarke:** Howe, *Sex and Education*, 32–51.

152 **called Clarke:** Howe, *Sex and Education*, 191–95.

152 **"regret that you":** Howe, *Sex and Education*, 192.

152 **Educator Anna Brackett:** Brackett, *The Education of American Girls*, 387–88.

152 **"In all books":** Howe, *Sex and Education*, 94–95.

153 **"She too requires":** Walsh, *Doctors Wanted*, 129.

153 **"One would think":** Howe, *Sex and Education*, 60.

153 **Clarke wrote back:** Edward H. Clarke, *The Building of a Brain* (Boston: James R. Osgood, 1874), 8.

154 **"duties are":** Clarke, *The Building of a Brain*, 15.

154 **"The best brains":** Clarke, *The Building of a Brain*, 20.

154 **reproduced in full:** Edward H. Clarke, "The Building of a Brain," *New York Times*, August 7, 1874.

154 **Holmes wrote:** Oliver Wendell Holmes, "The Americanized European," *Atlantic*, January 1875, https://www.theatlantic.com/magazine/archive/1875/01/the-americanized -european/631207/.

154 **"Many young women":** Holmes, "The Americanized European."

155 **coined the expression:** Andy Bowers, "Explainer: What's a Boston Brahmin?," *Slate*, March 1, 2004, https://slate.com/news-and-politics/2004/03/what-s-a-boston-brahmin.html.

155 **longing for eugenics:** Holmes, "The Americanized European."

156 **controversial changes:** "Charles Eliot," Harvard University, 2023, https://eliot.harvard .edu/about-charles-eliot; "A History of Harvard Medical School Part III: The Eliot Years," YouTube, uploaded by Harvard Medical School, May 12, 2016, https://www.youtube.com /watch?v=QFL6ayknjc4.

156 **When Susan Dimock and Sophia Jex-Blake:** Joint Committee on the Status of Women, "Matriculation of Women at Harvard Medical School," Harvard University, https://jcsw.hms. harvard.edu/matriculation-women-harvard-medical-school.

156 **"Neither the corporation":** "Female Medical Education: The Harvard University Re- fuses Admission to Women," *Chicago Evening Post*, April 26, 1867.

157 **Unwilling to accept:** Olivia Campbell, *Women in White Coats: How the First Women Doctors Changed the World of Medicine* (New York: Park Row Books, 2021), 105–6.

157 **society's founders:** Shin'ichi Kurihara, "The Boylston Medical Society of Harvard University and the Boylston Medical Prize," *Igaku Toshokan* 35, no. 2 (1988): 75–85.

157 **committee, whose:** Bittel, *Mary Putnam Jacobi*, 126.

Chapter 11: Fighting Back with Science

158 **fused closed:** Bittel, *Mary Putnam Jacobi*, 113; Jacobi, *Pathfinder*, 299.

158 **drug hypotheses:** Bittel, *Mary Putnam Jacobi*, 112.

158 **many forms:** Wells, *Out of the Dead House*, 141.

159 **sent a copy:** C. Alice Baker to Mary Putnam Jacobi, November 7, 1874, folder 10, Pa- pers of Mary Putnam Jacobi, Radcliffe Institute, Schlesinger Library.

159 **"In course of":** *History and Proceedings of the Pocumtuck Valley Memorial Association 1905–1911*: 354.

159 **writer and historian:** "C. Alice Baker," Frary Family Association, March 1897, updated 1909, https://www.fraryfamilyassociation.net/c-alice-baker.

160 **Wyman revealed:** Baker to Jacobi, November 7, 1874, Papers of Mary Putnam Jacobi.

160 **praised Jacobi's:** Baker to Jacobi, November 7, 1874, Papers of Mary Putnam Jacobi.

160 **Official rules:** "Editors' Notebook," *Unitarian Review and Religious Magazine* 6 (Bos- ton: Office of the Unitarian Review, 1876), 213.

161 **"that the honor":** Baker to Jacobi, November 7, 1874, Papers of Mary Putnam Jacobi.

161 **Baker volunteered:** Helen Lefkowitz Horowitz, "The Body in the Library," in *The "Woman Question" and Higher Education: Perspectives on Gender and Knowledge Production in America*, ed. Ann Mari May (Northampton, MA: Edward Elgar, 2008), 24–25.

161 *The undersigned:* Jacobi, *The Question of Rest*, 26.

162 **her colleagues:** Jacobi, *The Question of Rest*, introduction.

162 **visual graphic:** "Sphygmograph, 2004," Museum of Medicine and Health, University of Manchester Digital Collections, https://www.digitalcollections.manchester.ac.uk/view /MH-02004-00345/1.

162 **gauge the tractive:** Serge Nicolas and Vobořil Dalibor, "The Collin Dynamometer: History of the Development of an Instrument for Measuring Physical and Mental Strength,"

L'Année Psychologique 117, no. 2 (2017): 173–219, https://www.cairn.info/revue-l-annee-psychologique1-2017-2-page-173.htm.

163 **Her breakthrough:** "Contraception in America 1900–1950: Rhythm Method," Dittrick Medical History Center, Case Western Reserve University College of Arts and Sciences, accessed 8/22/23, https://artsci.case.edu/dittrick/online-exhibits/history-of-birth-control/contraception-in-america-1900–1950/rhythm-method/.

163 **urged her:** Bittel, *Mary Putnam Jacobi*, 164.

164 **"My Doctor":** Bittel, *Mary Putnam Jacobi*, 164.

164 **pushed the boat:** Truax, *The Doctors Jacobi*, 184.

164 **their late friend:** Truax, *The Doctors Jacobi*, 184.

164 **Abraham's delight:** Bittel, *Mary Putnam Jacobi*, 166.

164 **"loss of our":** Putnam, *Life and Letters*, 318.

165 **"baby is not":** Bittel, *Mary Putnam Jacobi*, 167.

165 **men had found:** Jacobi, *The Question of Rest*, 1.

165 **"have been portrayed":** Jacobi, *The Question of Rest*, 2.

166 **"Such indeed":** Jacobi, *The Question of Rest*, 1.

166 **"Menstruation in women":** Jacobi, *The Question of Rest*, 12.

166 **large female dog:** Thomas Laqueur, *Making Sex: Body and Gender from the Greeks to Freud* (Cambridge, MA: Harvard University Press, 1990), 213–18.

167 **human egg:** Laqueur, *Making Sex*, 211.

167 **menstruation corresponded:** Laqueur, *Making Sex*, 185.

167 **"bitch in heat":** Augustus K. Gardner, *The Causes and Curative Treatment of Sterility* (New York: De Witt and Davenport, 1856), 17.

167 **swelling and rupture:** "The Physiology of Menstruation," *Lancet* 39, no. 1013 (January 28, 1843): 645.

167 **doctors recommended:** "The Physiology of Menstruation," *Lancet*.

167 **"isolated menstruation":** Jacobi, *The Question of Rest*, 13.

168 **"Thus one of":** Jacobi, *The Question of Rest*, 15.

168 **gestation was:** Jacobi, *The Question of Rest*, 6.

168 **ancient concept:** Jacobi, *The Question of Rest*, 5.

169 **circulation of blood:** Bittel, *Mary Putnam Jacobi*, 91.

169 **female emotional:** S. Weir Mitchell, *Lectures on Diseases of the Nervous System, Especially in Women* (Philadelphia: Lea Brothers, 1885), 95–96.

169 **"afflux of blood":** Jacobi, *The Question of Rest*, 81.

169 **that ovulation:** Jacobi, *The Question of Rest*, 77.

170 **women experienced:** Jacobi, *The Question of Rest*, 115.

170 **268 were:** Jacobi, *The Question of Rest*, 21.

170 **the question about:** Jacobi, *The Question of Rest*, 26–63.

170 **found that immunity:** Jacobi, *The Question of Rest*, 62.

171 **"Rest during":** Jacobi, *The Question of Rest*, 62.

171 **a time of:** Jacobi, *The Question of Rest*, 109.

171 **"On the hypothesis":** Jacobi, *The Question of Rest*, 115.

171 **"Reproduction in":** Jacobi, *The Question of Rest*, 165.

171 **"Practically":** Jacobi, *The Question of Rest*, 202.

171 **"The menstrual flow":** Jacobi, *The Question of Rest*, 227.

172 **"do not in the least":** Jacobi, *The Question of Rest*, 230.

172 **Latin phrase:** Bittel, *Mary Putnam Jacobi*, 127.

172 **"willingly conferred":** Bittel, *Mary Putnam Jacobi*, 128.

173 **alerting her to:** Bittel, *Mary Putnam Jacobi*, 128.

173 **she was absolutely:** Bittel, *Mary Putnam Jacobi*, 128.

173 **praised Jacobi's book:** Bittel, *Mary Putnam Jacobi*, 133.

174 **"friends of the higher":** "'Sex in Education' Practically Refuted at Harvard," *Woman's Journal* (June 10, 1876): 189.

174 **approved of her:** Bittel, *Mary Putnam Jacobi*, 133.

Chapter 12: God's Gift to Women

175 **Benjamin Franklin:** Frank H. Lau and Kevin C. Chung, "Silas Weir Mitchell, M.D.: The Physician Who Discovered Causalgia," *Journal of American Hand Surgery* 29, no. 2 (2004): 181.

175 **"God's gift":** Nancy Cervetti, *S. Weir Mitchell, 1829–1914: Philadelphia's Literary Physician* (University Park: Pennsylvania State University Press, 2012), 141.

175 **typical patient:** For general patient descriptions, see Silas Weir Mitchell, *Fat and Blood: An Essay on the Treatment of Certain Forms of Neurasthenia and Hysteria* (Philadelphia: J. B. Lippincott, 1884), 33–48.

175 **tonics made of:** Mitchell, *Fat and Blood*, 39.

176 **experiment on himself:** W. Steven Metzer, "The Experimentation of S. Weir Mitchell with Mescal," *Neurology* 39, no. 2 (February 1989): 303; DOI: 10.1212/WNL.39.2.303.

176 **only person:** Cervetti, *Weir Mitchell*, 1.

176 **"You have no":** Cervetti, *Weir Mitchell*, 17.

176 **Mitchell insisted:** Cervetti, *Weir Mitchell*, 21.

176 **Meigs's reasoning:** Foster S. Kellogg, "Ether in Obstetrics," *Journal of the Michigan State Medical Society* 15 (1916): 277.

177 **"the neat foot":** Cervetti, *Weir Mitchell*, 33.

177 **received a letter:** Cervetti, *Weir Mitchell*, 44.

177 **reaction of a:** Silas Weir Mitchell, "The Poison of the Rattlesnake," *Atlantic*, April 1868, https://www.theatlantic.com/magazine/archive/1868/04/the-poison-of-the-rattlesnake/628656/.

178 **safely handle:** S. Weir Mitchell, *Researches Upon the Venom of the Rattlesnake; With an Investigation of the Anatomy and Physiology of the Organs Concerned* (Washington: Smithsonian Institution) 1860, chapter 1.

178 **"suffered terribly":** Mitchell, *Researches*, 71.

178 **so minute:** Mitchell, *Researches*, 64.

178 **150 animals:** Mitchell, "Chapter 7: Action of the Venom on the Tissues and Fluids," *Researches*, 76–97.

178 **"fully erected":** Mitchell, *Researches*, 25.

178 **so constructed:** Mitchell, *Researches*, 12.

179 **"ejaculated":** Mitchell, *Researches*, 6.

179 **"perfectly fresh":** Mitchell, *Researches*, 27.

179 ***Elsie Venner:*** Oliver Wendell Holmes, *Elsie Venner* (Cambridge, MA: Riverside Press, 1861).

179 **"commonly slender":** Holmes, *Elsie Venner*, 3.

179 **"physical statistics":** Cervetti, *Weir Mitchell*, 62

179 **In 1861:** Cervetti, *Weir Mitchell*, 67.

179 **"hell of pain":** Cervetti, *Weir Mitchell*, 69.

180 **"absence of all":** Mitchell, *Lectures on Diseases*, 275.

180 **"female invalidism":** Barbara Ehrenreich and Deirdre English, *Complaints and Disorders: The Sexual Politics of Sickness*, second edition (New York: Feminist Press, 2011), 49–50.

180 **featured stories:** Ehrenreich and English, *Complaints and Disorders*, 51.

181 **First, the patient:** Mitchell, *Fat and Blood*, chapters 4 through 8 describe the rest-cure treatment.

181 **"To lie abed":** Mitchell, *Fat and Blood*, 57.

181 **Each day until:** Mitchell, *Lectures on Diseases*, 260.

181 **milk-only diet:** Mitchell, *Fat and Blood*, 97–98.

182 **From ten to eleven:** Mitchell, *Fat and Blood*, 76.

182 **Letter-writing:** Mitchell, *Fat and Blood*, 60.

182 **exact home-life:** Cervetti, *Weir Mitchell*, 121.

182 **he had made:** S. Weir Mitchell, "The Evolution of the Rest Treatment," *Journal of Nervous and Mental Disease* (June 1904): 5.

182 **bed on fire:** Cervetti, *Weir Mitchell*, 112.

183 **"belief in his":** Mitchell, *Fat and Blood*, 55.

183 **could entice:** Mitchell, *Fat and Blood*, 157.

183 **he stated that:** "Female Physicians," *Times-Picayune*, New Orleans, April 14, 1878.

185 **openly scoffed:** Putnam, *Life and Letters*, 147.

185 **failed to properly:** "Mary Putnam Jacobi's Letter of Protest to S. Weir Mitchell, as Introduced and Transcribed by Nancy Cervetti," *Transactions and Studies of the College of Physicians of Philadelphia* 19, no. 5 (December 1997): 110.

185 **identical to:** Bittel, *Mary Putnam Jacobi*, 143.

185 **Jacobi's clinical studies:** Mary Putnam Jacobi and Victoria A. White, *On the Use of the Cold Pack Followed by Massage in the Treatment of Anaemia* (New York: G. P. Putnam's Sons, 1880).

186 **"Ernst is a":** Bittel, *Mary Putnam Jacobi*, 167.

187 **Hilton barred:** Lawrence Bush, "June 13: No Jews or Dogs Admitted," *Jewish Currents*, June 13, 2013, https://jewishcurrents.org/june-13-joseph-seligman-in-saratoga-springs.

187 **"shameful prejudice":** "Correspondence: New York Notes," *American Israelite* (Cincinnati, OH), June 11, 1880.

187 **called the incident:** "Ostracism of Hebrews," *New-York Tribune*.

188 **joined the faculty:** Joy Harvey, "Clanging Eagles: The Marriage and Collaboration Between Two Nineteenth-Century Physicians, Mary Putnam Jacobi and Abraham Jacobi," in *Creative Couples in the Sciences*, ed. Helena M. Pycior, Nancy G. Slack, and Pnina G. Abir-Am (New Brunswick, NJ: Rutgers University Press, 1996), 189.

188 **sparked a rivalry:** Harvey, "Clanging Eagles," 189.

Part Three: Breakthrough

189 **"as the bees":** Jacobi, *Pathfinder*, 498.

Chapter 13: Success, but at What Cost?

191 **"morbid nervous":** George J. Engelmann, *The American Girl of Today: Modern Education and Functional Health* (American Gynecological Society, 1900), 13–14.

191 **menstrual waves:** William Stephenson, "On the Menstrual Wave: Method of Analysis Case," *The American Journal of Obstetrics and Diseases of Women and Children (1819–1919)* (April 1, 1882): 287.

192 **kept proposing:** Martin Kaufman, "The Admission of Women to Nineteenth-Century American Medical Societies," *Bulletin of the History of Medicine* 50, no. 2 (1976): 251.

192 **First, the society:** Kaufman, "The Admission of Women," 252.

192 **"such nuisances":** Kaufman, "The Admission of Women," 253.

192 **"could not consent":** Kaufman, "The Admission of Women," 253.

193 **Flashing a:** Truax, *The Doctors Jacobi*, 84.

193 **"purchase direct":** Mary Putnam Jacobi, "Social Aspects of the Readmission of Women into the Medical Profession," *Papers and Letters Presented at the First Woman's Congress of the Association for the Advancement of Woman, October 1873* (New York, 1874), 177.

193 **suggested that:** Walsh, *Doctors Wanted*, 174.

193 **Emma Call:** Walsh, *Doctors Wanted*, 174.

194 **"Would you accept":** Zakrzewska, *A Woman's Quest*, 401–2.

194 **Enraged faculty:** Walsh, *Doctors Wanted*, 175.

194 **because women:** Morantz-Sanchez, *Sympathy and Science*, 72.

194 **admission of women to the Boston Medical Society:** Kaufman, "The Admission of Women," 254.

195 **"utilized its legacy":** Jacobi, "Woman in Medicine," 169.

195 **"quite as carefully":** Jacobi, "Woman in Medicine," 170.

195 **"When people":** Jacobi, "Woman in Medicine," 172.

195 **ninety-four women:** Jacobi, "Woman in Medicine," 168–69.

195 **Freedmen's Hospital:** Sterling M. Lloyd Jr., "History," Howard University College of Medicine, May 2006, https://medicine.howard.edu/about/history.

196 **women's smaller:** Zakrzewska, *A Woman's Quest*, 400.

196 **"no manner of doubt":** Jacobi, "Woman in Medicine," 176.

196 **"physician is summoned":** Jacobi, *Pathfinder*, 335.

197 **"But, before":** Jacobi, *Pathfinder*, 335–36.

197 **"have spoken of":** Jacobi, *Pathfinder*, 337.

197 **gain a foothold:** Jacobi, *Pathfinder*, 355.

197 **"Dear Madam":** Zakrzewska, *A Woman's Quest*, 402–3.

198 **approached the faculty:** Walsh, *Doctors Wanted*, 175.

199 **Abraham told parents:** Truax, *The Doctors Jacobi*, 192.

199 **"first family":** Truax, *The Doctors Jacobi*, 191.

199 **"Golden Decade":** Truax, *The Doctors Jacobi*, 192.

199 **"Everything that":** Truax, *The Doctors Jacobi*, 193.

199 **older and taciturn:** Harvey, "Clanging Eagles," 190.

199 **Carl Schurz:** Ernest K. Giese and Monique Bourque, "Carl Schurz," Historical Society of Pennsylvania, July 1990, http://www2.hsp.org/collections/Balch%20manuscript_guide/html/schurz.html.

200 **became inseparable:**, Harvey, "Clanging Eagles," 190.

200 **Mary arrived home:** Harvey, "Clanging Eagles," 190–91.

201 **"speak but not write":** Harvey, "Clanging Eagles," 190.

201 **"You will find":** Harvey, "Clanging Eagles," 190.

201 **Ernst complained:** Truax, *The Doctors Jacobi*, 196–97.

202 **patients with diphtheria:** For information about nineteenth-century diphtheria, see Hilda Parks, "Diphtheria in Blue Earth County," Blue Earth County Historical Society, September 2021, https://blueearthcountyhistory.com/2021/09/29/diphtheria/; "Diphtheria," Museum of Healthcare at Kingston, 2023, https://www.museumofhealthcare.ca/explore/exhibits/vaccinations/diphtheria.html; "Deadly Diphtheria: The Children's Plague," Dittrick Medical History Center, Case Western Reserve University, October 26, 2017, https://artsci.case.edu/dittrick/2014/04/29/deadly-diphtheria-the-childrens-plague/.

202 **Mary let him:** Bittel, *Mary Putnam Jacobi*, 172.

202 **might have included:** Annick Opinel et al., "Commentary: The Evolution of Methods to Assess the Effects of Treatments, Illustrated by the Development of Treatments for Diphtheria, 1825–1918," *International Journal of Epidemiology* 42, no. 3 (June 2013): 664.

203 **different things:** Bittel, *Mary Putnam Jacobi*, 182.

203 **The human organism:** Abraham Jacobi, *Dr. Jacobi's Works: Collected Essays, Addresses, Scientific Papers and Miscellaneous Writings* (New York: The Critic and Guide Company, 1909), 257.

203 **was derived:** Harvey, "Clanging Eagles," 192.

203 **"bacteriomania":** Bittel, *Mary Putnam Jacobi*, 186.

203 **the pathology:** Bittel, *Mary Putnam Jacobi*, 185.

204 **following notice:** Truax, *The Doctors Jacobi*, 197.

204 **"Do not ask":** Bittel, *Mary Putnam Jacobi*, 170.

204 **"The loss of this":** Bittel, *Mary Putnam Jacobi*, 170.

204 **buried Ernst:** Bittel, *Mary Putnam Jacobi*, 171.

204 **"This rooted":** Bittel, *Mary Putnam Jacobi*, 171.

205 **In 1883:** Perri Klass, "How Science Conquered Diphtheria, the Plague Among Children," *Smithsonian Magazine*, October 2021, https://www.smithsonianmag.com/science-nature/science-diphtheria-plague-among-children-180978572/.

205 **real "scourge":** Jacobi, *Dr. Jacobi's Works*, 446.

206 **"certain degree":** Jacobi, *Dr. Jacobi's Works*, 447.

206 **"the real basis":** Bittel, *Mary Putnam Jacobi*, 205.

206 **vowed her support:** "Letter from Dr. Mary Putnam Jacobi," *Woman's Journal* (February 7, 1885).

206 **first woman:** Bittel, *Mary Putnam Jacobi*, 143.

Chapter 14: The Agony of Her Mind

207 **First Citizen:** Anna Robeson Brown, *Weir Mitchell: His Life and Letters* (New York: Duffield, 1929), 117.

207 **with wards:** Cervetti, *Weir Mitchell*, 105.

208 **"wretched, wilted":** Mitchell, *Lectures on Diseases*, 84.

208 **"queer little":** Mitchell, *Lectures on Diseases*, 87.

208 **elegant study:** Cervetti, *Weir Mitchell*, 103; Brown, *Weir Mitchell*, 343.

209 **"Diana-like":** Cervetti, *Weir Mitchell*, 62.

209 **"tumbled heap":** S. Weir Mitchell, *The Hill of Stones and Other Poems* (Boston: Houghton, Mifflin and Company, 1883), 19.

209 **two categories:** Cervetti, *Weir Mitchell*, 147.

209 **treated two:** Ann J. Lane, *To Herland and Beyond: The Life and Work of Charlotte Perkins Gilman* (Charlottesville: University Press of Virginia, 1997), 113.

210 **Hamburg grapes:** Lane, *To Herland and Beyond*, 28.

211 **Providence Ladies:** Jane Lancaster, "'As Near to Flying as One Gets Outside a Circus': Charlotte Perkins Gilman and the Providence Ladies' Sanitary Gymnasium, 1881–1884," Small State Big History, http://smallstatebighistory.com/as-near-to-flying-as-one-gets-outside-a-circus-charlotte-perkins-gilman-and-the-providence-ladies-sanitary-gymnasium-1881–1884/.

211 **"I, Mary Perkins":** Lane, *To Herland and Beyond*, 63.

211 **proposed marriage:** Lane, *To Herland and Beyond*, 62.

212 **"lay all day":** Lane, *To Herland and Beyond*, 99.

212 **"Every morning":** Lane, *To Herland and Beyond*, 100.

212 **"first authority":** Cervetti, *Weir Mitchell*, 147.

212 **"Dear Sir":** Denise D. Knight, "'All the Facts of the Case': Gilman's Lost Letter to Dr. S. Weir Mitchell," *American Literary Realism* 37, no. 3 (2005): 271, http://www.jstor.org/stable/27747174.

213 **"Before marriage":** Knight, "'All the Facts of the Case,'" 273–74.

214 **"cerebral exhaustion":** Mitchell, *Wear and Tear*, 59.

214 **utterly useless:** Lane, *To Herland and Beyond*, 113.

215 **"moral reeducation":** Ellen L. Bassuk, "The Rest Cure: Repetition or Resolution of Victorian Women's Conflicts?," *Poetics Today* 6, nos. 1/2 (1985): 248–50, https://doi.org/10.2307/1772132.

216 **"Live as domestic"**: Lane, *To Herland and Beyond*, 121.

216 **overwhelming stress**: Lane, *To Herland and Beyond*, 121.

216 **"cast off"**: Lane, *To Herland and Beyond*, 123.

217 **"the fools are"**: Cervetti, *Weir Mitchell*, 114–15.

217 **Jane Addams**: Peter Gibbon, "Jane Addams: A Hero for Our Time," *Humanities* 42, no. 4, https://www.neh.gov/article/jane-addams-hero-our-time;GioiaDiliberto,"FromtheDepths," *Chicago Tribune*, June 6, 1999, https://www.chicagotribune.com/news/ct-xpm-1999-06-06 -9906060044-story.html.

218 **"mentally eager"**: S. Weir Mitchell, *Dr. North and His Friends* (New York: Century, 1905), 456.

219 **"bracing discipline"**: Cervetti, *Weir Mitchell*, 143.

219 **"If you could once"**: Cervetti, *Weir Mitchell*, 143.

220 **"fight the feeding"**: Cervetti, *Weir Mitchell*, 143.

220 **still very stubborn**: Cervetti, *Weir Mitchell*, 143.

220 **treatment centers**: Cervetti, *Weir Mitchell*, 144.

220 **"telegraphed you"**: Cervetti, *Weir Mitchell*, 143.

220 **autopsy on Winifred**: Cervetti, *Weir Mitchell*, 144.

220 **"You know perhaps"**: William Dean Howells, *Letters, Fictions, Lives: Henry James and William Dean Howells* (London: Oxford University Press, 1997), 274.

221 **"second mother"**: Lane, *To Herland and Beyond*, 178.

221 **"nervous depression"**: Charlotte Perkins Gilman, *The Yellow Wall Paper* (Boston: Small, Maynard, 1899), 2 (published under the name Charlotte Perkins Stetson).

222 **"physician of high standing"**: Gilman, *The Yellow Wall Paper*, 2.

222 **"have a schedule"**: Gilman, *The Yellow Wall Paper*, 6.

222 **"very careful and loving"**: Gilman, *The Yellow Wall Paper*, 6.

222 **"I'm really getting"**: Gilman, *The Yellow Wall Paper*, 13.

222 **"dull enough"**: Gilman, *The Yellow Wall Paper*, 8.

222 **"his darling"**: Gilman, *The Yellow Wall Paper*, 26.

222 **began to appear**: Gilman, *The Yellow Wall Paper*, 18.

223 **"all those strangled"**: Gilman, *The Yellow Wall Paper*, 51.

223 **dead babies**: Lane, *To Herland and Beyond*, 127.

223 **"'John dear'"**: Gilman, *The Yellow Wall Paper*, 54.

223 **Never again**: Lane, *To Herland and Beyond*, 127.

224 **"DEAR MADAM"**: Joanne B. Karpinski, "When the Marriage of True Minds Admits Impediments," in *Charlotte Perkins Gilman and Her Contemporaries: Literary and Intellectual Contexts*, ed. Cynthia J. Davis and Denise D. Knight (Tuscaloosa: University of Alabama Press, 2004), 17–18.

224 **right to vote**: Karpinski, "When the Marriage," 22.

224 **"Mr. Howells has"**: Karpinski, "When the Marriage," 26.

225 **"terrible and too"**: William Dean Howells, ed., *The Great Modern American Stories: An Anthology* (New York: Boni and Liveright, 1920), vii.

225 **"There is no doubt"**: Lilian Whiting, "Charlotte Perkins Stetson: A Young Literary Woman of Boston Town (Special Correspondence)," *Fall River Globe*, March 12, 1891.

225 **"There has been"**: Lane, *To Herland and Beyond*, 131.

225 **the story read**: *Fitchburg (MA) Sentinel*, January 8, 1892.

226 **more obsessed by**: Cervetti, *Weir Mitchell*, 138–40.

Chapter 15: Organizing to Win

227 **covertly investigating**: Truax, *The Doctors Jacobi*, 207.

227 **the shop clerks**: Anne M. Filiaci, "Organizing Retail Workers: The Working Woman's

Society and the New York City Consumers League," Lillian Wald—Public Health Progressive, March 2019, https://www.lillianwald.com/?page_id=1375.

228 **"humane and considerate":** Helen Campbell, *Women Wage-Earners: Their Past, Their Present, and Their Future* (Boston: Roberts Brothers, 1893), 263.

228 **$50,000 per year:** "Doctors' Incomes," *Columbus (NE) Sunday Telegram*, August 16, 1891.

228 **cures for anemia:** For example, "Mothers, Wives and Daughters," *Boston Evening Transcript*, July 1, 1891; *Portland Daily Press*, May 25, 1891; and *Boston Post*, June 24, 1891. On February 28, 1891, the Dodge City, Kansas, *Journal-Democrat* discouraged corset-wearing using a quote from Jacobi.

228 **"predominance of":** Mary Putnam Jacobi, *Essays on Hysteria, Brain-Tumor, and Some Other Cases of Nervous Disease* (New York: G. P. Putnam's Sons, 1888), 65–66.

229 **Allen claimed:** Grant Allen, "Woman's Place in Nature," *Forum* 7 (1889): 263.

229 **"Must she keep":** Hamlin, *From Eve to Evolution*, 113.

229 **"Mr. Allen's generalization":** "Woman's Kingdom: Mary Putnam Jacobi Meets Grant Allen on His Own Ground," *Inter Ocean*, June 1, 1889.

230 **In 1880, she:** Bittel, *Mary Putnam Jacobi*, 195.

231 **36 percent:** Solomon, *In the Company of Educated Women*, 63.

231 **Since the 1870s:** Smith-Rosenberg, *Disorderly Conduct*, 253.

231 **"The Deanery":** Helen Lefkowitz Horowitz, *The Power and Passion of M. Carey Thomas* (Champaign: University of Illinois Press, 1999), 202.

232 **"preach to the":** Horowitz, *The Power and Passion*, 226.

233 **uncluttered simplicity:** Ruth Levy Merriam, *A History of the Deanery* (Bryn Mawr, PA: The Deanery Committee, Bryn Mawr College, 1965).

233 **current state of medical:** M. Carey Thomas to Mary Elizabeth Garrett, March 16, 1890, M. Carey Thomas Papers, TriCollege Libraries Digital Collections, https://digitalcollections .tricolib.brynmawr.edu/object/bmc23299.

233 **"America is the only":** Bittel, *Mary Putnam Jacobi*, 223.

233 **Johns Hopkins had:** "History and Mission," Johns Hopkins University, 2023, https: //www.jhu.edu/about/history/.

234 **He wanted a hospital:** Morantz-Sanchez, *Sympathy and Science*, 85–86.

234 **thirteen years:** Morantz-Sanchez, *Sympathy and Science*, 86.

234 **forced Thomas:** Morantz-Sanchez, *Sympathy and Science*, 86.

234 **"rapture and fire":** Horowitz, *The Power and Passion*, xiii.

234 **Mary Elizabeth:** Leslie Mukau, "Johns Hopkins and the Feminist Legacy: How a Group of Baltimore Women Shaped American Graduate Medical Education," *American Journal of Clinical Medicine* 9, no. 3 (Fall 2012): 123, http://www.aapsus.org/wp-content /uploads/1fall20121.pdf; "Celebrating the Philanthropy of Mary Elizabeth Garrett," Alan Mason Chesney Medical Archives, Johns Hopkins University, 2023, https://exhibits.library .jhu.edu/exhibits/show/celebrating-the-philanthropy-o.

235 **Women's Medical School Fund:** For the Friday Evening group and the Women's Medical School Fund, see "The 'Friday Evening' Group," Alan Mason Chesney Medical Archives, Johns Hopkins University, 2023, https://exhibits.library.jhu.edu/exhibits /show/celebrating-the-philanthropy-o/the—friday-evening—group; "The Women's Medical School Fund," Alan Mason Chesney Medical Archives, Johns Hopkins University, 2023, https://exhibits.library.jhu.edu/exhibits/show/celebrating-the-philanthropy-o/the -women-s-medical-school-fun; William H. Jarrett II, "Raising the Bar: Mary Elizabeth Garrett, M. Carey Thomas, and the Johns Hopkins Medical School," *Baylor University Medical Center Proceedings* 24, no. 1 (January 2011), https://www.ncbi.nlm.nih.gov/pmc /articles/PMC3012286/; and Mukau, "Johns Hopkins and the Feminist Legacy."

235 **"She is such a":** Thomas to Garrett, M. Carey Thomas Papers.

236 **true lovers:** Horowitz, *The Power and Passion*, 227.

236 **"The Jews are":** Horowitz, *The Power and Passion*, 231.

236 **charged her with:** Horowitz, *The Power and Passion*, 232.

237 **Bessie King:** Jarrett, "Raising the Bar."

237 **"hasten the opening":** "Dear Girls" letters, Alan Mason Chesney Medical Archives, Johns Hopkins University, 2023, https://exhibits.library.jhu.edu/exhibits/show/celebrating -the-philanthropy-o/the-women-s-medical-school-fun/-dear-girls—letters.

237 **series of letters:** "Dear Girls" letters, Johns Hopkins University.

238 **those who joined:** Mukau, "Johns Hopkins and the Feminist Legacy," 125.

239 **led their chapter:** Bittel, *Mary Putnam Jacobi*, 222.

239 **expertise in gynecology:** Arlene Shaner, "Highlighting NYAM Women in Medical History: Elizabeth Martha Cushier, M.D.," NYAM History of Medicine and Public Health, October 15, 2020, https://nyamcenterforhistory.org/2020/10/15/highlighting-nyam-women -in-medical-history-elizabeth-martha-cushier-md/.

239 **"a remarkable lovely":** Pnina G. Abir-Am, *Uneasy Careers and Intimate Lives: Women in Science, 1789–1979* (New Brunswick, NJ: Rutgers University Press, 1987), 57.

240 **crowd of women:** "What Women Can Do. A Remarkable Gathering at the Johns Hopkins Hospital: The Medical School Fund Workers," *Baltimore Sun*, November 15, 1890.

240 **Bessie's father, Francis:** "What Women Can Do," *Baltimore Sun*.

241 **"It gives me":** "What Women Can Do," *Baltimore Sun*.

241 **"I do not think":** "What Women Can Do," *Baltimore Sun*.

242 **"However, I agree":** Zakrzewska, *A Woman's Quest*, 435–37.

Chapter 16: Combat Zones

243 **"Only a man":** "The Women's Medical School Fund," Johns Hopkins University.

243 **"seriously impair":** "The Temptation of Johns Hopkins," *Medical Record* (1890): 550.

243 **criticized the board:** A.C.K., "Correspondence: Women at Johns Hopkins," *Nation* 52, no. 1334 (January 22, 1891): 71.

244 **"Ranking easily":** "Famed as Physicians: New York's Leading Practitioners of the Healing Art," (Orangeburg, SC) *Times-Democrat*, April 3, 1891.

245 **"It will no longer":** Mary Putnam Jacobi, a response to "The Temptation of Johns Hopkins," *Medical Record* (1890): 588–89.

246 **"important to the":** Cardinal Gibbons et al., "The Opening of the Johns Hopkins Medical School to Women," *Century* (February 1891), https://collections.nlm.nih.gov/catalog/nlm: nlmuid-101204534-bk.

247 **second youngest:** "Biographical Overview, William Osler: The William Osler Papers," National Library of Medicine Profiles in Science, https://profiles.nlm.nih.gov/spotlight/gf /feature/biographical.

248 **international recognition:** Cervetti, *Weir Mitchell*, 166.

249 **to the facility:** Cervetti, *Weir Mitchell*, 167.

249 **coeducation was:** Cervetti, *Weir Mitchell*, 181.

249 **"This book is":** S. Weir Mitchell, *Characteristics*, author's definitive edition (New York: Century, 1910), 1.

250 **"of fortune":** Mitchell, *Characteristics*, 234.

250 **"wound this":** Mitchell, *Characteristics*, 250.

250 **"handsome":** Mitchell, *Characteristics*, 262

250 **"I never saw":** Mitchell, *Characteristics*, 251.

250 **"You cannot think":** Mitchell, *Characteristics*, 252.

251 **"a little bitter":** Cervetti, *Weir Mitchell*, 172.

251 **"You do not state"**: "Mary Putnam Jacobi's Letter of Protest," *Transactions*, 112.

252 **"Again, in 1876"**: "Mary Putnam Jacobi's Letter of Protest," *Transactions*, 113.

252 **her final paragraph:** "Mary Putnam Jacobi's Letter of Protest," *Transactions*, 113–14.

252 **exceptionally insulting:** Cervetti, *Weir Mitchell*, 178.

253 **"In the resolutions":** "Miss Garrett's Gift," *Baltimore Sun*, December 30, 1892.

253 **Garrett stipulated:** "Miss Garrett's Gift," *Baltimore Sun*.

254 **Osler joked:** "The Mary Elizabeth Garrett Fund," Alan Mason Chesney Medical Archives, Johns Hopkins University, 2023, https://exhibits.library.jhu.edu/exhibits/show/celebrating -the-philanthropy-o/the-mary-garrett-fund.

254 **"I often sat up":** Horowitz, *The Power and Passion*, 237.

254 **final letter:** "The Mary Elizabeth Garrett Fund," Johns Hopkins University.

256 **"Many of the leading":** William Osler, "Correspondence: American Medical Association," *Canada Medical and Surgical Journal* 8, no. 11 (June 1880): 503.

256 **"the clear, logical":** Osler, "Correspondence," 503.

Chapter 17: A Partnership of Women

257 **Susan B. Anthony:** Susan B. Anthony, Diaries: 1893, Susan B. Anthony Papers, Library of Congress, https://www.loc.gov/item/mss11049016.

257 **In Chicago:** Nan Robertson, "For Women, a Landmark Rediscovered," *New York Times*, July 12, 1981.

258 **age of seventy-five:** Anthony, Diaries: 1893.

258 **"sex most sensitive":** Bittel, *Mary Putnam Jacobi*, 200.

258 **that temperance:** Bittel, *Mary Putnam Jacobi*, 206.

258 *This shall be:* "This Shall Be the Land for Women: An Exhibit Examining Women's Suffrage in Colorado," Colorado Springs Pioneers Museum, accessed 10/24/23, https: //www.cspm.org/exhibits/this-shall-be-the-land-for-women/; "Woman's Suffrage Movement," History Colorado; Colorado Encyclopedia, https://coloradoencyclopedia.org/article /womens-suffrage-movement.

259 **Anthony asked Jacobi:** Ellen Carol DuBois, "Working Women, Class Relations, and Suffrage Militance: Harriot Stanton Blatch and the New York Woman Suffrage Movement, 1894–1909," *Journal of American History* 74, no. 1 (1987): 37, https://doi.org/10.2307/1908504.

259 **"such a canvass":** Joan Marie Johnson, *Funding Feminism: Monied Women, Philanthropy, and the Women's Movement, 1870–1967* (Chapel Hill: University of North Carolina Press, 2017), 26.

259 **total population:** Andy Mccarthy, "Manhattan Mistabulation: The Story of the 1890 New York City Police Census," New York Public Library, May 10, 2019, https://www.nypl.org /blog/2019/05/09/1890-new-york-city-police-census.

260 **35,000 prostitutes:** Lauren C. Santangelo, "'The Merry War Goes On': Elite Suffrage in Gilded Age Manhattan," *New York History* 98, nos. 3/4 (2017): 362, https://www.jstor.org /stable/26905067.

260 **let these ignorant:** Mary Putnam Jacobi, "Report of the 'Volunteer Committee' in New York City," in *Record of the New York Campaign of 1894* (New York: Charles Mann, 1895), 217.

260 **"hyenas in petticoats":** "Margaret Olivia Sage," Philanthropy Roundtable: Hall of Fame, 2023, https://www.philanthropyroundtable.org/hall-of-fame/margaret-olivia-sage/.

260 **She invited thirty:** Jacobi, "Report of the 'Volunteer Committee,'" 217–18.

261 **Lillie Devereux Blake:** "Lillie Devereaux Blake: Passionate Patriot," Glinda Factor, 2019, https://theglindafactor.com/lillie-blake/.

261 **Volunteer Committee:** Jacobi, "Report of the 'Volunteer Committee,'" 218; Santangelo, "'The Merry War Goes On,'" 349.

262 **especially Runkle:** Jacobi, "Report of the 'Volunteer Committee,'" 218.

262 **more than six hundred million:** "Now for Woman's Suffrage," *Sun*, April 15, 1894.

262 **spirited preaching:** Jacobi, "Report of the 'Volunteer Committee,'" 218.

263 **"You see, we":** Santangelo, "'The Merry War Goes On,'" 353.

263 **"piled up with":** Santangelo, "'The Merry War Goes On,'" 354.

263 **"political skill":** Santangelo, "'The Merry War Goes On,'" 354.

263 **"Dr. Mary Putnam Jacobi":** "Suffragists on the Warpath," *New York Times*, May 3, 1894.

263 **82 percent:** Santangelo, "'The Merry War Goes On,'" 353.

264 **anti-suffrage organization:** Santangelo, "'The Merry War Goes On,'" 353–55.

264 **As Jacobi stated:** Jacobi, "Report of the 'Volunteer Committee,'" 219.

264 **Jeering headlines:** Santangelo, "'The Merry War Goes On,'" 359; "Woman Against Woman," *New-York Tribune*, April 27, 1894.

264 **fairy-tale Cinderella:** "Now, Shall She Vote?," *Sun*, May 6, 1894.

265 **Denying that the "signature":** Santangelo, "'The Merry War Goes On,'" 358.

266 **"We believe in woman suffrage":** Santangelo, "'The Merry War Goes On,'" 360–61; "Women Ruled the Meeting," *New York Times*, May 8, 1894.

266 **"The State has":** "Women Ruled the Meeting," *New York Times*.

266 **yellow ribbon:** Jacobi, "Report of the 'Volunteer Committee,'" 8.

266 **numbers were impressive:** Jacobi, "Report of the 'Volunteer Committee,'" 141.

267 **"A small, dark":** "She Has a Logical Mind," *Fall River Daily Herald*, July 16, 1894.

267 **printed her entire address:** "Address of Mary Putnam Jacobi," *Woman's Journal* 25, no. 24 (June 16, 1894): 185–87.

269 **amendment would fail:** Putnam, *Life and Letters*, 378.

269 **failed in a vote:** Jacobi, "Report of the 'Volunteer Committee,'" 16.

269 **"I vote, not":** Jacobi, "Report of the 'Volunteer Committee,'" 11.

270 **as a "catechism":** Putnam, *Life and Letters*, 379.

270 **active girlhood:** Bittel, *Mary Putnam Jacobi*, 194.

270 **"indulge in a":** Jacobi, *Pathfinder*, 402.

271 **"allow your liberty":** Truax, *The Doctors Jacobi*, 234.

271 **offering to treat her:** Bittel, *Mary Putnam Jacobi*, 194; Charlotte Perkins Gilman, *The Living of Charlotte Perkins Gilman: An Autobiography* (1935, repr., Madison: University of Wisconsin Press, 1991), 290.

272 **Jacobi asked Gilman:** Gilman, *The Living of Charlotte Perkins Gilman*, 291.

272 **"years marked off":** Gilman, *The Living of Charlotte Perkins Gilman*, 291.

272 **study each case:** Jacobi, *Pathfinder*, 348.

273 **Jacobi was the:** Charlotte Perkins Gilman, "Addresses at the Unveiling of a Memorial Tablet," Woman's Medical College of Pennsylvania, 1907, 66.

273 **Like the child:** Mary Putnam Jacobi, *Physiological Notes on Primary Education and the Study of Language* (New York: G. P. Putnam's Sons, 1889), 7.

274 **to draw maps:** Jacobi, *Physiological Notes*, 8.

274 **more complex books:** Charlotte Perkins Gilman, "Dr. Clair's Place," in *The Yellow Wall-Paper and Other Stories*, ed. Robert Shulman (New York: Oxford University Press, 1995), 302.

274 **"all manner of easy things":** Gilman, *The Yellow Wall-Paper and Other Stories*, 298.

274 **wonderful people:** Gilman, *The Yellow Wall-Paper and Other Stories*, 303.

275 **farewell letter:** Zakrzewska, *A Woman's Quest*, 477.

Epilogue: The Last Victory

276 **"Vague longings":** Putnam, *Life and Letters*, 31 (see also footnote on page 30).

276 **"That settles the question":** "Emily Dunning Barringer," Changing the Face of Medicine, National Institutes of Health, last updated June 3, 2015, https://cfmedicine.nlm.nih.gov/physicians/biography_23.html?_gl=1*4nw5d7*_ga*MTUxNjkyNTQ1My4xNjUwOTEzNTA1*_ga_7147EPK006*MTY5MDIyNDYzMy40Mi4xLjE2OTAyMjQ2NjEuMC4wLjA.*_ga_P1FPTH9PL4*MTY5MDIyNDYzMy40My4xLjE2OTAyMjQ2NjEuMC4wLjA.

277 **keep applying at:** Putnam, *Life and Letters*, 375.

277 **Newspaper headlines announced:** "Woman on an Ambulance," *Brooklyn Citizen*, April 23, 1902; "Woman on an Ambulance: Exciting Experiences in Store for Surgeon Emily Dunning," *New York Times*, April 24, 1902.

278 **"Most frequently upon rising":** Jacobi, *Pathfinder*, 503.

278 **moved in with:** Putnam, *Life and Letters*, 376.

278 **Jacobi surprised Dunning:** Putnam, *Life and Letters*, 377.

278 **Helen Baldwin:** Bittel, *Mary Putnam Jacobi*, 226.

279 **"The heaviest blow":** Bittel, *Mary Putnam Jacobi*, 229.

279 **Women's Medical Association:** Truax, *The Doctors Jacobi*, 240–41.

279 **"emancipation of women":** "In Memory of Mary Putnam Jacobi," New York Academy of Medicine, January 4, 1907.

280 **Jacobi's life was dramatized:** Bittel, *Mary Putnam Jacobi*, 230.

280 **rarely publicly recognized:** Harvey, "Clanging Eagles," 194–95.

281 **seven thousand women:** Morantz-Sanchez, *Sympathy and Science*, xviii.

281 **accepting women in 1915:** Morantz-Sanchez, *Sympathy and Science*, 232.

281 **refused to hire women:** Morantz-Sanchez, *Sympathy and Science*, 246.

281 **By 1944:** "Women in Health Sciences: The Path to Medical Coeducation in the United States," Bernard Becker Medical Library Digital Collection, Washington University in St. Louis School of Medicine, 2009, http://beckerexhibits.wustl.edu/mowihsp/health/medcoedus.htm.

281 **remained open:** Peitzman, *A New and Untried Course*, 225.

281 **New England Hospital:** "About Dimock," The Dimock Center, https://dimock.org/about/.

281 **New York Infirmary:** Eve Heyn, "It Happened Here: Dr. Elizabeth Blackwell," NYP History, NewYork-Presbyterian, accessed November 16, 2023, https://healthmatters.nyp.org/happened-dr-elizabeth-blackwell/#:~:text=The%20New%20York%20Infirmary%20for,nurses%20soon%20joined%20the%20staff.

282 **rose to 6 percent:** Morantz-Sanchez, *Sympathy and Science*, 234.

282 **performed in 1966:** Ellen S. Moore, *Restoring the Balance: Women Physicians and the Profession of Medicine, 1850–1995* (Cambridge, MA: Harvard University Press, 1999), 217.

282 **"old-boy" hiring:** Moore, *Restoring the Balance*, 252.

282 **For Black women:** Lipi Roy, "'It's My Calling to Change the Statistics': Why We Need More Black Female Physicians," *Forbes*, February 25, 2020, https://www.forbes.com/sites/lipiroy/2020/02/25/its-my-calling-to-change-the-statistics-why-we-need-more-black-female-physicians/?sh=642c221d56a5.

282 **more than tripled:** Moore, *Restoring the Balance*, 219.

282 **more than 50 percent:** Kelley Piechowicz, "Women in Medicine: Challenges, Triumphs, and Change," GoodRx Health, March 17, 2022, https://www.goodrx.com/hcp/providers/history-women-in-medicine.

282 **Only 4.6 percent:** Ashley Hixson et al., "Understanding the Experiences of Black Women Medical Students and Residents: A Narrative Review," *Front Public Health*, June 14, 2022, https://www.ncbi.nlm.nih.gov/pmc/articles/PMC9237355/.

282 **60 percent of practicing:** "The Rise in Women Doctors and the Female Future of Medicine," Cassileth Plastic Surgery, April 2, 2021, https://www.drcassileth.com/blog/the

-rise-in-women-doctors-and-the-female-future-of-medicine/; "Healthcare Practitioner and Technical Industry: OB/GYN Demographics and Statistics in the US," Zippia Careers, 2023, https://www.zippia.com/ob-gyn-jobs/demographics/.

282 **roles of physician assistants:** "Healthcare Practitioner and Technical Industry: Physician Assistant Demographics and Statistics in the US," Zippia Careers, 2023, https://www.zippia.com/physician-assistant-jobs/demographics/; "Nurse Practitioners and Nurse Midwives," Data USA, 2021, https://datausa.io/profile/soc/nurse-practitioners-nurse-midwives.

282 **follow in her footsteps:** Bittel, *Mary Putnam Jacobi*, 232.

283 **"Procuring an abortion":** "Explaining SCOTUS's Abortion Decision in *Dobbs v. Jackson Women's Health Organization*," League of Women Voters of the US, 2022, https://my.lwv.org/lwvus/article/explaining-scotuss-abortion-decision-dobbs-v-jackson-womens-health-organization.

283 **"A woman's ovaries":** Ely Van De Warker, "The Fetich of the Ovary," *American Journal of Obstetrics and Gynecology* 3 (1907): 364.

Index

About the Author

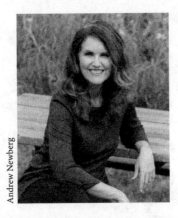

Andrew Newberg

LYDIA REEDER's research and writing brings to light the stories of little-known or forgotten pioneers. Her first book, *Dust Bowl Girls*, was a Junior Library Guild Selection and a finalist for the Oklahoma Book Award and the WILLA Literary Award. A regional bestseller in Oklahoma and Colorado, it was named a 2017 top nonfiction book by Amazon, *Bustle, Romper,* and *Bookbub,* and optioned for a film five times. A native of Oklahoma, Lydia now lives in Denver, Colorado.